Nutrition: An Applied Approach

Nutrition: An Applied Approach

Edited by Kristen Foley

STATES
ACADEMIC PRESS
www.statesacademicpress.com

Published by States Academic Press,
109 South 5th Street,
Brooklyn, NY 11249, USA
www.statesacademicpress.com

Nutrition: An Applied Approach
Edited by Kristen Foley

International Standard Book Number: 978-1-63989-390-4 (Hardback)

Cataloging-in-Publication Data

Nutrition : an applied approach / edited by Kristen Foley.
p. cm.
Includes bibliographical references and index.
ISBN 978-1-63989-390-4
1. Nutrition. 2. Physiology. 3. Food. I. Foley, Kristen.
QP141 .N88 2022
613.2--dc23

TABLE OF CONTENTS

PREFACE

The science of interpretation of various substances and nutrients in food is referred to as nutrition. Human nutrition is the study of nutrients present in food that are important to sustain human life and health. It studies the processes of growth, reproduction, maintenance, health and disease of an individual in relation to food. Nutrients are of two types. These are macronutrients and micronutrients. Macronutrients are comparatively taken in large quantities and are used to generate energy whereas micronutrients are taken in smaller quantities and have physiological and biochemical effects in cellular processes. The most common nutrients are fats, proteins, carbohydrates, minerals, fiber, water and vitamins. Lack of nutrients in an individual's diet can lead to diseases like blindness, scurvy, stillbirth, anemia and other chronic diseases like diabetes, osteoporosis, etc. This book includes some of the vital pieces of work being conducted across the world, on various topics related to nutrition. It elucidates the concepts and innovative models around prospective developments with respect to this discipline. Students, researchers, experts and all associated with this field will benefit alike from this book.

All of the data presented henceforth, was collaborated in the wake of recent advancements in the field. The aim of this book is to present the diversified developments from across the globe in a comprehensible manner. The opinions expressed in each chapter belong solely to the contributing authors. Their interpretations of the topics are the integral part of this book, which I have carefully compiled for a better understanding of the readers.

At the end, I would like to thank all those who dedicated their time and efforts for the successful completion of this book. I also wish to convey my gratitude towards my friends and family who supported me at every step.

Editor

The influence of prenatal exposure to trans-fatty acids for development of childhood haematopoietic neoplasms (EnTrance): a natural societal experiment and a case-control study

Ina Olmer Specht[1*], Inge Huybrechts[2], Peder Frederiksen[1], Eva Steliarova-Foucher[3], Veronique Chajes[2] and Berit Lilienthal Heitmann[1,4,5]

Abstract

Background: Little is known about the causes of childhood cancer, partly as not many children develop cancer, although childhood cancer is a leading cause of death by disease in the young. The young age of the children suggests that risk factors for childhood cancer may be present during pregnancy. Previous studies have shown that exposure to trans-fat, a type of unsaturated fat common in industrially produced foods (iTFA), has adverse health effects in adults, including the risk of developing cancer. Haematopoietic neoplasms are the most common cancer types among European children under the age of 15 years. This study will bring new knowledge as to whether trans-fat and other fatty acids may also increase the risk of developing haematopoietic neoplasms during childhood.

Methods: We will investigate if the Danish iTFA legislation ban, which radically reduced the use of iTFA in foodstuffs, influenced the risk of childhood haematopoietic neoplasms in children born either before or after the change in legislation, adjusting for relevant secular trends. Further, in a case-control study, we will examine if levels of fatty acids in dried blood spots from newborns can predict the risk of developing childhood haematopoietic neoplasms. Permission from the Danish Data Protection Agency and the Ethical Committee has been granted.

Discussion: The results from this study will provide important information about fatty acids in the mother's diet as a contributor to development of haematopoietic neoplasms during childhood, which may result in relevant preventive action.

Keywords: Trans fatty acids, Childhood leukemia, Childhood cancer, In utero, Prenatal, Haematopoietic neoplasms

* Correspondence: Ina.olmer.specht@regionh.dk
[1]Parker Institute, Research Unit for Dietary Studies, Frederiksberg and Bispebjerg Hospital, Frederiksberg, Denmark
Full list of author information is available at the end of the article

Background

Although childhood cancer is relatively rare, it is a leading cause of death by disease in children under the age of 15 years in Western populations [1], and the incidence is rising [2]. Among the 12 major groups of childhood cancer, leukemia has the highest incidence, with age standardized rate of 49 per million in the age 0–14 years in Northern Europe [3].

The etiology of malignant tumors in the young is mostly unknown. A small proportion of childhood cancers seems inherited [4] or has a viral origin [5, 6]. A few environmental risk factors, such as high-dose radiation and some chemicals are currently recognized as causes of a small proportion of childhood neoplasms [6]. The role of diet in relation to childhood cancers has only sparsely been investigated [7], despite increasing evidence pointing towards diet as a main modifiable risk factor for cancers among adults [8]. Chromosomal translocations noticed in blood samples at birth of children subsequently diagnosed with leukemia, suggest that initiating molecular events in childhood cancer development occur as early as in utero [9]. This emphasizes the need to investigate exposure to potential risk factors already during fetal development. It has been shown that during 'critical time windows' of fetal development fetuses are especially vulnerable to environmental exposures. This suggests that lack off, or excess of specific nutritional elements (maternal diet) may program permanent changes in the genome directly by oxidative DNA damage or by epigenetic mechanisms (such as DNA methylation), and in this way modulate later disease risk [10–12].

Trans-fats are a type of unsaturated fatty acids and can be classified as naturally/ruminant (rTFAs) occurring or industrially produced (iTFAs). Industrially produced trans-fats are formed when fats and oils are hydrogenated by industrial processing techniques. The proportions of iTFAs in food are generally much higher than those of rTFAs and in most European countries they are the main dietary source of trans-fats. Examples of foods commonly high in iTFA are baked goods (e.g. pies, biscuits, pastries, sweet rolls) in which shortenings such as margarine are used, and fried foods (e.g. French fries, chicken nuggets), while the counterpart rTFA naturally occurs in low levels in diary and meat products.

Evidence of adverse health effects of iTFAs has been increasing over the past three decades, however rTFA seems to have a less potent effect on cardio metabolic outcomes [13, 14]. The WHO stated that intake of trans-fats should be as low as possible (<1% of total energy intake). Yet intake remains high in most countries worldwide [15–17]. An example of an iTFA high diet could be; one doughnut (3.2 g iTFA), one large portion French fries (6.8 g iTFA) and a bag of microwave popcorn (10 g iTFA), corresponding to overall 23 g iTFA. Guidance to minimize trans-fat intake is based predominantly on evidence that trans-fat consumption significantly increases the risk of coronary heart disease (CHD), where an increase of 2% in total energy derived from iTFA is shown to be associated with an increased risk of death from CHD or myocardial infarction of 23% [14]. In addition, trans-fat intake seems associated with the development of other non-communicable diseases like central adiposity, diabetes, Alzheimer's disease, endometriosis, cholelithiasis and total mortality [18]. Furthermore, among adults, iTFAs is found to be directly associated with cancer of stomach, multiple myeloma, lung (in never smoking men), mouth/pharynx, breast cancer [19, 20], non-aggressive prostate cancer [21, 22] and colorectal cancer [23].

A case-control study investigating dietary fat and protein intake showed increased risk of non-Hodgkin lymphoma among adults with a diet high in iTFA [24]. TFA has pro-inflammatory properties which might be the mechanism explaining carcinogenesis. A randomized controlled trial in women showed that industrially produced iTFA induced low-grade systemic inflammation by elevating circulating concentrations of tumor necrosis factor (TNF) α and its receptors [25]. TFA exposure in mice during pregnancy and lactation has shown to affect the global DNA methylation in the dams, thus TFA intake may exert long-term effects on the epigenome following maternal exposure [26].

Studies demonstrating relationships between trans-fat intake and cancer in childhood are lacking. However, evidence has shown some possible negative effects on other health outcomes among children. Bouwstra and colleagues have shown that neonates with high TFA umbilical levels have a less favorable neurologic condition at 18 months [27]. Furthermore, a recent review (including human and animal studies) concluded that fetal exposure to trans-fat appears to increase the offspring risk for developing metabolic diseases throughout life [28]. TFAs also interfere in the metabolism of long-chain polyunsaturated fatty acids which might result in a negative impact on infant growth and development [29, 30]. Lifelong, including prenatal, consumption of a diet rich in polyunsaturated fatty acids (PUFA, contained in nuts, seeds and fish) has been shown to protect against tumor growth and to modify glucose metabolism in Walker tumor cells and lymphocytes in Wistar rats [31]. Therefore, the inhibitory effect of PUFA and their interference with trans fatty acids might also be relevant in the fetal programming of childhood cancers.

Despite a general reduction in the iTFA use in food production, Denmark, as the first EU country, legislated against the use of iTFA in all Danish and imported human foodstuffs [32]. The order came into effect on March 31st, 2003, with a transition period until January

1st, 2004. The order imposed a maximum of 2 g of iTFA/100 g oils and fats. During the transition period a maximum level of 5% iTFA was allowed in foodstuffs also containing ingredients other than oils and fats [32]. This legislation led to a radical reduction of iTFA from margarine and shortenings which resulted in a rapid decline in products with trans-fat followed by a decrease in population-level CVD mortality rates [33].

Despite the alarming evidence of increased risk of several diseases caused by TFA consumption and the fact that millions of people still have a too high iTFA intake in Europe, currently no EU legislation regulates the content of iTFA in food products [34].

Given the direct associations found between high TFA intakes and some cancer types among adults, and the deleterious health effects associated with higher TFA intakes among the fetus and offspring, other detrimental effects of an early life exposure to trans-fats, such as childhood cancer, could be envisaged. The health effects of TFA during gestation have never previously been followed in large populations, in part because large-scale interventions are needed to examine how TFA exposure during pregnancy affects long-term health outcomes of offspring, and in particular the risk of developing childhood cancer. However, such interventions may never be conducted due to the associated high financial and logistical costs and ethical aspects. Therefore, alternative study designs should be used to explore associations between early life trans-fat exposure and childhood cancers.

Hypotheses and objectives

We hypothesize that high TFA exposures, and in particular iTFA exposures, during the critical phase of fetal development increase the risk of developing childhood cancers in general and haematopoietic neoplasms in particular.

We investigate this in two broad designs and study objectives:

1) We will examine if the legislatively reduced use of iTFA in the production of human foodstuff for the Danish market has shown any beneficial effect on population level in preventing childhood haematopoietic neoplasms. Thus we will compare the incidence of childhood haematopoietic neoplasms between all Danish children born in the years before and after the law came into effect. The specific hypothesis is that individuals born in 2004–2008 were exposed to reduced iTFA during fetal development and will have a lower risk of developing childhood haematopoietic neoplasms compared to individuals born in 1988–2003, before the policy was implemented, while taking into account the underlying secular trends in these cancers.
2) We aim to compare neonatal levels of TFA in children with and without a later diagnosis of childhood haematopoietic neoplasm in a matched case-control study. As a secondary aim, we wish to investigate the interactions between TFA and polyunsaturated fatty acids, and their impact on risk of haematopoietic neoplasms in children, since TFA have been shown to inhibit the metabolism of polyunsaturated fatty acids.

The aim of this protocol is to describe the methods and analyses that will be used in this study to investigate the influence of prenatal exposure to trans-fatty acids for development of haematopoietic neoplasms (EnTrance). If deviations from this initial study protocol occur during data analyses, we will update the protocol.

Methods

As childhood cancers are histologically and etiologically very diverse, investigating effects of prenatal TFA intake on each type of the childhood cancer would require very large sample sizes given the low incidence rates of different tumour types. Therefore, we restrict our study to investigating the potential adverse effects of a high TFA exposure on risk of haematopoietic neoplasms (ICD-10 codes: DC81-C96), the most frequent cancer types in children.

The two objectives of this study reinforce each other by first investigating effects of the trans-fat order on fetal programming of haematopoietic neoplasms on population level and second by investigating variations in biomarkers of TFA and risk of haematopoietic neoplasms, based on measurements of individual exposures. Therefore, null findings in the first objective would not necessarily imply null findings in the second objective.

Study population

The cancer registry is complete until December 31st 2015. To secure equal time of follow-up for cancer diagnosis in all individuals we censor at 7 years of age, which is the longest follow-up time in which we have information on possible cancer outcomes for all individuals.

We will exclude all children born with a Down's Syndrome (DS) diagnoses due to their increased risk of childhood leukemia [35] and due to secular trends in DS incidence, because of a new screening practice for DS and other chromosomal aberrations introduced in 2004.

In the first objective, national birth cohorts of individuals born between January 1st, 1988 and December 31st, 2008 in Denmark will be included (Fig. 1). This is a register based study using the Danish civil registration number which will be linked to the Danish National

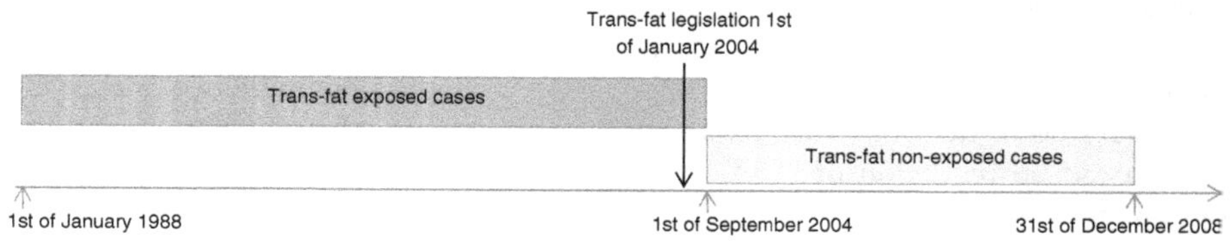

Fig. 1 Constitution of the exposed versus non-exposed groups of cases who developed haematological malignancy before the age of 7 years and registered in The Danish Cancer Registry (Objective 1)

Cancer Register, where the cancer patients are followed-up until December 31st, 2015.

The incidence of childhood haematopoietic neoplasms among 1,101,055 individuals from the period before the iTFA legislation born between January 1st, 1988 and August 31st, 2004, will be compared to the incidence of childhood haematopoietic neoplasms among 276,422 individuals from the period after the iTFA legislations born between September 1st, 2004 and December 31st, 2008, as a proxy of iTFA gestationally exposed or not exposed, respecitvely. In this overall time period approximately 740 incident haematopoietic neoplasms cases occurred in children before the age of 7 years.

The second objective is a case-control study investigating biomarkers of neonatal trans-fatty acid concentrations from stored DBS [34] from individuals who developed childhood haematopoietic neoplasms before the age of 7 years and born in the period 1988–2008 compared to matched controls (Fig. 2).

Since 1981, routinely collected DBS samples taken by heel prick 48–72 h after birth have been collected for all newborn in Denmark. DBS cards are stored in the Biological Specimen Bank for Neonatal Screening at Statens Serum Institute and have been made available to the project [36].

For each case with haematopoietic neoplasms, a control, individually matched for gender, exact date and year of birth, mother's parity, place of birth, being alive and with no diagnosis of cancer, will be selected and fatty acids isomers measured in the DBS. A case is defined as a child, less than 7 years, with a cancer diagnosis (ICD-10 DC81-C96) and without a DS diagnosis [37]. If more than one participant meets the matching criteria a random control from the eligible participants will be selected. If no participant meets the matching criteria the

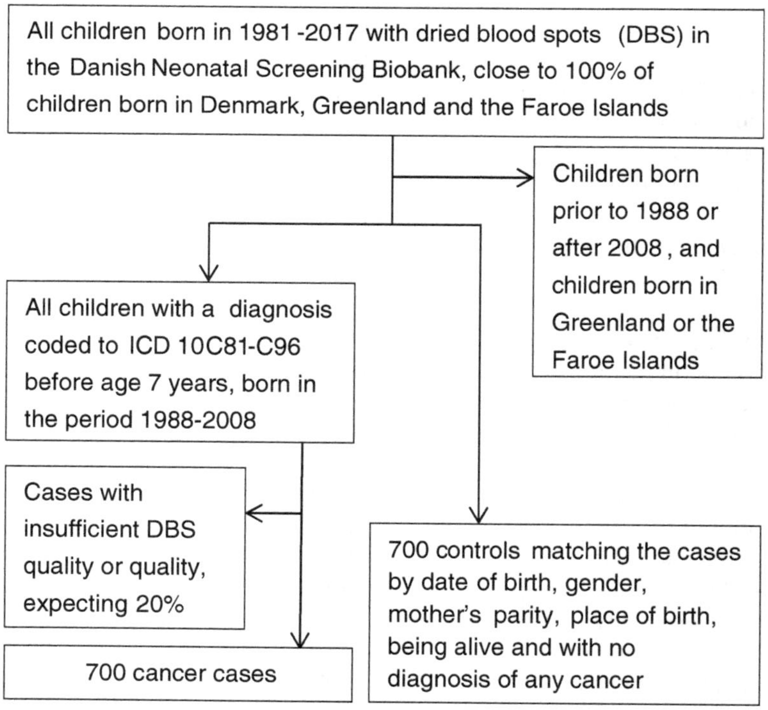

Fig. 2 Flow chart of the matched case-control study (Objective 2)

criteria for exact date of birth or place of birth will be relaxed as needed to match controls to cases and the adjustments made will be reported.

Previous studies have confirmed that storage time of DBS as long as 20 years do not bias inter-individual variation in concentrations of vitamin D and possible other fat soluble substances [38]. Furthermore, as date of birth is used as matching criterion for the controls, potential degradation of TFA would affect equally cases and controls and is therefore unlikely to bias the results.

The methodology for measuring biomarkers of fatty acids in DBS has been set up at the International Agency of Research of Cancer (IARC) in Lyon, France, a specialized WHO and UN organization. The DBS will securely be transported from Denmark to IARC, Lyon, France, where they will be kept in a – 80 °C freezer until analysis. Our validated gas chromatography methodology allows a complete separation, identification and quantification of sixty fatty acids from short-chain saturated to long-chain polyunsaturated fatty acids, including fifteen individual isomers of industrial trans fatty acids (elaidic acid, trans n-6 and n-3 PUFA) separated from natural trans fatty acids (CLA, vaccenic acid) in one-hour runs. The laboratory involved in the set up at IARC is at the cutting edge of lipidomic technologies and have developed sound and innovative high-throughput methods for fatty acid measurements [20]. Fatty acid concentrations will be determined in plasma phospholipids, as some specific fatty acids measured in this lipid fraction have been shown to be reliable biomarkers of specific dietary intakes, as well as fatty acid metabolism [39–41]. Samples from cases and their matched controls will be analysed within the same daily batch, with two quality controls in each batch. The technical staff will not have any information on the case/control status. Total lipids will be extracted from plasma samples with chloroform-methanol containing antioxidant butylated hydroxytoluene and L-A-phosphatidylcholine-dimyristoyl-d as an internal standard. Phospholipids will be purified by adsorption chromatography; fatty acid methyl esters will be separated through gas chromatography. The relative amount of each fatty acid, expressed as percent of total fatty acids, will be quantified by integrating the area under the peak and dividing the result by the total area. Fatty acids will also be expressed as absolute concentrations in plasma (μmol/l) based on the quantity of the methyl deuterated internal standard.

Based on this methodology, coefficients of variation (CVs) for fatty acids have been calculated for 60 samples. CVs ranged from 0.013% for large peaks to 7.75% for the smallest peaks (less than 0.10% of total fatty acids). Overall CVs (within-batch and between batch CVs) are very good for iTFA isomers, mainly for elaidic acid (CV = 0.137%). Overall CV is 0.122% for total iTFA. CVs for rTFAs are also good, mainly for vaccenic acid, the main iTFA isomer (CV = 0.282%). CV for total iTFA is 0.123%.

Because the TFA levels in the new-born blood also reflects the TFA status of the mother at the end of pregnancy, measurement of iTFA levels in DBS will furthermore serve as validation for the effect of trans-fat elimination for incident cases.

To take into account different cohort effects or changes in life-style in the period 1988 to 2008, we will merge the cohort data with information from the Danish Medical Birth Registry on trends in co-variates which might have changed during the time period, e.g. smoking during pregnancy and age of the mother.

Power calculation

Using the command stpower for the log-rank test for comparison of two survival functions in Stata 14 we calculated the least detectable hazard ratio (exposed versus unexposed) to be 1.35 assuming 80% power and a significance level of 5% in objective 1 (the cohort study) [42].

In objective 2 (the case-control study) we have a sample size of 700 cancer cases and 700 controls, and assuming 80% power, the least detectable OR will be between 1.35 and 1.75, depending on the exposure among the controls (10–90%). The power analysis for the matched 1:1 case-control study was performed using the power mcc command in Stata 14 [43].

Statistical analysis

In objective 1 we will use a Cox proportional hazard model with age as the underlying timescale to investigate the hazard of childhood haematopoietic neoplasms in children born before and after the iTFA ban, as a proxy for iTFA exposed or not exposed in fetal life. Observations will be censored in case of death, immigration or at 7 years of age. To take the potential secular trend in the incidence of haematopoietic neoplasms into account we will model the variation in cancer risk across birth cohorts by a piecewise linear spline with a knot at 1st of September 2004. Further, we will investigate incidence trends over time.

By examining *all* children from the entire national birth cohorts it is reasonable to assume that all confounding variables will be equally distributed among the exposed and non-exposed individuals, but still we will investigate potential influence of secular variation or possible confounding effects which might have changed during the time period and which might be associated with both TFA exposure and haematopoietic neoplasms. Such potential confounders could be age of the mother at the time of giving birth, assuming accumulation of TFA with age and an older age for first time pregnancies over time. The median gestational age might have increased during the investigated time period, which would increase the average intrauterine exposure to TFA over the study period [44]. Smoking status during pregnancy might have decreased over time and smoking might be associated with increased cancer risk, smoking is also associated with gestational age and thereby with the length of the TFA exposure during pregnancy.

As sub-analysis we will exclude cancer cases diagnosed before the 90 day of life since the origin most likely is due to chromosomal alterations leading to oncogene activation [37]. If feasible we will investigate the first born only since some studies have shown higher risk of childhood cancers in the first born compared to their younger siblings [45] and sensitivity analysis of sub-types of haematopoietic neoplasms (leukemia and lymphoma). Further, we will investigate children with early diagnosis, e.g. before age 4 years.

Conditional logistic regression analyses will be used in the 2nd objective to compare blood spot fatty acid levels between subjects with haematopoietic neoplasms and matched subjects who have not developed cancer. We will investigate industrial as well as ruminant TFA independently and mutually adjusted. Based on a priori consideration we will adjust for maternal and paternal age, smoking during pregnancy, birth weight and gestational age. Also, there might be regional and urban/rural differences in iTFA intake. Place of residence is available from Statistics Denmark, and can be included into analyses. Diets are usually different between families with higher and lower socioeconomic status and maternal socioeconomic status may influence intake of certain food products rich in trans-fat. Information on socioeconomic status, education and ethnicity is available from Statistics Denmark and can be controlled for.

As mentioned in the methods description, other fatty acids potentially related to haematopoietic neoplasms in children will be analysed in the DBS since our methodology allows a complete separation, identification and quantification of sixty fatty acids. We will therefore also investigate interactions between TFA and polyunsaturated fatty acids, and risk of haematopoietic neoplasms in children as well as association between polyunsaturated fatty acids and risk of cancer stratified by trans fatty acids.

Discussion

Our main goal for this study is to strengthen the scientific basis for understanding idiopathic haematopoietic neoplasms in children. By presenting the protocol before undertaking the actual analyses, we intend to improve the quality, integrity and transparency of the study.

Strengths of the first objective include the unselected national cohort, the prospective design and the register-based measure of outcome. This explorative study takes advantage of the iTFA elimination policy implemented in Denmark almost fifteen years ago, and nests this "societal experiment" in a setting where the effect of conditions from conception (and before) for development of certain diseases can be followed among individuals from birth and onwards. The study is possible due to complete identification of every resident in Denmark via a civil registration number. This number can be linked, on an individual level, to Danish birth, patient and medical registries; social and ethnic registries; and clinical and other national databases. The comprehensive linkage of datasets for both aims makes it possible to study mediation, confounding and/or modification of effects of iTFA for childhood haematopoietic neoplasms.

For the first objective we do not collect any individual data on iTFA intake. In contrast, all individuals are unselected in relation to iTFA exposure and later disease occurrence. This may be considered a very strong feature of the present study, as neither confounding from external or internal factors, nor the lack of individual data on iTFA intake, is a prerequisite for the study, as the influences of lifestyle differences (e.g. use of infant formula, individual diet intake, use of supplements), or biological (adipose tissue stores, weight changes during pregnancy and post-partum) which we would not be able to adjust for, are all independent of the iTFA legislation.

Nevertheless, the proposed study design, especially in the first objective, also implies some uncertainties, including a potential ecological fallacy. The exposure measure is applied equally to all members of the cohort before and after the ban, while the individual exposures have probably differed. However, a previous study has shown a marked decline of average iTFA intake resulting in elimination after the ban [32]. In the case-control study we investigate TFA exposure individually in all cases from 1988 to 2008. The variations in the exposure observed in the case-control study will then inform our assumptions taken in the cohort study.

Any societal changes preceding 1988 or succeeding 2008 will influence the exposed and control groups similarly, while results will be confounded by any potential societal changes occurring around the time where the trans-fat ban was implemented (e.g. 2003/04). However, we are unaware of such changes except for a screening for DS which we have taken into account by excluding children with DS.

Potentially exposure to TFA from maternal adipose stores could affect the "unexposed" group (born after the ban of iTFA) and postnatal influences like maternal feeding practice and weight gain, may also influence cancer risk through a non-TFA mechanism. Although this may indeed seem a possible limitation, since literature has shown that weight loss of the mother (e.g. during lactation) liberates TFA fat deposits [44], proper randomization in our societal experiment study is mimicked by separating exposed and non-exposed individuals by one point in time with a minimum of selection bias. Thus, it is an obvious strength to the present research design, that the individuals will be unselected, and generally representative of the Danish population, in relation to exposed vs. non-exposed to the trans-fat legislation, as well as to the development of haematopoietic neoplasms. However, since we do not know the exact mechanism between TFA and childhood neoplasms, we cannot account for a residual confounding which might affect observed associations. Residual confounding could be caused by additional components in food products with high contents of TFA. We are not able to investigate TFA levels at specific developmental stages during gestation, but since no knowledge exist on specific target windows for childhood cancers, this may not be relevant.

Other health outcomes in children, which will not be described in this protocol, will be investigated in future studies using the same study designs, include: negative birth outcomes, cognitive function, epilepsy, asthma, heart disease, eye diseases, bone fracture, and metabolic diseases like type 1 diabetes and childhood obesity.

Abbreviations

DBS: Dried blood spots; DS: Down's syndrome; IARC: The International Agency of Research of Cancer; iTFA: Industrially produced trans fatty acids; PUFA: Polyunsaturated fatty acids; rTFA: Ruminant trans fatty acids; TFA: Trans fatty acids; TNF: Tumor necrosis factor α

Acknowledgements

We would like to acknowledge Dagny Yrsa Eythorsdottir for her contribution in writing the initial study protocol.

Funding

The first objective of this study is funded by the Danish Børnecancerfonden (The Danish Child Cancer Foundation). The Danish Child Cancer Foundation has no influence on the interpretation of the results. Funding is still pending for the second objective.

Authors' contributions

BLH is the principal investigator in charge of the project and IH is the co-principal investigator. BLH, IH and VC designed the initial study. IOS is managing the daily activities in the project. PF is the responsible statistician, ESF advises on the relevant childhood cancers and VC is managing the analysis of fatty acids in the dried blood spots. IOS prepared the initial draft of the manuscript and all other authors have contributed. All authors have critically reviewed and approved the final version of the manuscript.

Competing interests

The authors declare that they have no competing interests.

Author details

[1]Parker Institute, Research Unit for Dietary Studies, Frederiksberg and Bispebjerg Hospital, Frederiksberg, Denmark. [2]International Agency for Research on Cancer (IARC), Nutrition and Metabolism Section, Lyon, France. [3]International Agency for Research on Cancer (IARC), Cancer Surveillance Section (CSU), Lyon, France. [4]Department of Public Health, Section for general Medicine, University of Copenhagen, Copenhagen, Denmark. [5]National Institute of Public health, University of Southern Denmark, Odense, Denmark.

References

1. Ward E, DeSantis C, Robbins A, Kohler B, Jemal A. Childhood and adolescent cancer statistics, 2014. CA Cancer J Clin. 2014;64:83–103.
2. Kaatsch P. Epidemiology of childhood cancer. Cancer Treat Rev. 2010;36:277–85.
3. Steliarova-Foucher E, Colombet M, Ries LAG, Moreno F, Dolya A, Bray F, Hesseling P, Shin HY, Stiller CA. International incidence of childhood cancer, 2001-10: a population-based registry study. Lancet Oncol. 2017;18:719–31.
4. Narod SA, Stiller C, Lenoir GM. An estimate of the heritable fraction of childhood cancer. Br J Cancer. 1991;63:993–9.
5. Kinlen LJ. Epidemiological evidence for an infective basis in childhood leukaemia. Br J Cancer. 1995;71:1–5.
6. Buka I, Koranteng S, Osornio Vargas AR. Trends in childhood cancer incidence: review of environmental linkages. Pediatr Clin N Am. 2007;54:177–203. x
7. Dessypris N, Karalexi MA, Ntouvelis E, Diamantaras AA, Papadakis V, Baka M, Hatzipantelis E, Kourti M, Moschovi M, Polychronopoulou S, et al. Association of maternal and index child's diet with subsequent leukemia risk: a systematic review and meta analysis. Cancer Epidemiol. 2017;47:64–75.
8. Mosby TT, Cosgrove M, Sarkardei S, Platt KL, Kaina B. Nutrition in adult and childhood cancer: role of carcinogens and anti-carcinogens. Anticancer Res. 2012;32:4171–92.
9. Hjalgrim LL, Madsen HO, Melbye M, Jorgensen P, Christiansen M, Andersen MT, Pallisgaard N, Hokland P, Clausen N, Ryder LP, et al. Presence of clone-specific markers at birth in children with acute lymphoblastic leukaemia. Br J Cancer. 2002;87:994–9.
10. Anderson LM, Diwan BA, Fear NT, Roman E. Critical windows of exposure for children's health: cancer in human epidemiological studies and neoplasms in experimental animal models. Environ Health Perspect. 2000;108(Suppl 3):573–94.
11. Kleinjans J, Botsivali M, Kogevinas M, Merlo DF. Fetal exposure to dietary carcinogens and risk of childhood cancer: what the NewGeneris project tells us. BMJ. 2015;351:h4501.
12. Lee HS. Impact of maternal diet on the epigenome during in utero life and the developmental programming of diseases in childhood and adulthood. Nutrients. 2015;7:9492–507
13. Gayet-Boyer C, Tenenhaus-Aziza F, Prunet C, Marmonier C, Malpuech-Brugere C, Lamarche B, Chardigny JM. Is there a linear relationship between the dose of ruminant trans-fatty acids and cardiovascular risk markers in healthy subjects: results from a systematic review and meta-regression of randomised clinical trials. Br J Nutr. 2014;112:1914–22.
14. de Souza RJ, Mente A, Maroleanu A, Cozma AI, Ha V, Kishibe T, Uleryk E, Budylowski P, Schunemann H, Beyene J, Anand SS. Intake of saturated and trans unsaturated fatty acids and risk of all cause mortality, cardiovascular disease, and type 2 diabetes: systematic review and meta-analysis of observational studies. BMJ. 2015;351:h3978.
15. Craig-Schmidt MC. World-wide consumption of trans fatty acids. Atheroscler Suppl. 2006;7:1–4.
16. Teegala SM, Willett WC, Mozaffarian D. Consumption and health effects of trans fatty acids: a review. J AOAC Int. 2009;92:1250–7.
17. Hendry VL, Almiron-Roig E, Monsivais P, Jebb SA, Neelon SE, Griffin SJ, Ogilvie DB. Impact of regulatory interventions to reduce intake of artificial trans-fatty acids: a systematic review. Am J Public Health. 2015;105:e32–42.
18. Kiage JN, Merrill PD, Robinson CJ, Cao Y, Malik TA, Hundley BC, Lao P, Judd SE, Cushman M, Howard VJ, Kabagambe EK. Intake of trans fat and all-cause mortality in the reasons for geographical and racial differences in stroke (REGARDS) cohort. Am J Clin Nutr. 2013;97:1121–8.

19. Laake I, Carlsen MH, Pedersen JI, Weiderpass E, Selmer R, Kirkhus B, Thune I, Veierod MB. Intake of trans fatty acids from partially hydrogenated vegetable and fish oils and ruminant fat in relation to cancer risk. Int J Cancer. 2013;132:1389–403.
20. Chajes V, Thiebaut AC, Rotival M, Gauthier E, Maillard V, Boutron-Ruault MC, Joulin V, Lenoir GM, Clavel-Chapelon F. Association between serum trans-monounsaturated fatty acids and breast cancer risk in the E3N-EPIC study. Am J Epidemiol. 2008;167:1312–20.
21. King IB, Kristal AR, Schaffer S, Thornquist M, Goodman GE. Serum trans-fatty acids are associated with risk of prostate cancer in beta-carotene and retinol efficacy trial. Cancer Epidemiol Biomark Prev. 2005;14:988–92.
22. Chavarro JE, Stampfer MJ, Campos H, Kurth T, Willett WC, Ma J. A prospective study of trans-fatty acid levels in blood and risk of prostate cancer. Cancer Epidemiol Biomark Prev. 2008;17:95–101.
23. Vinikoor LC, Schroeder JC, Millikan RC, Satia JA, Martin CF, Ibrahim J, Galanko JA, Sandler RS. Consumption of trans-fatty acid and its association with colorectal adenomas. Am J Epidemiol. 2008;168:289–97.
24. Charbonneau B, O'Connor HM, Wang AH, Liebow M, Thompson CA, Fredericksen ZS, Macon WR, Slager SL, Call TG, Habermann TM, Cerhan JR. Trans fatty acid intake is associated with increased risk and n3 fatty acid intake with reduced risk of non-hodgkin lymphoma. J Nutr. 2013;143:672–81.
25. Bendsen NT, Stender S, Szecsi PB, Pedersen SB, Basu S, Hellgren LI, Newman JW, Larsen TM, Haugaard SB, Astrup A. Effect of industrially produced trans fat on markers of systemic inflammation: evidence from a randomized trial in women. J Lipid Res. 2011;52:1821–8.
26. Flores-Sierra J, Arredondo-Guerrero M, Cervantes-Paz B, Rodriguez-Rios D, Alvarado-Caudillo Y, Nielsen FC, Wrobel K, Wrobel K, Zaina S, Lund G. The trans fatty acid elaidate affects the global DNA methylation profile of cultured cells and in vivo. Lipids Health Dis. 2016;15:75.
27. Bouwstra H, Dijck-Brouwer J, Decsi T, Boehm G, Boersma ER, Muskiet FA, Hadders-Algra M. Neurologic condition of healthy term infants at 18 months: positive association with venous umbilical DHA status and negative association with umbilical trans-fatty acids. Pediatr Res. 2006;60:334–9.
28. Mennitti LV, Oliveira JL, Morais CA, Estadella D, Oyama LM, Oller do Nascimento CM, Pisani LP. Type of fatty acids in maternal diets during pregnancy and/or lactation and metabolic consequences of the offspring. J Nutr Biochem. 2015;26:99–111.
29. Dalainas I, Ioannou HP. The role of trans fatty acids in atherosclerosis, cardiovascular disease and infant development. Int Angiol. 2008;27:146–56.
30. Larque E, Zamora S, Gil A. Dietary trans fatty acids in early life: a review. Early Hum Dev. 2001;65(Suppl):S31–41.
31. Aikawa J, Moretto KD, Denes F, Yamazaki RK, Freitas FA, Hirabara SM, Tchaikovski O Jr, Kaelher MA, Brito GA, Curi R, Fernandes LC. Glucose metabolism by lymphocytes, macrophages, and tumor cells from Walker 256 tumor-bearing rats supplemented with fish oil for one generation. Cell Biochem Funct. 2008;26:874–80.
32. Leth T, Jensen HG, Mikkelsen AA, Bysted A. The effect of the regulation on trans fatty acid content in Danish food. Atheroscler Suppl. 2006;7:53–6.
33. Restrepo BJ, Rieger M. Denmark's policy on artificial trans fat and cardiovascular disease. Am J Prev Med. 2016;50:69–76.
34. European Parliament EPRS: Trans fats - Overwiew of recent developments. 2016.
35. Hasle H, Clemmensen IH, Mikkelsen M. Risks of leukaemia and solid tumours in individuals with Down's syndrome. Lancet. 2000;355:165–9.
36. Norgaard-Pedersen B, Hougaard DM. Storage policies and use of the Danish newborn screening biobank. J Inherit Metab Dis. 2007;30:530–6.
37. Isaacs H Jr. Fetal and neonatal leukemia. J Pediatr Hematol Oncol. 2003;25:348–61.
38. Eyles D, Almeras L, Benech P, Patatian A, Mackay-Sim A, McGrath J, Feron F. Developmental vitamin D deficiency alters the expression of genes encoding mitochondrial, cytoskeletal and synaptic proteins in the adult rat brain. J Steroid Biochem Mol Biol. 2007;103:538–45.
39. Chajes V, Biessy C, Ferrari P, Romieu I, Freisling H, Huybrechts I, Scalbert A, Bueno de Mesquita B, Romaguera D, Gunter MJ, et al. Plasma elaidic acid level as biomarker of industrial trans fatty acids and risk of weight change: report from the EPIC study. PLoS One. 2015;10:e0118206.
40. Saadatian-Elahi M, Slimani N, Chajes V, Jenab M, Goudable J, Biessy C, Ferrari P, Byrnes G, Autier P, Peeters PH, et al. Plasma phospholipid fatty acid profiles and their association with food intakes: results from a cross-sectional study within the European prospective investigation into cancer and nutrition. Am J Clin Nutr. 2009;89:331–46.
41. Chajes V, Joulin V, Clavel-Chapelon F. The fatty acid desaturation index of blood lipids, as a biomarker of hepatic stearoyl-CoA desaturase expression, is a predictive factor of breast cancer risk. Curr Opin Lipidol. 2011;22:6–10.
42. Dupont WD. Power calculations for matched case-control studies. Biometrics. 1988;44:1157–68.
43. Freedman LS. Tables of the number of patients required in clinical trials using the logrank test. Stat Med. 1982;1:121–9.
44. Chappell JE, Clandinin MT, Kearney-Volpe C. Trans fatty acids in human milk lipids: influence of maternal diet and weight loss. Am J Clin Nutr. 1985;42:49–56.
45. Von Behren J, Spector LG, Mueller BA, Carozza SE, Chow EJ, Fox EE, Horel S, Johnson KJ, McLaughlin C, Puumala SE, et al. Birth order and risk of childhood cancer: a pooled analysis from five US states. Int J Cancer. 2011;128:2709–16.

Nutrient intake disparities in the US: modeling the effect of food substitutions

Zach Conrad[1*], LuAnn K. Johnson[1], James N. Roemmich[1], WenYen Juan[2] and Lisa Jahns[1]

Abstract

Background: Diet quality among federal food assistance program participants remains low, and little research has assessed the diet quality of food insecure non-participants. Further research is needed to assess the extent to which food substitutions can improve the nutritional status of these vulnerable populations. Substituting egg dishes for other commonly consumed dishes at certain eating occasions may be an effective strategy for improving the daily nutrient intake among these groups. Eggs are rich in many important nutrients, and are low-cost and part of a wide range of cultural food menus, which are important considerations for low-income and ethnically diverse populations. To help guide the focus of targeted nutrition interventions and education campaigns for vulnerable populations, the present work begins by 1) estimating the prevalence of nutrient inadequacy among these groups, and then models the effect of consuming egg dishes instead of commonly consumed dishes at each eating occasion on 2) the prevalence of nutrient inadequacy, and 3) the mean intake of nutrients.

Methods: Dietary data from 34,741 adults ≥ 20 y were acquired from the National Health and Nutrition Examination Survey, 2001–2014. Diet pattern modeling was used to substitute commonly consumed egg dishes for commonly consumed main dishes at breakfast, lunch, and dinner. National Cancer Institute usual intake methods were used to estimate the prevalence of inadequate intake of 31 nutrients pre- and post-substitution, and a novel index was used to estimate change in intake of all nutrients collectively.

Results: Substituting eggs for commonly consumed main dishes at lunch or dinner did not change total daily nutrient intake for each group ($P > 0.05$), but decreased the prevalence of vitamin D inadequacy by 1–4 percentage points ($P < 0.01$). Substituting eggs for commonly consumed foods at breakfast increased the prevalence of folate inadequacy by 8–12 percentage points among each group ($P < 0.01$).

Conclusions: When making food substitutions to increase nutrient intake, eating occasion should be an important consideration. Further research is needed to better understand how food substitutions affect diet costs, which may be an important driver of food purchasing decisions among low income individuals with limited food budgets.

Keywords: Diet quality, Nutrient intake, Food security, Food assistance, Diet model

Background

Federal food assistance programs in the US have expanded in scale and number over the past century, and are now a cornerstone of the national nutrition agenda. These programs represent essential tools to reduce food insecurity and improve the diet quality of low-income individuals and households across the country.

* Correspondence: zach.conrad@ars.usda.gov
[1]Grand Forks Human Nutrition Research Center, US Department of Agriculture, Agricultural Research Service, 2420 2nd Ave. N, Grand Forks, ND 58203, USA
Full list of author information is available at the end of the article

The largest of these programs, in federal financial outlays and the number of individuals participating, are the Supplemental Nutrition Assistance Program (SNAP) and Special Supplemental Nutrition Program for Women, Infants, and Children (WIC). SNAP, formerly known as the "Food Stamp Program", provides financial benefits to eligible households to purchase foods for at-home consumption. Eligibility is determined primarily by household income at or below 130% of the poverty level [1]. Over 45 million individuals participated in SNAP in 2016, [2] with annual program costs exceeding $80 billion [3]. In contrast to SNAP, WIC provides financial benefits to eligible individuals to purchase a select suite of approved foods [4]. Eligibility is determined by a categorical requirement (pregnant, post-partum, or breastfeeding women; infants; and children), income requirement (state-specific income-to-poverty ratio threshold), and nutrition risk requirement (individuals deemed to be at risk of nutrition-related poor health outcomes). Approximately 9.5 million individuals participated in WIC in 2016, [4] with a program cost of $6.6 billion [3].

Low diet quality is the leading cause of mortality in the US [5]. Income is an important moderator of diet quality, with lower income individuals exhibiting lower quality diets than their higher income counterparts [6, 7]. SNAP and WIC participants, in particular, generally exhibit low quality diets [8, 9] and high rates of cardio-metabolic mortality [10]. Yet little research has assessed the diet quality of food insecure individuals who are not participating in either SNAP or WIC. Further efforts are needed to address this important research gap and to assess interventions to improve the nutritional status of these vulnerable populations.

Evidence suggests that moderate diet and lifestyle changes can be more easily adopted and sustained than more drastic changes, and can ultimately elicit meaningful health improvements [11–13]. Following this principle, one approach to improving diet quality is to counsel individuals to make healthier food choices one meal at a time. Several studies have found that the greatest amount of calories is consumed at dinner, yet the intake of micronutrients at each eating occasion was not examined [14–16]. Others have examined the micronutrient contribution of individual foods to daily nutrient intakes, such as beef, [17] dairy, [18–20] breakfast cereal, [21] orange juice, [22] potatoes, [23] avocados, [24] and canned fruits and vegetables, [25] yet evidence is lacking on how specific food choices at each eating occasion (i.e. breakfast, lunch, and dinner) contribute to daily nutrient intake.

Substituting egg dishes for other commonly consumed dishes at certain eating occasions may be an effective strategy for improving the daily nutrient intake among vulnerable populations. Eggs are rich in many important nutrients, [26–28] increase the bioavailability of co-consumed carotenoids [29] and vitamin E, [30] and promote positive health outcomes at all ages and all stages of life [30, 31]. In a recent study, pregnant egg consumers were much more likely to meet daily choline intake recommendations than pregnant non-egg consumers [32]. And eggs are low-cost and part of a wide range of cultural food menus, [31] which are important considerations for low-income and ethnically diverse populations.

To help guide the focus of targeted nutrition interventions and education campaigns for individuals participating in federal food assistance programs and those with low food security, the present work begins by 1) estimating the prevalence of nutrient inadequacy among these groups, and then models the effect of consuming egg dishes instead of commonly consumed dishes at each eating occasion on 2) the prevalence of nutrient inadequacy, and 3) the mean intake of nutrients.

Methods

Dietary data

Data on individual-level food and nutrient intake, SNAP and WIC participation, food security status, and other characteristics were acquired from the National Health and Nutrition Examination Survey (NHANES), waves 2001–2002, 2003–2004, 2005–2006, 2007–2008, 2009–2010, 2011–2012, and 2013–2014 [33]. NHANES is a continuous, cross-sectional survey that collects data on demography and health behaviors from a sample of ~ 5000 individuals per year, and data are released in two-year cycles. Data on food and nutrient intake were acquired from What We Eat In America (WWEIA), the dietary component of NHANES. Individuals complete a 24-h recall (24HR) administered by a trained interviewer using United States Department of Agriculture's (USDA) Automated Multiple Pass Method, [34] and a subset of the study population (~ 80%) completes a subsequent 24HR by telephone on a non-consecutive day. Food security status was assessed by trained NHANES staff using the US Food Security Module [35].

Study populations

All individuals 20+ y with dietary recalls that were considered reliable by trained NHANES staff were included in this study (n = 34,741). Respondents were categorized as SNAP participants, WIC participants, food insecure non-participants, and food secure non-participants. SNAP participants were identified as individuals who reported that someone in their household was participating in SNAP at the time of the survey (n = 4020), and WIC participants were identified as individuals who reported that they were participating in WIC at the time of the survey (n = 636). Individuals who reported participating in SNAP and WIC at the time of the survey (n = 209) were categorized as WIC participants in order to maintain the relative homogeneity of this group compared to the SNAP group (due to the more restrictive eligibility requirements of WIC). Individuals who did not report participating in SNAP or WIC but reported low or very low food security were categorized as food insecure non-participants (n = 3631), and individuals who did not report participating in SNAP or WIC and reported marginal or full food security were categorized as food secure non-participants (n = 26,454).

Identifying main dishes at each eating occasion

For each individual food reported consumed in WWEIA 2001–2014, the eating occasion and time of day each food was consumed was reported in either English or Spanish. Foods reported consumed at breakfast, lunch, or dinner were grouped into main dish categories primarily according to the categorization scheme used in the Food and Nutrient Database for Dietary Studies (FNDDS; Additional file 1: Table S1) [36]. A total of 17 main dish categories were identified: beef dishes, pork dishes, bacon, poultry dishes, other meat dishes, seafood dishes, sandwiches, sausages, soups, breads, sweet baked goods, pancakes and waffles, oatmeal, breakfast cereal, pasta, Mexican dishes, and pizzas and calzones. Additionally, six egg dishes were identified: whole eggs, scrambled eggs and omelets, egg sandwiches, egg soups, frozen egg dishes, and quiches. A composite nutrient profile was created for each main dish and each egg dish by averaging the nutrient content per gram weight of each of the foods in each dish category.

Diet modeling

A diet model was constructed to estimate the effects on daily nutrient intake if egg dishes were substituted for commonly consumed main dishes at each eating occasion (i.e. breakfast, lunch, and dinner). Commonly consumed dishes at each eating occasion among each group (i.e. SNAP participants, WIC participants, food insecure non-participants, and food secure non-participants) were identified by frequency of reported consumption (i.e. percent of individuals reporting consumption of each dish). The diet model replaced the most commonly consumed main dish with the most commonly consumed egg dish at each eating occasion for each individual in each group, on a gram weight basis. For example, if the most commonly consumed main dish among SNAP participants at breakfast was bread, and the most commonly consumed egg dish among SNAP participants at breakfast was scrambled eggs, then for each SNAP participant the amount of bread consumed (in grams) was replaced with the same gram weight of scrambled eggs.

Total nutrient index

A total nutrient index was developed to provide a summary estimate of how much nutrient intake changed (for all nutrients collectively) when egg dishes were consumed instead of the most commonly consumed dishes at each eating occasion. This index is interpreted as the mean percent change in nutrient intake from baseline intake to modeled intakes. The total nutrient index was calculated in two steps: first, by estimating the percent change in intake from baseline for each individual nutrient, and then 2) computing the mean percent change in nutrient intake across all nutrients. Nutrients which Americans are encouraged to limit, including sodium and saturated fat, were reverse scored prior to computing the total nutrient index so that greater values represented lower percent change from baseline. To ensure that more accurately measured nutrient intakes had greater influence on the index, the total nutrient index was weighted by the standard error of each nutrient, so that nutrients with greater standard errors received less weight in the index. The total nutrient index can be expressed as:

$$\textit{Total nutrient index} = \frac{\sum_{i=1}^{N} C_i/se_i}{\sum_{i=1}^{N} se_i}$$

where C is the percent change in the intake of a given nutrient (i) weighted by its standard error (se), and N is the number of nutrients included in the index.

Sensitivity analyses were used to test the sensitivity of the total nutrient index to potentially influential individual nutrients. In these analyses, nutrients with the greatest change from baseline were iteratively removed from the index and compared against the original index.

Statistical analyses

Daily nutrient intake was estimated at baseline (i.e. reported daily intake) and for three modeled intakes: substituting egg dishes for the most commonly consumed main dishes at breakfast, lunch, and dinner. The percent of individuals in each group not meeting age-and sex-specific daily intake recommendations, as well as the mean daily intake of each nutrient, were estimated using the National Cancer Institute's (NCI) usual intake methodology [37]. The NCI method uses information from two 24HRs to estimate within-person variation using the SAS macros MIXTRAN and DISTRIB. MIXTRAN uses logistic regression with a person-specific random effect to estimate the probability of consumption, accounting for the day of intake and whether it was a weekday or weekend; DISTRIB estimates daily intake; and the results from both macros are linked with a correlated person-specific random effects model.

The percent of individuals not meeting daily intake recommendations was estimated for the 16 nutrients with an Estimated Average Requirement (EAR; vitamins A, B_6, B_{12}, C, D, E; thiamin; riboflavin; niacin; folate; calcium; iron; magnesium; and zinc), an Upper Limit (UL; sodium), or a Dietary Guidelines for Americans 2015–2020 (DGA) recommendation (saturated fatty acids; Additional file 2: Table S2). Mean nutrient intakes were estimated for all nutrients, additionally including 12 nutrients without a recommended intake amount: fiber, eicosapentanoic acid, docosahexaenoic acid, α-linolenic acid, vitamin K, choline, potassium, α-carotene, β-carotene, β-cryptoxanthin, lutein and zeaxanthin, and lycopene. Mean intakes were also estimated for total protein, carbohydrate, and fat. The balanced repeated replication method was used to estimate standard errors while accounting for the complex sampling design of NHANES.

All analyses were adjusted for age (20–30, 31–50, 51–70, 71+), gender, race-ethnicity (non-Hispanic white, non-Hispanic black, Mexican-American), education (less than high school, high school or equivalent, some college, college graduate), marital status (single and never married; married or living with a partner; widowed, divorced, or separated), household size (1, 2, 3–4, 5+), currently participating in a health insurance plan (yes, no), body mass index (less than 18.5, 18.5–24.9, 25–29.9, 30+), income-to-poverty ratio (less than 0.5, 0.51–1.0, 1.01–1.3, greater than 1.3), and whether the dietary recall was completed on a weekday or weekend. Differences in baseline nutrient intake across groups, and differences between baseline intake and each of the modeled intakes within each group were tested using z-scores, with significance at $P < 0.05$ with Bonferroni adjustment for multiple comparisons. Stata 14 was used for data management and SAS 9.4 was used for all analyses. This study was deemed exempt by the University of North Dakota Institutional Review Board.

Results

Sociodemographic characteristics

WIC participants were younger (26.3 y, 95% CI: 25.6–26.9 y) than all other groups (Table 1), and food secure non-participants were older (48.0 y, 47.5–48.5 y). All WIC participants were female, and between 50 and 60% of food insecure non-participants, SNAP participants, and food secure non-participants were female. Most individuals in each group were non-Hispanic white, with the greatest proportion in the food secure non-participant group (82.7%, 80.7–84.6%). All groups had a similar distribution of educational attainment except for food secure non-participants, which had higher educational attainment compared to the other groups. Most individuals in each group were married or living with a partner, with the greatest proportion in the WIC participant group (67.8%, 61.9–73.2%) and food secure non-participant group (65.9%, 64.6–67.1%). WIC participants reported the greatest household size (4.3, 4.2–4.5), and food secure non-participants reported the lowest household size (2.9, 2.8–2.9). Food secure non-participants reported the highest prevalence (84.9%, 83.9–85.8%) of currently participating in a health insurance plan, followed by WIC participants (74.6%, 69.0–79.4%), SNAP participants (67.3%, 64.7–70.0%), and food insecure non-participants (58.0%, 55.3–60.6%). Overweight and obese individuals accounted for 67–76% of each group, yet food secure non-participants had the highest proportion of normal weight individuals (31.2%, 30.2–32.2%). Most (87.2%, 86.2–88.1%) food secure non-participants had an income-to-poverty ratio greater than 1.3, compared with 46.9% (43.9–50.0%) of food insecure non-participants, 35.5% (30.0–41.4%) of WIC participants, and 24.7% (21.7–28.1%) of SNAP participants.

Most commonly consumed dishes at each eating occasion

Among each group, the most commonly consumed main dishes at breakfast, lunch, and dinner were breakfast cereal, sandwiches (including hotdogs and sausages), and poultry dishes (including mixed dishes with poultry and vegetables), respectively (Additional file 3: Table S3). Whole eggs and scrambled eggs were the most commonly consumed egg dishes at breakfast, lunch, and dinner among each group (Additional file 4: Table S4). Mean consumption amounts and nutrient profiles are presented in Additional file 5: Table S5 and Additional file 6: Table S6, respectively.

Reported nutrient intake

Table 2 displays reported daily nutrient intakes among each group, with food insecure non-participants as the reference group. The percent not meeting recommendations for vitamin C and calcium was lower, and the percent not meeting recommendations for vitamin E was higher, among WIC participants compared to food insecure non-participants ($P < 0.001$ for vitamin C, and $P < 0.01$ for vitamin E and calcium). WIC participants also had higher mean intakes of energy ($P = 0.023$), protein ($P = 0.009$), and carbohydrates ($P = 0.007$) compared to food insecure non-participants. The percent not meeting recommendations for vitamin D among food insecure non-participants (98.0%, 97.8–98.2%) was higher than SNAP participants (96.0%, 95.8–96.2%; $P < 0.001$); and the percent not meeting recommendations for folate (30.9%, 28.4–33.5%) and zinc (47.0%, 44.7–49.3%) among food insecure non-participants was lower than SNAP participants (folate: 35.7%, 33.2–38.1%; $P < 0.05$ and zinc: 52.4%, 49.7–55.2%; $P < 0.01$). Compared to food insecure non-participants, the percent not meeting recommendations was lower among food secure non-participants for all nutrients ($P < 0.01$ or $P < 0.001$ for all comparisons) except for saturated fatty acids (higher, $P < 0.01$), sodium (higher, $P < 0.001$), niacin (no difference, $P = 0.251$), and folate (no difference, $P = 0.036$).

No difference in mean intake was observed between food insecure non-participants and WIC participants (Table 2) for total fatty acids ($P = 0.045$), fiber ($P = 0.808$), α-linolenic acid ($P = 0.776$), vitamin K ($P = 0.373$), choline ($P = 0.033$), potassium ($P = 0.557$), α-carotene ($P = 0.455$), β-carotene ($P = 0.846$), β-cryptoxanthin ($P = 0.109$), lutein and zeaxanthin ($P = 0.557$), and lycopene ($P = 0.620$). Compared to food insecure non-participants, SNAP participants had lower mean intake of fiber and lycopene ($P < 0.01$ for both comparisons), and higher mean intake of α-carotene ($P < 0.001$) and β-carotene ($P < 0.01$). Food secure non-participants had lower mean

Table 1 Sociodemographic characteristics of participants in federal food assistance programs, food insecure individuals, and other individuals 2001–2014 ($n = 34{,}741$)

Characteristic	n	Food insecure, non-participants (n = 3631)		WIC participants (n = 636)		SNAP participants (n = 4020)		Food secure, non-participants (n = 26,454)	
					% (95% CI)[a]				
Age (y)	34,741	41.5	(40.5–42.4)	26.3	(25.6–26.9)	42.9	(42.1–43.7)	48.0	(47.5–48.5)
Female	34,741	50.0	(47.8–51.4)	100.0	(NA)	59.0	(57.1–60.9)	50.7	(50.1–51.3)
Race-ethnicity	29,696								
Non-Hispanic white		56.9	(52.0–61.6)	43.0	(35.4–50.8)	55.7	(50.7–62.4)	82.7	(80.7–84.6)
Non-Hispanic black		20.3	(17.5–23.5)	28.3	(22.6–34.9)	30.6	(26.3–25.4)	10.0	(8.8–11.3)
Mexican American		22.8	(19.3–26.8)	28.7	(22.8–35.4)	12.7	(9.7–16.4)	7.3	(6.1–8.6)
Education	34,704								
Less than high school		33.9	(31.1–36.7)	34.0	(28.8–40.0)	39.5	(37.0–42.1)	13.6	(12.6–14.7)
High school or equivalent		27.0	(24.8–29.2)	34.1	(26.7–36.5)	28.4	(26.1–31.0)	22.9	(21.8–24.0)
Some college		31.4	(28.8–34.2)	29.0	(24.2–34.2)	27.1	(25.1–29.1)	31.8	(30.8–32.7)
College graduate		7.7	(6.4–9.3)	5.6	(3.7–8.5)	5.0	(3.9–6.3	31.7	(30.1–33.4)
Marital status	34,723								
Single, never married		25.0	(22.3–27.9)	26.6	(21.6–32.1)	29.5	(26.3–32.4)	16.7	(15.5–18.0)
Married or living with partner		50.5	(47.6–53.4)	67.8	(61.9–73.2)	39.7	(37.1–42.5)	65.9	(64.6–67.1)
Widowed, divorced, or separated		24.5	(22.4–26.8)	5.7	(3.5–9.0)	30.7	(28.3–33.2)	17.4	(16.7–18.1)
Household size (n)	34,741	3.3	(3.2–3.4)	4.3	(4.2–4.5)	3.6	(3.46–3.78)	2.9	(2.8–2.9)
Health insurance[b]	34,620	58.0	(55.3–60.6)	74.6	(69.0–79.4)	67.3	(64.7–70.0)	84.9	(83.9–85.8)
Weight status	34,066								
Underweight		2.6	(1.9–3.5)	0.9	(0.3–2.5)	2.7	(2.1–3.6)	1.5	(1.3–1.7)
Normal weight		28.5	(26.2–31.0)	22.9	(18.3–28.2)	25.5	(23.5–27.5)	31.2	(30.2–32.2)
Overweight		30.0	(27.7–32.4)	32.2	(26.7–38.3)	27.7	(25.7–29.3)	34.6	(33.6–35.6)
Obese		38.9	(36.4–41.5)	44.0	(38.6–49.7)	44.[illegible]	(41.3–46.3)	32.7	(31.6–33.8)
Income-to-poverty ratio	32,247								
Less than or equal to 0.50		11.3	(9.5–13.3)	19.9	(15.2–25.5)	21.1	(18.9–23.5)	2.3	(1.9–2.7)
0.51 to 1.00		22.0	(19.6–24.6)	30.9	(26.2–36.1)	40.3	(37.0–43.7)	5.1	(4.7–5.6)
1.01 to 1.30		19.9	(17.4–22.5)	13.7	(10.3–18.1)	13.8	(12.5–15.3)	5.4	(4.9–6.0)
> 1.30		46.9	(43.9–50.0)	35.5	(30.0–41.4)	24.7	(21.7–28.1)	87.2	(86.2–88.1)

[a]Does not apply to age or household size
[b]Participated in health insurance plan at time of survey
Some SNAP participants may have income-to-poverty ratios greater than 1.3 because income test are the primary, but not the only, criterion of program eligibility. For example, Income tests are relaxed if all family members participate in Temporary Assistance for Needy Families (TANF) or receive Supplemental Security Income (SSI). Additionally, individuals move in and out of SNAP on a monthly basis whereas income data were collected on an annual basis

intake of potassium, and higher mean intake of protein, fiber, α-linolenic acid, vitamin K, choline, α-carotene, β-carotene, β-cryptoxanthin, and lutein and zeaxanthin compared to food insecure non-participants ($P < 0.001$ for all comparisons except protein: $P = 0.012$).

Modeled nutrient intake: substituting eggs as the main dish

Tables 3, 4, 5 and 6 display the results of models that substituted the most commonly consumed egg dish for the most commonly consumed main dish at each eating occasion among food insecure non-participants (Table 3), WIC participants (Table 4), SNAP participants (Table 5), and food secure non-participants (Table 6).

Among food insecure non-participants, no changes in the percent not meeting recommended nutrient intakes were observed when eggs were substituted at breakfast (Table 3). At lunch, substituting eggs decreased the percent not meeting daily recommendations for saturated fatty acids ($P < 0.001$), vitamin D ($P < 0.01$), and magnesium ($P < 0.001$). When eggs were substituted as the main dish at dinner, the percent not meeting recommendations decreased for vitamin A ($P < 0.01$) and vitamin D ($P < 0.01$). Among WIC participants (Table 4), substituting eggs at breakfast increased the percent not meeting folate recommendations ($P < 0.01$); at lunch, the percent not meeting recommendations decreased for saturated fatty acids ($P < 0.01$) and magnesium ($P < 0.001$), and mean intake of choline increased

Table 2 Reported daily nutrient intakes among federal food assistance program participants, food insecure non-participants, and food secure non-participants, 2001–2014 (n = 34,741)

Nutrient	Food insecure non-participants[a] (n = 3631)		WIC participants (n = 636)		SNAP participants (n = 4020)		Food secure non-participants (26,454)	
	Percent not meeting recommendations (95% CI)[d]							
Saturated fatty acids[c]	55.3	(52.1–58.5)	57.5	(50.4–64.7)	58.9	(55.5–62.2)	62.1	(60.6–63.6)**
Vitamin A[d]	67.5	(64.7–70.2)	60.9	(53.3–68.6)	66.4	(62.8–70.0)	46.9	(45.4–48.4)***
Vitamin C	58.7	(55.9–61.4)	47.3	(39.2–55.3)***	60.3	(57.4–55.3)	45.9	(44.3–47.5)***
Vitamin D	98.0	(97.8–98.2)	96.0	(94.0–98.0)	96.0	(95.8–96.2)***	95.0	(94.8–95.2)***
Vitamin E	94.9	(93.9–95.8)	97.3	(95.9–98.6)**	95.1	(94.1–96.1)	88.1	(87.0–89.2)***
Thiamin	12.0	(10.5–13.6)	15.8	(12.6–18.9)	11.6	(10.2–13.0)	9.5	(8.8–10.2)***
Riboflavin	12.5	(10.9–14.0)	12.7	(9.8–15.6)	11.6	(10.2–13.0)	9.7	(9.0–10.4)***
Niacin	10.2	(8.8–11.6)	9.6	(6.9–12.3)	9.6	(8.2–10.9)	9.3	(8.5–10.0)
Vitamin B_6	22.6	(20.5–24.6)	25.7	(20.6–30.9)	23.8	(21.9–25.8)	18.8	(17.6–19.9)***
Folate[e]	30.9	(28.4–33.5)	27.3	(22.3–32.2)	35.7	(33.2–38.1)*	27.9	(26.8–29.0)
Vitamin B_{12}	13.6	(12.0–15.3)	11.3	(8.7–13.9)	12.3	(10.7–13.9)	10.8	(10.0–11.6)**
Calcium	54.7	(52.0–57.4)	44.6	(37.8–51.4)**	55.5	(52.7–58.2)	47.4	(46.2–48.6)***
Iron	15.7	(14.1–17.4)	62.6	(50.6–74.6)***	17.2	(15.4–19)	12.7	(11.9–13.5)***
Magnesium	83.1	(81.3–84.9)	86.9	(83.5–90.4)	85.8	(84.1–87.6)	72.1	(70.9–73.3)***
Sodium[f]	78.7	(76.9–80.5)	81.4	(76.6–86.2)	76.5	(74.5–78.5)	81.4	(80.5–82.3)***
Zinc	47.0	(44.7–49.3)	44.2	(38.5–49.9)	52.4	(49.7–55.2)**	39.4	(38.2–40.6)**
	Mean intake (95% CI)							
Energy (kcal)	2171	(2119–2224)	2309	(2202–2416)*	2192	(2144–2239)	2176	(2159–2192)
Protein, total (g)	81	(79–83)	88	(83–92)*	81	(80–83)	84	(83–84)*
Carbohydrate, total (g)	267	(260–274)	289	(275–304)*	270	(263–277)	262	(260–264)
Fatty acids, total (g)	81	(78–83)	87	(81–92)	81	(79–83)	83	(82–84)
Fiber (g)	14	(13–14)	14	(13–15)	13	(12–13)**	16	(16–16)***
Eicosapentaenoic acid (g)	0.02	(0.02–0.02)	0.02	(0.02–0.03)	0.02	(0.02–0.02)	0.03	(0.03–0.03)**
Docosahexaenoic acid (g)	0.07	(0.06–0.08)	0.07	(0.06–0.08)	0.06	(0.06–0.06)**	0.08	(0.08–0.08)*
α-linolenic acid (g)	1.40	(1.35–1.44)	1.38	(1.26–1.5)	1.35	(1.31–1.4)	1.53	(1.5–1.55)***
Vitamin K (μg)	76	(72–79)	72	(65–80)	72	(68–76)	100	(97–103)***
Choline (mg)	291	(282–300)	269	(251–287)	294	(285–302)	317	(312–322)***
Potassium (mg)	2586	(2555–2618)	2252	(2113–2392)	2586	(2555–2618)	2222	(2159–2286)***
α-carotene (μg)	320	(292–349)	352	(274–430)	516	(488–544)***	516	(488–544)***
β-carotene (μg)	1417	(1331–1504)	1395	(1187–1603)	2136	(2054–2218)**	2136	(2054–2218)***
β-cryptoxanthin (μg)	84	(78–90)	102	(81–123)	78	(73–83)	112	(108–116)***
Lutein and zeaxanthin (μg)	998	(938–1058)	1040	(914–1166)	931	(875–987)	1418	(1362–1473)***
Lycopene (μg)	7514	(6764–8264)	7939	(6436–9442)	6184	(5627–6742)**	8218	(7838–8598)

All estimates adjusted for age, gender, race-ethnicity, education, marital status, household size, health insurance, BMI, income-to-poverty ratio, and whether the dietary recall was on a weekday or weekend

[a]Reference group

[b]Daily nutrient recommendations are Estimated Average Requirements (EAR) unless otherwise specified. National Academy of Sciences. Institute of Medicine. 2006. Dietary reference intakes: The essential guide to nutrient requirements. Jennifer J. Otten, Jennifer Pitzi Hellwig, Linda D. Meyers (eds.). National Academies Press, Washington, DC

[c]Recommendation is less than 10% of total energy. US Department of Health and Human Services & US Department of Agriculture. 2015–2020. Dietary Guidelines for Americans 2015–2020. U.S. Government Printing Office, Washington, DC. Available at: http://health.gov/dietaryguidelines/ (verified 29 March 2016)

[d]Retinol Activity Equivalent (RAE)

[e]Dietary Folate Equivalent (DFE)

[f]Tolerable upper intake level limit (UL). National Academy of Sciences, Institute of Medicine. 2006. Dietary reference intakes: The essential guide to nutrient requirements. Jennifer J. Otten, Jennifer Pitzi Hellwig, Linda D. Meyers (eds.). National Academies Press, Washington, DC

*Different than food insecure non-participants at $P < 0.017$ (Bonferroni adjusted for multiple comparisons)

**Different than food insecure non-participants at $P < 0.003$ (Bonferroni adjusted for multiple comparisons)

***Different than food insecure non-participants at $P < 0.0003$ (Bonferroni adjusted for multiple comparisons)

Table 3 Reported daily nutrient intakes and modeled nutrient intakes if eggs were consumed as the main dish at each eating occasion among food insecure non-participants, 2001–2014 ($n = 3631$)

Nutrient	Reported daily intake[b,c]		Modeled daily intake[a]					
			Eggs consumed as main dish at breakfast		Eggs consumed as main dish at lunch		Eggs consumed as main dish at dinner	
	Percent not meeting recommendations (95% CI)[d]							
Saturated fatty acids[e]	55.3	(52.1–58.5)	57.4	(54.0–60.7)	44.2	(41.0–47.4)***	59.2	(56.1–62.4)
Vitamin A[f]	67.5	(64.7–70.2)	70.0	(67.4–72.7)	63.3	(60.5–66.2)	61.3	(58.1–64.4)**
Vitamin C	58.7	(55.9–61.4)	59.2	(56.5–61.9)	58.8	(56.0–61.5)	58.9	(56.3–61.6)
Vitamin D	98.0	(97.8–98.2)	98.0	(97.8–98.2)	94.0	(93.8–94.2)**	94.0	(93.8–94.2)**
Vitamin E	94.9	(93.9–95.8)	95.4	(94.4–96.3)	94.1	(93.0–95.1)	94.0	(92.9–95.0)
Thiamin	12.0	(10.5–13.6)	12.3	(10.7–13.8)	11.5	(10.0–13.0)	10.7	(9.2–12.2)
Riboflavin	12.5	(10.9–14.0)	12.8	(11.2–14.3)	11.9	(10.3–13.4)	11.0	(9.5–12.5)
Niacin	10.2	(8.8–11.6)	10.7	(9.3–12.1)	10.6	(9.1–12.1)	10.2	(8.8–11.6)
Vitamin B_6	22.6	(20.5–24.6)	24.6	(22.6–26.7)	22.7	(20.8–24.7)	24.8	(22.8–26.8)
Folate[g]	30.9	(28.4–33.5)	34.8	(32.1–37.5)	31.0	(28.5–33.6)	29.9	(27.4–32.4)
Vitamin B_{12}	13.6	(12.0–15.3)	13.8	(12.1–15.5)	13.4	(11.8–15.0)	12.0	(10.5–13.5)
Calcium	54.7	(52.0–57.4)	55.1	(52.4–57.9)	55.3	(52.6–58.0)	53.6	(50.8–56.3)
Iron	15.7	(14.1–17.4)	15.7	(14.1–17.3)	15.7	(14.1–17.4)	15.3	(13.7–17.0)
Magnesium	83.1	(81.3–84.9)	84.2	(82.4–85.9)	71.8	(69.4–74.2)***	83.7	(82.0–85.4)
Sodium[h]	78.7	(76.9–80.5)	78.5	(76.7–80.2)	77.8	(76.0–79.6)	78.5	(76.7–80.3)
Zinc	47.0	(44.7–49.3)	49.7	(47.3–52.0)	48.0	(45.8–50.3)	47.1	(44.8–49.4)
	Mean intake (95% CI)							
Energy (kcal)	2171	(2119–2224)	2157	(2104–2210)	2162	(2110–2215)	2167	(2114–2220)
Protein, total (g)	81	(79–83)	80	(78–83)	79	(76–81)	75	(73–78)**
Carbohydrate, total (g)	267	(260–274)	262	(255–269)	267	(260–274)	270	(263–277)
Fatty acids, total (g)	81	(78–83)	81	(78–83)	79	(76–81)	78	(76–81)
Fiber (g)	14	(13–14)	14	(13–14)	14	(13–14)	14	(13–14)
Eicosapentaenoic acid (g)	0.02	(0.02–0.02)	0.02	(0.02–0.02)	0.02	(0.02–0.02)	0.02	(0.02–0.02)
Docosahexaenoic acid (g)	0.07	(0.06–0.08)	0.07	(0.06–0.07)	0.07	(0.07–0.08)	0.08	(0.07–0.08)
α-linolenic acid (g)	1.40	(1.35–1.44)	1.40	(1.35–1.44)	1.38	(1.34–1.43)	1.40	(1.35–1.44)
Vitamin K (μg)	76	(72–79)	76	(72–79)	76	(72–79)	75	(72–79)
Choline (mg)	291	(282–300)	302	(292–312)	324	(314–335)***	346	(334–358)***
Potassium (mg)	2586	(2555–2618)	2569	(2539–2599)	2566	(2536–2596)	2561	(2530–2592)
α-carotene (μg)	320	(292–349)	282	(260–304)	283	(198–368)	268	(156–379)
β-carotene (μg)	1417	(1331–1504)	1418	(1333–1504)	1411	(1326–1496)	1389	(1306–1472)
β-cryptoxanthin (μg)	84	(78–90)	77	(72–82)	82	(76–87)	80	(75–85)
Lutein and zeaxanthin (μg)	998	(938–1058)	996	(936–1055)	1064	(1004–1125)	1110	(1046–1175)
Lycopene (μg)	7514	(6764–8264)	7403	(6717–8088)	7775	(7005–8545)	7578	(6818–8338)

All estimates adjusted for age, gender, race-ethnicity, education, marital status, household size, health insurance, BMI, income-to-poverty ratio, and whether the dietary recall was on a weekday or weekend

[a]Modeled daily nutrient intake if eggs were consumed as the main dish at each eating occasion

[b]Mean, 2001–2014

[c]Referent

[d]Daily nutrient recommendations are Estimated Average Requirements (EAR) unless otherwise specified. National Academy of Sciences, Institute of Medicine. 2006. Dietary reference intakes: The essential guide to nutrient requirements. Jennifer J. Otten, Jennifer Pitzi Hellwig, Linda D. Meyers (eds.). National Academies Press, Washington, DC

[e]Less than 10% of total energy. US Department of Health and Human Services & US Department of Agriculture. 2015–2020. Dietary Guidelines for Americans 2015–2020. U.S. Government Printing Office, Washington, DC. Available at: http://health.gov/dietaryguidelines/ (verified 29 March 2016)

[f]Retinol Activity Equivalent (RAE)

[g]Dietary Folate Equivalent (DFE)

[h]Tolerable upper intake level limit. National Academy of Sciences, Institute of Medicine. 2006. Dietary reference intakes: The essential guide to nutrient requirements. Jennifer J. Otten, Jennifer Pitzi Hellwig, Linda D. Meyers (eds.). National Academies Press, Washington, DC

*Different than food insecure non-participants at $P < 0.017$ (Bonferroni adjusted for multiple comparisons)

**Different than food insecure non-participants at $P < 0.003$ (Bonferroni adjusted for multiple comparisons)

Table 4 Reported daily nutrient intakes and modeled nutrient intakes if eggs were consumed as the main dish at each eating occasion among participants in the Special Supplemental Nutrition Program for Women, Infants, and Children (WIC), 2001–2014 ($n = 636$)

Nutrient	Reported daily intake[b,c]		Modeled daily intake[a]					
			Eggs consumed as main dish at breakfast		Eggs consumed as main dish at lunch		Eggs consumed as main dish at dinner	
	Percent not meeting recommendations (95% CI)[d]							
Saturated fatty acids[e]	57.5	(50.4–64.7)	62.1	(55.5–68.7)	40.9	(34.1–47.7)**	63.1	(56.5–69.7)
Vitamin A[f]	60.9	(53.3–68.6)	66.3	(58.8–73.8)	54.5	(47.7–61.2)	54.6	(46.8–62.5)
Vitamin C	47.3	(39.2–55.3)	48.9	(40.8–57.0)	48.9	(40.8–57.0)	47.8	(39.9–55.8)
Vitamin D	96.0	(94.0–98.0)	97.0	(96.8–97.2)	95.0	(94.0–98.0)	96.0	(95.8–96.2)
Vitamin E	97.3	(95.9–98.6)	97.6	(96.5–98.8)	96.7	(95.2–98.3)	96.9	(95.4–98.3)
Thiamin	15.8	(12.6–18.9)	19.0	(15.3–22.6)	15.4	(12.3–18.4)	14.8	(11.6–18.1)
Riboflavin	12.7	(9.8–15.6)	14.3	(11.1–17.4)	11.6	(8.9–14.4)	11.1	(8.3–13.8)
Niacin	9.6	(6.9–12.3)	11.6	(8.4–14.7)	10.9	(7.9–13.8)	9.7	(7.0–12.4)
Vitamin B_6	25.7	(20.6–30.9)	33.6	(27.3–39.8)	26.4	(21.2–31.6)	29.4	(23.9–34.9)
Folate[j]	27.3	(22.3–32.2)	38.9	(31.8–46.1)**	28.0	(22.9–33.1)	26.6	(21.6–31.6)
Vitamin B_{12}	11.3	(8.7–13.9)	12.2	(9.4–15.1)	10.9	(8.4–13.4)	10.0	(7.6–12.5)
Calcium	44.6	(37.8–51.4)	44.92	(38.3–51.6)	45.49	(38.3–52.7)	42.4	(35.8–49.0)
Iron	62.6	(50.6–74.6)	67.4	(56.0–78.9)	62.1	(50.1–74.2)	61.9	(49.8–73.9)
Magnesium	86.9	(83.5–90.4)	88.7	(85.3–92.0)	63.3	(57.1–69.4)***	87.5	(84.1–90.9)
Sodium[h]	81.4	(76.6–86.2)	80.7	(75.6–85.8)	80.9	(75.9–85.9)	81.2	(76.4–85.9)
Zinc	44.2	(38.5–49.9)	51.2	(45.1–57.2)	46.3	(40.1–52.4)	45.5	(39.5–51.5)
	Mean intake (95% CI)							
Energy (kcal)	2309	(2202–2416)	2279	(2172–2387)	2300	(2193–2408)	2304	(2198–2410)
Protein, total (g)	88	(83–92)	88	(83–92)	85	(80–89)	78	(77–79)**
Carbohydrate, total (g)	289	(275–304)	256	(254–258)**	289	(275–304)	298	(283–313)
Fatty acids, total (g)	87	(81–92)	88	(82–93)	85	(79–90)	88	(82–93)
Fiber (g)	14	(13–15)	13	(13–14)	14	(13–15)	14	(13–15)
Eicosapentaenoic acid (g)	0.02	(0.02–0.03)	0.02	(0.02–0.03)	0.023	(0.02–0.02)	0.019	(0.02–0.02)
Docosahexaenoic acid (g)	0.07	(0.06–0.08)	0.07	(0.06–0.08)	0.079	(0.06–0.08)	0.069	(0.06–0.08)
α-linolenic acid (g)	1.38	(1.26–1.5)	1.40	(1.28–1.51)	1.36	(1.24–1.48)	1.41	(1.29–1.52)
Vitamin K (μg)	72	(65–80)	72	(65–80)	71	(63–78)	71	(64–79)
Choline (mg)	269	(251–287)	286	(267–305)	316	(294–337)**	308	(285–331)***
Potassium (mg)	2252	(2113–2392)	2233	(2092–2373)	2215	(2070–2360)	2222	(2083–2362)
α-carotene (μg)	352	(274–430)	309	(252–367)	307	(200–414)	314	(174–453)
β-carotene (μg)	1395	(1187–1603)	1386	(1176–1596)	1368	(1158–1578)	1390	(1181–1599)
β-cryptoxanthin (μg)	102	(81–123)	92	(75–110)	100	(82–118)	96	(80–113)
Lutein and zeaxanthin (μg)	1040	(914–1166)	1034	(916–1151)	1158	(1038–1279)	1141	(1013–1268)
Lycopene (μg)	7939	(6436–9442)	8249	(6743–9756)	8078	(6402–9754)	9180	(7504–10,857)

All estimates adjusted for age, race-ethnicity, education, marital status, household size, health insurance, BMI, income-to-poverty ratio, and whether the dietary recall was on a weekday or weekend

[a]Modeled daily nutrient intake if eggs were consumed as the main dish at each eating occasion

[b]Mean, 2001–2014

[3]Referent

[d]Daily nutrient recommendations are Estimated Average Requirements (EAR) unless otherwise specified. National Academy of Sciences, Institute of Medicine. 2006. Dietary reference intakes: The essential guide to nutrient requirements. Jennifer J. Otten, Jennifer Pitzi Hellwig, Linda D. Meyers (eds.). National Academies Press, Washington, DC

[e]Less than 10% of total energy. US Department of Health and Human Services & US Department of Agriculture. 2015–2020. Dietary Guidelines for Americans 2015–2020. U.S. Government Printing Office, Washington, DC. Available at: http://health.gov/dietaryguidelines/ (verified 29 March 2016)

[f]Retinol Activity Equivalent (RAE)

[j]Dietary Folate Equivalent (DFE)

[h]Tolerable upper intake level limit. National Academy of Sciences, Institute of Medicine. 2006. Dietary reference intakes: The essential guide to nutrient requirements. Jennifer J. Otten, Jennifer Pitzi Hellwig, Linda D. Meyers (eds.). National Academies Press, Washington, DC

*Different than food insecure non-participants at $P < 0.017$ (Bonferroni adjusted for multiple comparisons)

**Different than food insecure non-participants at $P < 0.003$ (Bonferroni adjusted for multiple comparisons)

***Different than food insecure non-participants at $P < 0.0003$ (Bonferroni adjusted for multiple comparisons)

Table 5 Reported daily nutrient intakes and modeled nutrient intakes if eggs were consumed as the main dish at each eating occasion among participants in the Supplemental Nutrition Assistance Program (SNAP), 2001–2014 (n = 4020)

Nutrient	Reported daily intake[b,c]		Modeled daily intake[a]					
			Eggs consumed as main dish at breakfast		Eggs consumed as main dish at lunch		Eggs consumed as main dish at dinner	
	Percent not meeting recommendations (95% CI)[d]							
Saturated fatty acids[e]	58.9	(55.5–62.2)	61.9	(58.5–65.3)	40.1	(36.8–43.4)***	63.5	(60.2–66.8)
Vitamin A[f]	66.4	(62.8–70.0)	70.1	(66.7–73.6)	62.5	(58.8–66.3)	59.4	(55.7–63.1)**
Vitamin C	60.3	(57.4–55.3)	61.4	(58.6–64.2)	60.0	(57.3–62.7)	60.4	(57.6–63.1)
Vitamin D	96.0	(95.8–96.2)	97.0	(96.8–97.2)**	96.0	(95.8–96.2)	95.0	(94.8–95.2)**
Vitamin E	95.1	(94.1–96.1)	95.6	(94.7–96.5)	94.6	(93.5–95.6)	94.3	(93.2–95.4)
Thiamin	11.6	(10.2–13.0)	12.3	(10.9–13.8)	11.1	(9.6–12.5)	10.1	(8.7–11.4)
Riboflavin	12.0	(10.6–13.5)	12.6	(11.1–14.1)	11.4	(9.9–12.8)	10.1	(8.7–11.4)
Niacin	9.6	(8.2–10.9)	10.6	(9.2–12.0)	10.1	(8.7–11.4)	9.5	(8.1–10.9)
Vitamin B_6	23.8	(21.9–25.8)	28.3	(26.1–30.4)**	24.6	(22.6–26.5)	27.1	(25.0–29.1)
Folate[g]	35.7	(33.2–38.1)	43.4	(41.0–45.8)**	36.0	(33.5–38.6)	34.4	(31.8–36.9)
Vitamin B_{12}	12.3	(10.7–13.9)	13.0	(11.3–14.6)	12.1	(10.5–13.8)	10.6	(9.1–12.1)
Calcium	55.5	(52.7–58.2)	55.61	(52.8–58.4)	55.18	(52.5–57.9)	54.2	(51.5–56.9)
Iron	17.2	(15.4–19)	18.71	(16.9–20.5)	17.44	(15.6–19.3)	16.5	(14.7–18.3)
Magnesium	85.8	(84.1–87.6)	87.1	(85.4–88.9)	74.1	(71.6–76.6)***	86.4	(84.7–88.0)
Sodium[h]	76.5	(74.5–78.5)	76.2	(74.2–78.2)	75.2	(73.2–77.3)	76.1	(74.1–78.2)
Zinc	52.4	(49.7–55.2)	56.5	(53.7–59.2)	53.5	(50.8–56.3)	52.6	(49.9–55.2)
	Mean intake (95% CI)							
Energy (kcal)	2192	(2144–2239)	2173	(2125–2220)	2183	(2135–2230)	2183	(2136–2231)
Protein, total (g)	81	(80–83)	81	(80–83)	81	(79–82)	84	(80–88)
Carbohydrate, total (g)	270	(263–277)	281	(266–296)	273	(266–280)	272	(265–279)
Fatty acids, total (g)	81	(79–83)	82	(80–84)	82	(80–84)	79	(77–81)
Fiber (g)	13	(12–13)	12	(12–13)	13	(12–14)	13	(12–13)
Eicosapentaenoic acid (g)	0.02	(0.02–0.02)	0.02	(0.02–0.02)	0.02	(0.02–0.02)	0.021	(0.02–0.02)
Docosahexaenoic acid (g)	0.06	(0.06–0.06)	0.06	(0.05–0.06)	0.06	(0.06–0.07)	0.071	(0.07–0.08)
α-linolenic acid (g)	1.35	(1.31–1.4)	1.36	(1.32–1.41)	1.35	(1.31–1.4)	1.35	(1.3–1.39)
Vitamin K (μg)	72	(68–76)	72	(69–76)	72	(68–76)	71	(68–75)
Choline (mg)	294	(285–302)	304	(296–313)	322	(312–331)***	351	(340–361)***
Potassium (mg)	2586	(2555–2618)	2569	(2539–2599)	2566	(2536–2596)	2561	(2530–2592)
α-carotene (μg)	246	(218–274)	227	(204–250)	226	(157–295)	214	(124–305)
β-carotene (μg)	1231	(1133–1329)	1234	(1139–1329)	1241	(1142–1339)	1213	(1120–1306)
β-cryptoxanthin (μg)	78	(73–83)	72	(68–77)	75	(70–79)	76	(71–81)
Lutein and zeaxanthin (μg)	931	(875–987)	925	(871–979)	986	(928–1044)	1053	(995–1111)**
Lycopene (μg)	6184	(5627–6742)	6386	(5811–6961)	6833	(6206–7461)	6274	(5693–6855)

All estimates adjusted for age, gender, race-ethnicity, education, marital status, household size, health insurance, EMI, income-to-poverty ratio, and whether the dietary recall was on a weekday or weekend

[a]Modeled daily nutrient intake if eggs were consumed as the main dish at each eating occasion

[b]Mean, 2001–2014

[c]Referent

[d]Daily nutrient recommendations are Estimated Average Requirements (EAR) unless otherwise specified. National Academy of Sciences, Institute of Medicine. 2006. Dietary reference intakes: The essential guide to nutrient requirements. Jennifer J. Otten, Jennifer Pitzi Hellwig, Linda D. Meyers (eds.). National Academies Press, Washington, DC

[e]Less than 10% of total energy. US Department of Health and Human Services & US Department of Agriculture. 2015–2020. Dietary Guidelines for Americans 2015–2020. U.S. Government Printing Office, Washington, DC. Available at: http://health.gov/dietaryguidelines/ (verified 29 March 2016)

[f]Retinol Activity Equivalent (RAE)

[f]Dietary Folate Equivalent (DFE)

[j]Tolerable upper intake level limit. National Academy of Sciences, Institute of Medicine. 2006. Dietary reference intakes: The essential guide to nutrient requirements. Jennifer J. Otten, Jennifer Pitzi Hellwig, Linda D. Meyers (eds.). National Academies Press, Washington, DC

*Different than food insecure non-participants at $P < 0.017$ (Bonferroni adjusted for multiple comparisons)

**Different than food insecure non-participants at $P < 0.003$ (Bonferroni adjusted for multiple comparisons)

***Different than food insecure non-participants at $P < 0.0003$ (Bonferroni adjusted for multiple comparisons)

Table 6 Reported daily nutrient intakes and modeled nutrient intakes if eggs were consumed as the main dish at each eating occasion among food secure non-participants, 2001–2014 ($n = 26{,}454$)

Nutrient	Reported daily intake[b,c]		Modeled daily intake[a]					
			Eggs consumed as main dish at breakfast		Eggs consumed as main dish at lunch		Eggs consumed as main dish at dinner	
			Percent not meeting recommendations (95% CI)[d]					
Saturated fatty acids[e]	62.1	(60.6–63.6)	65.6	(64.2–67.1)*	37.0	(35.4–38.5)***	66.3	(64.8–67.8)**
Vitamin A[f]	46.9	(45.4–48.4)	50.1	(48.6–51.6)**	42.7	(41.2–44.2)***	40.4	(38.9–41.9)**
Vitamin C	45.9	(44.3–47.5)	47.2	(45.6–48.8)	46.1	(44.5–47.7)	46.4	(44.8–48.0)
Vitamin D	95.0	(94.8–95.2)	95.0	(94.8–95.2)	94.0	(93.8–94.2)**	94.0	(93.8–94.2)**
Vitamin E	88.1	(87.0–89.2)	89.7	(88.7–90.6)	87.0	(85.9–88.1)	86.5	(85.4–87.6)
Thiamin	9.5	(8.8–10.2)	9.7	(9.0–10.5)	9.3	(8.5–10.0)	8.9	(8.1–9.6)
Riboflavin	9.7	(9.0–10.4)	9.9	(9.2–10.7)	9.4	(8.6–10.1)	8.9	(8.2–9.6)
Niacin	9.3	(8.5–10.0)	10.2	(9.4–10.9)	9.6	(8.8–10.3)	9.3	(8.5–10.0)
Vitamin B_6	18.8	(17.6–19.9)	22.6	(21.3–23.9)***	19.1	(18.0–20.3)	20.8	(19.6–21.9)
Folate[j]	27.9	(26.8–29.0)	35.8	(34.6–37.0)**	27.9	(26.7–29.0)	27.1	(25.9–28.2)
Vitamin B_{12}	10.8	(10.0–11.6)	11.4	(10.5–12.3)	10.6	(9.8–11.4)	9.9	(9.1–10.6)
Calcium	47.4	(46.2–48.6)	48.32	(47.1–49.5)	47.55	(46.4–48.7)	46.3	(45.1–47.5)
Iron	12.7	(11.9–13.5)	13.62	(12.8–14.4)	12.61	(11.8–13.4)	12.3	(11.6–13.1)
Magnesium	72.1	(70.9–73.3)	74.7	(73.5–75.8)*	58.8	(57.3–60.3)***	73.1	(71.9–74.3)
Sodium[h]	81.4	(80.5–82.3)	81.1	(80.2–82.0)	80.5	(79.6–81.4)	81.3	(80.5–82.2)
Zinc	39.4	(38.2–40.6)	44.0	(42.8–45.3)***	40.1	(38.9–41.3)	39.5	(38.2–40.7)
			Mean intake (95% CI)					
Energy (kcal)	2176	(2159–2192)	2158	(2142–2175)	2170	(2153–2186)	2171	(2154–2187)
Protein, total (g)	84	(83–84)	83	(82–84)	81	(81–82)***	76	(74–78)***
Carbohydrate, total (g)	262	(260–264)	264	(258–271)	262	(260–264)	265	(262–267)
Fatty acids, total (g)	83	(82–84)	83	(82–83)	81	(80–82)*	80	(79–81)
Fiber (g)	16	(16–16)	15	(15–15)***	16	(15–16)	16	(15–16)
Eicosapentaenoic acid (g)	0.03	(0.03–0.03)	0.03	(0.03–0.03)	0.03	(0.02–0.03)	0.03	(0.02–0.03)
Docosahexaenoic acid (g)	0.08	(0.08–0.08)	0.08	(0.08–0.08)	0.08	(0.08–0.09)	0.09	(0.09–0.09)
α-linolenic acid (g)	1.53	(1.50–1.55)	1.53	(1.51–1.55)	1.52	(1.50–1.54)	1.53	(1.50–1.55)
Vitamin K (μg)	100	(97–103)	100	(97–103)	100	(97–103)	99	(96–102)
Choline (mg)	317	(312–322)	336	(331–341)	353	(348–358)***	382	(376–388)***
Potassium (mg)	2222	(2159–2286)	2219	(2158–2279)	2207	(2145–2269)	2205	(2143–2267)
α-carotene (μg)	516	(488–544)	426	(405–446)	425	(300–551)	403	(236–570)
β-carotene (μg)	2136	(2054–2218)	2134	(2053–2214)	2138	(2057–2219)	2104	(2022–2186)
β-cryptoxanthin (μg)	112	(108–116)	103	(99–107)	107	(103–111)	105	(101–109)
Lutein and zeaxanthin (μg)	1418	(1362–1473)	1436	(1383–1490)	1489	(1435–1543)	1544	(1491–1598)**
Lycopene (μg)	8218	(7838–8598)	8096	(7759–8433)	8653	(8242–9065)	8290	(7920–8660)

All estimates adjusted for age, gender, race-ethnicity, education, marital status, household size, health insurance, BMI, income-to-poverty ratio, and whether the dietary recall was on a weekday or weekend

[a]Modeled daily nutrient intake if eggs were consumed as the main dish at each eating occasion

[b]Mean, 2001–2014

[c]Referent

[d]Daily nutrient recommendations are Estimated Average Requirements (EAR) unless otherwise specified. National Academy of Sciences, Institute of Medicine. 2006. Dietary reference intakes: The essential guide to nutrient requirements. Jennifer J. Otten, Jennifer Pitzi Hellwig, Linda D. Meyers (eds.). National Academies Press, Washington, DC

[e]Less than 10% of total energy. US Department of Health and Human Services & US Department of Agriculture. 2015–2020. Dietary Guidelines for Americans 2015–2020. U.S. Government Printing Office, Washington, DC. Available at: http://health.gov/dietaryguidelines/ (verified 29 March 2016)

[f]Retinol Activity Equivalent (RAE)

[j]Dietary Folate Equivalent (DFE)

[h]Tolerable upper intake level limit. National Academy of Sciences, Institute of Medicine. 2006. Dietary reference intakes: The essential guide to nutrient requirements. Jennifer J. Otten, Jennifer Pitzi Hellwig, Linda D. Meyers (eds.). National Academies Press, Washington, DC

*Different than food insecure non-participants at $P < 0.017$ (Bonferroni adjusted for multiple comparisons)

**Different than food insecure non-participants at $P < 0.003$ (Bonferroni adjusted for multiple comparisons)

***Different than food insecure non-participants at $P < 0.0003$ (Bonferroni adjusted for multiple comparisons)

($P < 0.001$). No changes in nutrient intake were observed when eggs were substituted at dinner, except a decrease in mean intake of protein ($P < 0.001$) and an increase in mean intake of choline ($P < 0.01$). Among SNAP participants (Table 5), substituting eggs at breakfast increased the percent not meeting recommendations for vitamin D ($P < 0.01$), vitamin B_6 ($P < 0.01$), and folate ($P < 0.01$), and substituting eggs at lunch decreased the percent not meeting recommendations for saturated fatty acids ($P < 0.001$) and magnesium ($P < 0.001$). Substituting eggs at dinner decreased the percent not meeting recommendations for vitamin A ($P < 0.01$) and vitamin D ($P < 0.01$). Among food secure non-participants (Table 6), substituting eggs at breakfast increased the percent of individuals not meeting recommendations for saturated fatty acids ($P < 0.05$), vitamin A ($P < 0.01$), vitamin B_6 ($P < 0.001$), folate ($P < 0.01$), magnesium ($P < 0.05$), and zinc ($P < 0.001$), and decreased the mean intake of fiber ($P < 0.001$). Substituting eggs at lunch decreased the percent not meeting recommendations for saturated fatty acids ($P < 0.001$), vitamin A ($P < 0.001$), vitamin D ($P < 0.01$), and magnesium ($P < 0.001$), and decreased the mean intake of protein and total fatty acids ($P < 0.001$). Substituting eggs at dinner increase the percent not meeting recommendations for saturated fatty acids ($P < 0.001$), but decreased the percent not meeting recommendations for vitamins A and D ($P < 0.01$).

Total nutrient index

Figure 1a-d display the results of the total nutrient index, which represents the percent change from the reported intake of all 31 nutrients collectively when eggs are substituted for the most commonly consumed main dish at each eating occasion. Among each group (i.e., food insecure non-participants, SNAP participants, WIC participants, and food secure non-participants), total nutrient intake did not change at breakfast, lunch, or dinner ($P > 0.05$). Sensitivity analyses demonstrated that individual nutrients have minimal effect on the reliability of the total nutrient index (Additional file 7: Table S7).

Discussion

In this nationally representative sample of nearly 35,000 adults surveyed over 14 years, meaningful disparities in daily intake of several key nutrients were observed between distinct populations differentiated by food security status and participation in federal food assistance programs. Importantly, using dietary modeling techniques, we demonstrated that well-defined, moderate dietary changes at the population-level can increase intake of some, but not all, nutrients, and can reduce the prevalence of nutrient inadequacy among these nutritionally vulnerable populations.

Diet modeling has become a popular tool for estimating the impact of food substitutions on nutrient adequacy at the population level [18, 19, 23, 38]. Yet to the best of our knowledge, the present study is the first to use diet modeling to examine the effects of food substitutions at multiple eating occasions on meeting daily nutrient intake recommendations among distinct groups of nutritionally vulnerable populations.

Consistent with our findings, a review by Andreyeva et al. [9] indicated lower nutrient intake among SNAP participants compared to higher income non-participants. Leung et al. [39] analyzed NHANES (1998–2008) dietary data from 918 SNAP participants and reported that 52 and 67% did not meet recommendations for folate and calcium, respectively, which are higher than our estimates (36% for folate and 56% for calcium). These disagreements may stem from differences in sample size ($n = 3724$ SNAP participants in the present study) resulting from different inclusion criteria. In contrast to Leung et al., [39] we categorized SNAP participants regardless of age or income, which allowed for greater sample size and improved generalizability to the target population. To the best of our knowledge, no previous studies have examined nutrient adequacy among adult WIC participants, although several studies have observed an overall improvement in the healthfulness of food choices among WIC participants since 2009 [8, 40]. Our results for the proportion of food insecure non-participants meeting individual nutrient recommendations are largely consistent with others [41].

In the present study, we demonstrated that consuming eggs as the main dish at lunch or dinner did not have an effect on total nutrient intake among nutritionally vulnerable populations (i.e., food insecure non-participants, WIC participants, and SNAP participants) or their food secure non-participant counterparts. However, our findings for several specific nutrients warrant particular mention. Importantly, we observed a meaningful reduction in the prevalence of food insecure non-participants not meeting daily vitamin D recommendations when eggs were consumed as the main dish at lunch or dinner. The 2015–2020 Dietary Guidelines for Americans proclaimed vitamin D a nutrient of public health concern [42] given the strikingly high prevalence of intake inadequacy (92–97%) [43] and its relationship to chronic disease patterns [42]. Yet, when eggs were consumed as the main dish at breakfast, the prevalence of folate inadequacy increased for WIC participants and SNAP participants, which is concerning. Folate is a critical nutrient for fetal neural tube development, which is the reason for elevated intake recommendations during pregnancy [44]. This is of particular concern for adult WIC participants, over 40% of whom are pregnant and, of those, over half enrolled during their first trimester [4] when adequate folate intake is most critical [45]. We estimated that breakfast cereal, much

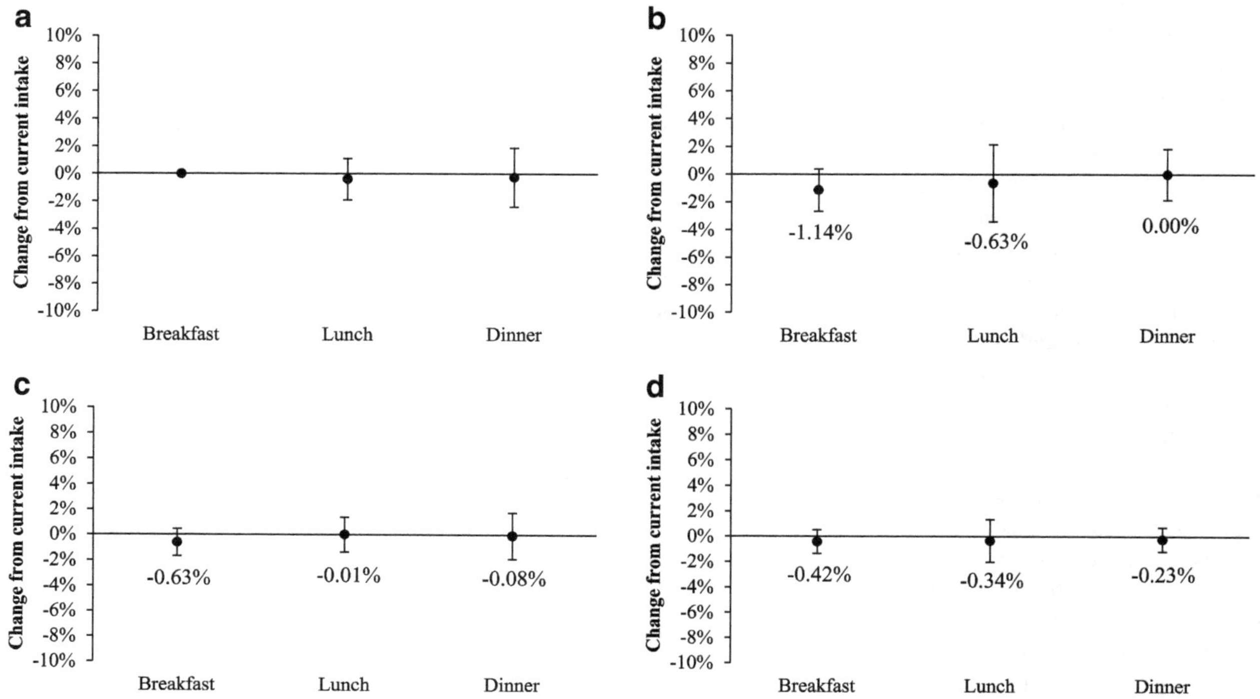

Fig. 1 Percent change from reported daily intake of all nutrients if eggs were consumed as the main dish at each eating occasion among **a**) food insecure non-participants ($n = 3631$), **b**) WIC participants ($n = 636$), **c**) SNAP participants ($n = 4020$), and **d**) food secure non-participants ($n = 26{,}454$), 2001–2014. Adjusted for age, gender, race-ethnicity, education, marital status, household size, currently participating in a health insurance plan, body mass index, income-to-poverty ratio, and whether the dietary recall was on a weekday or weekend

of which is fortified with folic acid, was the most commonly consumed main dish at breakfast among all groups, so it is not surprising that consuming eggs instead of breakfast cereal resulted in reduced folate (i.e. dietary folate equivalent) intake. Although others have recently reported successful innovations in the development of folate-enriched eggs, [46] more research is needed before these products can be successfully introduced to consumers on a large scale.

Several important strengths of this study warrant mention. To the best of our knowledge this is the first study to assess nutrient intake among distinct nutritionally vulnerable populations simultaneously, for a diverse array of 31 nutrients including macronutrients, vitamins, minerals, and carotenoids. NCI methods and macros were used to estimate usual intake distributions, which represent the gold standard for addressing the foremost statistical challenges when assessing nutrient intake among populations [47]. We also used a novel approach, the total nutrient index, to assess intake of all 31 nutrients collectively, which accounts for relative differences in the standard errors of each nutrient. Finally, and importantly, the large sample size ($n > 34{,}000$) and national representation of our data make our findings generalizable to each of our study populations.

This study is also not without limitations. We conducted our food substitution analyses on a gram basis, ensuring that equal grams of dishes were being substituted; other approaches include using a serving basis or calorie basis. In the present study our data represented main dishes as they were reported consumed, which included a combination of individual foods with distinct serving sizes, thus it was not possible to use the serving basis for this analysis. We tested using the calorie basis for food substitutions and observed that it provided essentially the same results as the gram basis (~ 1% difference in calories between food substitutions). It is also possible that pooling data across NHANES waves may have masked changes in nutrient intake among some groups, particularly WIC participants [8, 40]. Yet it was necessary to pool these data, especially for WIC participants, due to small sample sizes in individual waves, in order to observe clinically and statistically meaningful results.

Regular assessment of nutrient inadequacy at the population level is a crucial component of the public health nutrition agenda in the US, and nutritional monitoring of low income and other vulnerable populations is of particular importance. On the one hand, it is reassuring that populations with a high prevalence of nutrient inadequacy for key nutrients are participating in federal food assistance programs. On the other hand, more research is needed to better understand why many income-eligible food insecure individuals do not participate in these vital programs (over 50% in this study), given their high prevalence of nutrient inadequacy. Continued efforts are needed to ensure that nutritionally vulnerable populations have access to healthy foods, and that at-risk individuals are counseled to make food choices that promote nutrient adequacy. Additional research is needed to better understand how food substitutions affect diet costs, which may be an important driver of food purchasing decisions among low income individuals with limited food budgets [6, 7].

Conclusions

This study is the first to use diet modeling to examine the effects of food substitutions at multiple eating occasions on meeting daily nutrient intake recommendations among distinct groups of nutritionally vulnerable populations. A novel total nutrient index was also used to estimate changes in the intake of a broad array of diverse nutrients collectively. Regular assessment of nutrient inadequacy at the population level is a crucial component of the public health nutrition agenda in the US, and nutritional monitoring of low income and other vulnerable populations is of particular importance. Clinically meaningful disparities in nutrient intake remain between distinct populations differentiated by food security status and participation in federal food assistance programs. Well-defined and moderate dietary changes at the population-level have the potential to increase nutrient intake and reduce the prevalence of nutrient inadequacy among these nutritionally vulnerable populations, particularly at lunch and dinner. However, careful consideration should be awarded to food substitutions at breakfast, particularly among individuals who are pregnant or trying to become pregnant, in order to maintain adequate folate status. Further research is needed in two key areas: to better understand why many income-eligible food insecure individuals do not participate in federal food assistance programs, and to better understand how food substitutions affect diet costs among low income individuals with limited food budgets.

Additional files

Additional file 1: Table S1. Foods included in main dish groups.

Additional file 2: Table S2. Daily nutrient intake recommendations.

Additional file 3: Table S3. Percent of individuals consuming types of main dishes at each eating occasion, 2001–2014 ($n = 34{,}741$).

Additional file 4: Table S4. Percent of individuals consuming types of egg dishes at each eating occasion, 2001–2014 ($n = 34{,}741$).

Additional file 5: Table S5. Amount of each dish used in substitution modeling.

Additional file 6: Table S6. Nutrient content of dishes used in substitution modeling.

Additional file 7: Table S7. Sensitivity analysis for total nutrient index.

Abbreviations

24HR: 24-h recall; DGA: Dietary guidelines for Americans; FNDDS: Food and nutrient database for dietary studies; NCI: National Cancer Institute; NHANES: National Health and Nutrition Examination Survey; SNAP: Supplemental Nutrition Assistance Program; USDA: United States Department of Agriculture; WIC: Special Supplemental Nutrition Program for Women, Infants, and Children; WWEIA: What we eat in America

Funding

This research was funded by the Egg Nutrition Center of the American Egg Board. The funding body did not have any role in the design of the study, data collection, data analysis, and interpretation of the data, and in writing the manuscript. Partial funding was also received from USDA-ARS 3062-51000-051-00D.

Authors' contributions

ZC, JNR, and LJ designed the research; ZC conducted the research; ZC and LKJ provided essential materials; ZC, LKJ, and WJY analyzed the data and performed statistical analyses; ZC wrote the paper; ZC and LJ had primary responsibility for final content; all authors have read and approved the final manuscript.

Competing interests

The authors declare that they have no competing interests.

Author details

[1]Grand Forks Human Nutrition Research Center, US Department of Agriculture, Agricultural Research Service, 2420 2nd Ave. N, Grand Forks, ND 58203, USA. [2]Center for Food Safety and Applied Nutrition, US Department of Health and Human Services, Food and Drug Administration, 5001 Campus Drive, College Park, MD 20740, USA.

References

1. Supplemental Nutrition Assistance Program (SNAP) eligibility [Available at: http://www.fns.usda.gov/snap/eligibility (verified 16 June 2017)].
2. US Department of Agriculture, Food and Nutrition Service: Supplemental Nutrition Assistance Program (SNAP) national level annual summary. 2016.
3. US Department of Agriculture: FY 2016 Budget Summary and Performance Plan. 2015.
4. US Department of Agriculture, Food and Nutrition Service: WIC Participant and Program Characteristics Final Report. 2015.
5. U S Burden of Disease Collaborators. The state of U.S. health, 1990-2010: burden of diseases, injuries, and risk factors. JAMA. 2013;310:591–606.
6. Kirkpatrick SI, Dodd KW, Reedy J, Krebs-Smith SM. Income and Race/Ethnicity Are Associated with Adherence to Food-Based Dietary Guidance among US Adults and Children. J Acad Nutr Diet. 2012;112:624–35.
7. Hiza HAB, Casavale KO, Guenther PM, Davis CA. Diet Quality of Americans Differs by Age, Sex, Race/Ethnicity, Income, and Education Level. J Acad Nutr Diet. 2013;113:297–306.
8. Tester JM, Leung CW, Crawford PB. Revised WIC Food Package and Children's Diet Quality. Pediatrics. 2016;137
9. Andreyeva T, Tripp AS, Schwartz MB. Dietary quality of Americans by Supplemental Nutrition Assistance Program participation status: a systematic review. Am J Prev Med. 2015;49:594–604.
10. Conrad Z, Rehm CD, Wilde P, Mozaffarian D. Cardiometabolic Mortality by Supplemental Nutrition Assistance Program Participation and Eligibility in the United States. Am J Public Health. 2017:e1–9.

11. Damschroder LJ, Lutes LD, Kirsh S, Kim HM, Gillon L, Holleman RG, Goodrich DE, Lowery JC, Richardson CR. Small-Changes Obesity Treatment Among Veterans: 12-Month Outcomes. Am J Prev Med. 2014;47:541–53.
12. Lutes LD, DiNatale E, Goodrich DE, Ronis DL, Gillon L, Kirsh S, Richardson CR, Damschroder LJ. A randomized trial of a small changes approach for weight loss in veterans: Design, rationale, and baseline characteristics of the ASPIRE-VA trial. Contemp Clin Trials. 2013;34:161–72.
13. Hills AP, Byrne NM, Lindstrom R, Hill JO. 'Small changes' to diet and physical activity behaviors for weight management. Obesity Facts. 2013;6:228–38.
14. de Castro JM: The time of day of food intake influences overall intake in humans. J Nutr 2004, 134:104–111.
15. Howarth NC, Huang TT, Roberts SB, Lin BH, McCrory MA. Eating patterns and dietary composition in relation to BMI in younger and older adults. Int J Obesity. 2007;31:675–84.
16. Berner LA, Becker G, Wise M, Doi J. Characterization of dietary protein among older adults in the United States: amount, animal sources, and meal patterns. J Acad Nutr Diet. 2013;113:809–15.
17. Nicklas TA, O'Neil CE, Zanovec M, Keast DR, Fulgoni VL 3rd. Contribution of beef consumption to nutrient intake, diet quality, and food patterns in the diets of the US population. Meat Sci. 2012;90:152–8.
18. Quann EE, Fulgoni VL 3rd, Auestad N. Consuming the daily recommended amounts of dairy products would reduce the prevalence of inadequate micronutrient intakes in the United States: diet modeling study based on NHANES 2007-2010. Nutr J. 2015;14:90.
19. Fulgoni VL III, Keast DR, Auestad N, Quann EE. Nutrients from dairy foods are difficult to replace in diets of Americans: Food pattern modeling and an analyses of the National Health and Nutrition Examination Survey 2003-2006. Nutr Res. 2011;31:759–65.
20. Nicklas TA, O'Neil CE, Fulgoni VL 3rd. The nutritional role of flavored and white milk in the diets of children. J Sch Health. 2013;83:728–33.
21. Fulgoni VL, Buckley RB. The Contribution of Fortified Ready-to-Eat Cereal to Vitamin and Mineral Intake in the U.S. Population, NHANES 2007-2010. Nutrients. 2015;7:3949–58.
22. O'Neil CE, Nicklas TA, Rampersaud GC, Fulgoni VL 3rd. 100% orange juice consumption is associated with better diet quality, improved nutrient adequacy, decreased risk for obesity, and improved biomarkers of health in adults: National Health and Nutrition Examination Survey, 2003-2006. Nutr J. 2012;11:107.
23. Nicklas TA, Liu Y, Islam N, O'Neil CE. Removing Potatoes from Children's Diets May Compromise Potassium Intake. Adv Nutr. 2016;7:247s–53s.
24. Fulgoni VL 3rd, Dreher M, Davenport AJ. Avocado consumption is associated with better diet quality and nutrient intake, and lower metabolic syndrome risk in US adults: results from the National Health and Nutrition Examination Survey (NHANES) 2001-2008. Nutr J. 2013;12:1.
25. Freedman MR, Fulgoni VL 3rd. Canned Vegetable and Fruit Consumption Is Associated with Changes in Nutrient Intake and Higher Diet Quality in Children and Adults: National Health and Nutrition Examination Survey 2001-2010. J Acad Nutr Diet. 2016;116:940–8.
26. Griffin BA. Eggs: good or bad? Proc Nutr Soc. 2016;75:259–64.
27. US Department of Agriculture, Agricultural Research Service: National Nutrient Database for Standard Reference, Release 28. Nutrient Data Laboratory. 2016.
28. Abdel-Aal EM, Akhtar H, Zaheer K, Ali R. Dietary Sources of Lutein and Zeaxanthin Carotenoids and Their Role in Eye Health. Nutrients. 2013;5:1169–85.
29. Kim JE, Gordon SL, Ferruzzi MG, Campbell WW. Effects of egg consumption on carotenoid absorption from co-consumed, raw vegetables. Am J Clin Nutr. 2015;102:75–83.
30. Kim JE, Ferruzzi MG, Campbell WW. Egg Consumption Increases Vitamin E Absorption from Co-Consumed Raw Mixed Vegetables in Healthy Young Men. J Nutr. 2016;146:2199–205.
31. Miranda JM, Anton X, Redondo-Valbuena C, Roca-Saavedra P, Rodriguez JA, Lamas A, Franco CM, Cepeda A. Egg and egg-derived foods: effects on human health and use as functional foods. Nutrients. 2015;7:706–29.
32. Lewis ED, Subhan FB, Bell RC, McCargar LJ, Curtis JM, Jacobs RL, Field CJ. Estimation of choline intake from 24 h dietary intake recalls and contribution of egg and milk consumption to intake among pregnant and lactating women in Alberta. Br J Nutr. 2014;112:112–21.
33. US Department of Health and Human Services, Centers for Disease Control and Prevention (CDC): About the National Health and Nutrition Examination Survey. 2017.
34. Moshfegh AJ, Rhodes DG, Baer DJ, Murayi T, Clemens JC, Rumpler WV, Paul DR, Sebastian RS, Kuczynski KJ, Ingwersen LA, et al. The US Department of Agriculture Automated Multiple-Pass Method reduces bias in the collection of energy intakes. Am J Clin Nutr. 2008;88:324–32.
35. Bickel G, Nord M, Price C, Hamilton W, Cook J. Guide to measuring household food security: US Department of Agriculture; 2000.
36. US Department of Agriculture, Agricultural Research Service. Food and Nutrient Database for Dietary Studies. 2001–2014.
37. Usual Dietary Intakes: SAS Macros for Analysis of a Single Dietary Component, version 2.1 [Available at: http://epi.grants.cancer.gov/diet/usualintakes/macros_single.html#ver2 (verified 16 June 2017)].
38. Houchins JA, Cifelli CJ, Demmer E, Fulgoni Iii VL. Diet Modeling in Older Americans: The Impact of Increasing Plant-Based Foods or Dairy Products on Protein Intake. J Nutr Health Aging. 2017;21:673–80.
39. Leung CW, Ding EL, Catalano PJ, Villamor E, Rimm EB, Willett WC. Dietary intake and dietary quality of low-income adults in the Supplemental Nutrition Assistance Program. Am J Clin Nutr. 2012;96:977–88.
40. Schultz DJ, Byker Shanks C, Houghtaling B. The Impact of the 2009 Special Supplemental Nutrition Program for Women, Infants, and Children Food Package Revisions on Participants: A Systematic Review. J Acad Nutr Diet. 2015;115:1832–46.
41. Leung CW, Epel ES, Ritchie LD, Crawford PB, Laraia BA. Food Insecurity Is Inversely Associated with Diet Quality of Lower-Income Adults. J Acad Nutr Diet. 2014;114:1943–U1329.
42. US Department of Health and Human Services and US Department of Agriculture. Dietary Guidelines for Americans 2015–2020, Chapter 2. 8th ed. edition. Washington, DC2015–2020.
43. Dietary Guidelines Advisory Committee. Scientific Report of the 2015 Dietary Guidelines Advisory Committee: Advisory Report to the Secretary of Health and Human Services and the Secretary of Agriculture. Appendix E-2. 1. Washington, DC2015.
44. National Academy of Sciences, Institute of Medicine. Dietary Reference Intakes: The Essential Guide to Nutrient Requirements. Washington, DC: Jennifer J. Otten, Jennifer Pitzi Hellwig, Linda D. Meyers (eds.); 2006.
45. McNulty B, McNulty H, Marshall B, Ward M, Molloy AM, Scott JM, Dornan J, Pentieva K. Impact of continuing folic acid after the first trimester of pregnancy: findings of a randomized trial of Folic Acid Supplementation in the Second and Third Trimesters. Am J Clin Nutr. 2013;98:92–8.
46. Altic L, McNulty H, Hoey L, McAnena L, Pentieva K. Validation of Folate-Enriched Eggs as a Functional Food for Improving Folate Intake in Consumers. Nutrients. 2016;8
47. Tooze JA, Midthune D, Dodd KW, Freedman LS, Krebs-Smith SM, Subar AF, Guenther PM, Carroll RJ, Kipnis V. A new statistical method for estimating the usual intake of episodically consumed foods with application to their distribution. J Am Diet Assoc. 2006;106:1575–87.

3

User-documented food consumption data from publicly available apps: an analysis of opportunities and challenges for nutrition research

Marcus Maringer[1*], Pieter van't Veer[1], Naomi Klepacz[2], Muriel C. D. Verain[3], Anne Normann[4], Suzanne Ekman[4], Lada Timotijevic[2], Monique M. Raats[2] and Anouk Geelen[1]

Abstract

Background: The need for a better understanding of food consumption behaviour within its behavioural context has sparked the interest of nutrition researchers for user-documented food consumption data collected outside the research context using publicly available nutrition apps. The study aims to characterize the scientific, technical, legal and ethical features of this data in order to identify the opportunities and challenges associated with using this data for nutrition research.

Method: A search for apps collecting food consumption data was conducted in October 2016 against UK Google Play and iTunes storefronts. 176 apps were selected based on user ratings and English language support. Publicly available information from the app stores and app-related websites was investigated and relevant data extracted and summarized. Our focus was on characteristics related to scientific relevance, data management and legal and ethical governance of user-documented food consumption data.

Results: Food diaries are the most common form of data collection, allowing for multiple inputs including generic food items, packaged products, or images. Standards and procedures for compiling food databases used for estimating energy and nutrient intakes remain largely undisclosed. Food consumption data is interlinked with various types of contextual data related to behavioural motivation, physical activity, health, and fitness. While exchange of data between apps is common practise, the majority of apps lack technical documentation regarding data export. There is a similar lack of documentation regarding the implemented terms of use and privacy policies. While users are usually the owners of their data, vendors are granted irrevocable and royalty free licenses to commercially exploit the data.

Conclusion: Due to its magnitude, diversity, and interconnectedness, user-documented food consumption data offers promising opportunities for a better understanding of habitual food consumption behaviour and its determinants. Non-standardized or non-documented food data compilation procedures, data exchange protocols and formats, terms of use and privacy statements, however, limit possibilities to integrate, process and share user-documented food consumption data. An ongoing research effort is required, to keep pace with the technical advancements of food consumption apps, their evolving data networks and the legal and ethical regulations related to protecting app users and their personal data.

Keywords: Food consumption data, Dietary intake assessment, Diet apps, User-documented data, Contextual data, Technological innovations, Data management, Legal and ethical governance, Research infrastructure

* Correspondence: m.maringer@seedmobi.com
[1]Division of Human Nutrition, Wageningen University & Research, Wageningen, The Netherlands
Full list of author information is available at the end of the article

Background

With the widespread use of mobile phones and tablets, there has been an increase in the number of software applications that record and aim to improve people's food consumption behaviour [1–4]. The need for more suitable and effective methods for measuring, understanding and influencing food consumption behaviours has sparked interest amongst behavioural and nutrition researchers for these digital solutions. Smartphones and their implemented technologies such as barcode scanners, image processors, microphones, databases, and wireless network interfaces have the potential to enhance the accuracy and efficiency of data collection and reduce the costs and inconvenience of assessing diets in real time [1, 5–7]. Previous research provides vital insights regarding features and functionalities of publicly available food consumption apps [1, 2, 8], their effectiveness for weight loss interventions and improving nutrition related behaviours [4, 6, 9–11], the quality of the provided information and implemented behavioural change techniques [12–16], user adherence [6, 10, 17], app usability and perceived usefulness [2, 18].

Accompanied by the growing interest in new and efficient technologies for recording and improving people's food consumption behaviours, there is growing interest in the collection and investigation of the large stream of food consumption data, which is generated by the vast amount of users of these technologies. Investigating such *user-documented* food consumption data, which is data that has already been collected by users of apps (e.g., for self-monitoring purposes), is in itself highly efficient because such secondary data usage reduces the costs for collecting data and reduces the burden on respondents [19, 20]. More importantly, food-related consumer behaviours are most often studied in isolation, in short time frames and in a relatively limited social and physical context [21]. Every day, users of diet apps generate "big data" - large volumes of information, that offer detailed descriptions of food consumptions, including time and place (e.g., using Global Positioning Systems; GPS). If these data-rich sources could be linked and analyzed, they have the potential to contribute greatly towards answering key questions regarding food and health (e.g., obesity, cardiovascular disease) and to a better understanding of food consumption behaviour including its drivers and barriers [22]. In order to advance health and nutrition research, the European Union (EU) funded RICHFIELDS project (http://www.richfields.eu) aims to design an EU-wide research infrastructure (RI) and distributed open access data platform for the collection, integration, and sharing of food consumption data from various sources including the increasing stream of food consumption data documented by users of nutrition apps.

The use of user-documented data, however, creates new challenges, which go beyond the type and quality of implemented app features. These challenges involve procedures of finding and retrieving relevant data, the methods and purposes of data collection, informed consent, confidentiality, and data ownership [20, 23]. It was our aim to investigate the characteristics and qualities of user-documented food consumption data in order to learn more about its *scientific relevance* in regarding its potential for estimating habitual food intake and for providing a better understanding of the determinants of food consumption behaviours. In addition, we focused on characteristics relevant for *data management* practices including data access and data integration. This information is important for implementing data processing strategies that rely on effective and reliable data exchange protocols. Finally, we focused on characteristics of the data relevant to its *legal and ethical governance.* The rights, obligations, and expectations regarding data usage are important since failure to adhere to these regulations might compromise data integrity [24]. In sum, in the present research we focused on evaluating characteristics of apps, which relate to the secondary usage of data generated by regular "users" of publicly available apps, which we refer to as user-documented data. Our aim was to provide an overview of important scientific, technical, legal and ethical aspects of user-documented food consumption data that should inform researchers about the opportunities and challenges associated with collecting and investigating this type of data for nutrition research.

Methods

App identification

The iTunes and Google Play stores were searched between 15 and 23 October 2016 in order to identify apps which allow the user to collect food consumption data. A set of search terms created by Franco et al. in their review of popular nutrition apps [1] were adopted. Search terms included: calorie(s), diet, diet tracker, dietician, dietitian, eating, fit, fitness, food, food diary, food tracker, health, lose weight, nutrition, nutritionist, weight, weight loss, weight management, weight watcher, and ww calculator. Automated data collection techniques were used for both apps stores. Each search term was queried separately without combining individual search terms. For the iTunes store, app data was queried from the public iTunes Search application programming interface (API) [25]. For the Google Play Store, app data was extracted by a web data crawling software [26]. The open source Nodejs module itunes-search[1] (version 1.0.1) was used to collect data from the iTunes search API, and the open source Nodejs module google-play-scraper[2] (version 0.2.1) was used to collect data from the Google Play Store. For more detailed documentation regarding the usage of these two Nodejs modules for conducting searches against the Google Play Store and the iTunes search API, please refer to the documentation and examples provided in their public repositories. Our aim was to limit the number of apps to only the most relevant with an already established user-base and a certain degree of app quality. To limit the apps identified, the modules were configured to retrieve only the first 100 applications for each search term. Search results were further limited by means of app user ratings. Both iTunes and Google Play stores provide app users with a function to rate their liking of the apps on a 5-point scale. Apps from the returned searches that had a mean user rating of more than 2 (based on a minimum of 10 user ratings) were retained for use in this study. To ensure the retrieval of English language apps, United Kingdom (UK) storefronts were searched only. No affiliate account or token was used at the iTunes Search API. This search strategy resulted in the collection of 176 unique apps (see Fig. 1).

User-documented data characterization

Information sources

Descriptions of apps and services were taken from publicly available information for each app published by the app vendors. This information included the technical details, app descriptions and screenshots provided in the respective app stores (iTunes and Google Play Store) and, where available, feature and service descriptions, documentation, and frequently asked questions on associated homepages. Terms of use and privacy statements were reviewed to identify information relevant to legal and ethical governance.

Data characteristics

A list of characteristics related to user-documented data was generated for the extraction of information from the

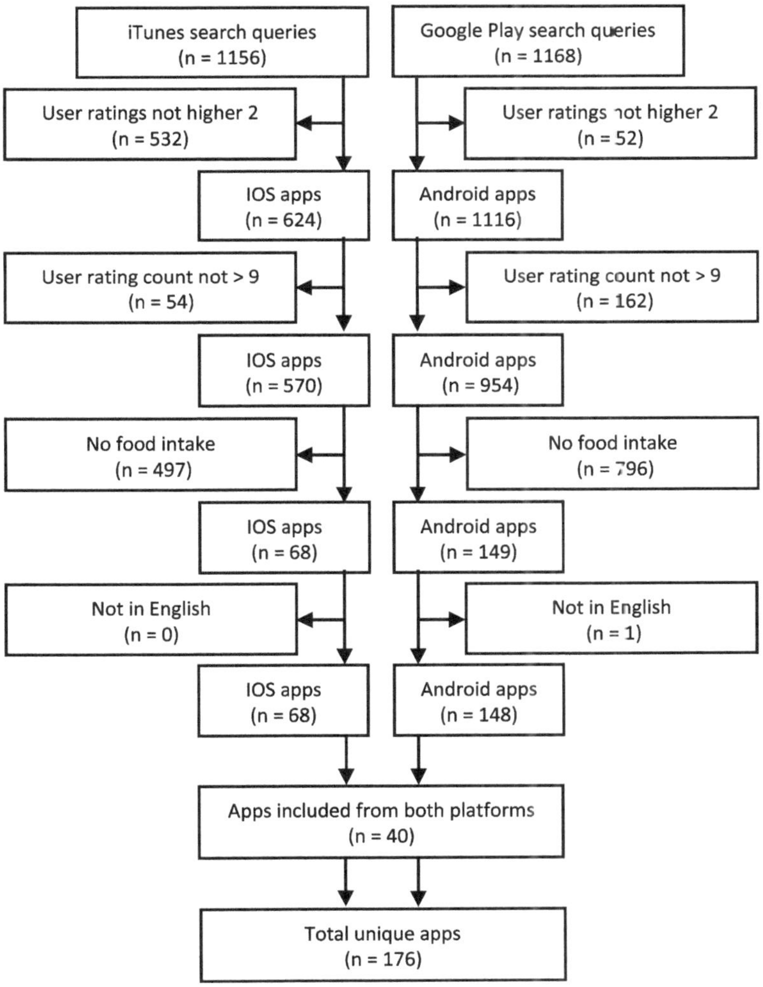

Fig. 1 Flow diagram of app search and selection

defined information sources. The criterion for inclusion of a characteristic was based on whether information regarding the characteristic could be expected to be publicly available, without the need to install and use the app. Specifically, there is a vast array of quality criteria which have been discarded because they require the installation and usage of the apps, including criteria related to the functionality of the tools or the resulting user experience, such as feasibility, intuitiveness, learnability, efficiency, engagement, etc. The following paragraphs provide a brief explanation of the chosen characteristics with some examples. See Table 1-3 for complete lists of characteristics and their descriptions.

Scientific relevance characteristics

This was defined as how well the collected data meets the needs and standards of researchers in terms of the concepts measured [27]. The information collected reflected the methods and standards used for dietary intake assessments and the estimations of habitual food intake behaviours [28]. Information extraction properties included implemented methods for collecting food intake data, types of food data collected (e.g., generic foods, labeled products, images), and estimations of portion sizes and nutrient values. Information related to the collection of contextual data (e.g., activity, health, sleep) was collected as it offers the potential to better understand the determinants of food consumption behaviours [29]. Scientific relevance does not refer to testing the reliability and validity of the collected dietary assessment data. Rather by investigating these characteristics of the apps we aimed at getting indications about the potential usefulness of the data they generate for investigating habitual food intake and its determinants.

Data management characteristics

The FAIR data principles act as an international guideline for enhancing the ability to find, access and use scholarly data. FAIR stands for 'Findable, Accessible, Interoperable, and Reusable'. In the present research we focused mainly on data access and data interoperability characteristics, including methods for data export, exchanged data formats and references to other relevant data.

Legal and ethical governance characteristics

These characteristics were based on some of the existing literature on the legal and ethical issues related to data collected by commercial mobile health apps [30–35] and ethics of secondary data analysis and big data [19, 23, 36]. We included criteria such as data ownership, data sharing, data usage, personally identifiable information, privacy and informed consent.

Data collection

A web-based data collection tool was built using the open source Nodejs content management system Keystonejs (version 0.3.17) as an application framework. The tool consisted of a set of branched web forms for data input and data editing. The content and structure of the web form were based on the data characteristics defined for collecting information from the defined sources. The web form implemented various answering formats (widgets) including open format text and number input fields, as well as closed format input fields with predefined and selectable answering options. The tool was designed to allow for the management of these closed format input options and their definitions (except for the yes-no format). This had the advantage of providing the flexibility needed for explorative data collection, while at the same time applying a certain degree of standardization by making previously provided inputs and their definitions reusable. The tool also supports the visualization of app relevant information sources (e.g., screenshots, app descriptions, etc.) and for aggregations and visualizations of the extracted information. All collected information from app stores and online resources contained in the database have been exported and imported into an Excel file (see Additional file 1).

Results

The app sample

Most apps (90 and 91%) were listed in the category "Health and Fitness" in their respective app stores. The purpose of the majority of apps was to support some form of behavioural change, with weight management being the most commonly stated purpose. Since we selected apps based on mean user ratings (on a 5-point rating scale), user ratings of included apps were high, with a mean of $M = 3.8$ ($SD = 0.7$) for IOS apps and $M = 4.0$ ($SD = 0.4$) for Android apps. In 70% of the cases, apps included from the iTunes store were free of charge with the remaining paid apps ranging in price from £0.79 to £3.99. Apps included from the Android store were, in 87% of the cases, free of charge and the paid apps ranged in price from £0.55 to £7.61. Additional paid services or in app purchases were offered by 46% of all apps. The Android platform was supported by 88% of apps in our sample. IOS devices were supported by 109 apps (63%). Apps which also supported Windows and Blackberry devices accounted for 2% of our sample. Only 1 of the apps, the mySugr Diabetes Diary, was registered as a medical device as defined by the quality regulations and standards associated with that status [37]. In addition to monitoring blood glucose levels, this app supported the monitoring of daily carbohydrate intakes. In 80% of the cases, a website was available, which allowed for further investigation of the apps publicly

Table 1 Investigated characteristics of user documented food consumption data related to scientific relevance and extracted information ($n = 176$)

Characteristic	Description	Extracted information (n)
Dietary assessment method	The dietary assessment method used by the app for collecting food consumption data	Food diary (166), No information (8), Incidental food logging (2)
Food consumption inputs[a]	The type of food consumption data inputs supported	Generic input (91), Custom input (74), Labeled or packaged food products (44), Barcodes (scanned) (39), Water (30), Food images (21), Recipes (20), Restaurant dishes (19), Nutrient/Energy input (19), Diet plans (9), Voice input (4), Food log reminder (2), No information (2)
Precompiled food database	Whether the food consumption logging is supported by selecting foods from precompiled databases	Yes (93), No (83)
Food database compilation	The official food database the apps use for calculating nutrition and energy estimations	USDA (7)
User compiled databases[a]	The type of user compiled databases the app generates for logging references	Favorite eaten foods (29), Recently eaten foods input (15), Frequently eaten foods (14)
Nutrient/Energy estimation[a]	The unit or level of detail nutrient and energy consumption is estimated	Calorie (94), Macronutrients (78), Carbohydrates (49), Protein (49), Food score (26), Micronutrients (25), No information (20)
Portion size	Whether the app collect portion size estimations	Yes (96), No information (57), No (23)
Method portion size[a]	The methods that was used to collect portion size estimations	Standard serving sizes (59), Weight estimation (26), Volume estimation (9), Manual energy/nutrient input (5), Custom serving sizes (4)
Location	Whether the app collects information about where the consumptions took place	No (162), Yes (14)
Occasion	Whether the app collects information about the occasion or event of the consumptions	No (175), Yes (1)
Contextual data[a]	Data parameters the app collects about users other than food intake data	Motivation (107): Nutrition goals (59), Diet plans (38), Weight goals (32), Food preferences (29), Fitness goals (10), Fitness plan (10), Emotions (9), Health goals (7), Hydration goals (7), Stress level (5), Muscle building goals (3), Sleep goal (3), Health (108): Body weight (76), BMI (22), Medications (11), Symptoms (12), Body composition (11), Body measurements (9), Body image (8), Blood sugar (8). Blood pressure (8), Heart rate (7), BMR (7), Cholesterol (4), Physical fitness (4), Oxygen saturation (2) Physical activity (90): Exercise (59), Activity type (29), Steps (19), Activity level (14), Sleep (13) Uncategorized (34): Posts (27), Notes (22), Comments (6), Lifelogging data (3)
Interventional influences type[a]	The type of interventional influences the app contains that might have an direct influence on the recorded food intake behavior	Reminders/Notifications (54), Advices (53), Social support (23), Connected users (21), Coaching (19), Challenges (17), Personal feedback (14), Rewards (6), Encouragements (6), Allowance badge (4)
Sensors type[a]	The type of own external devices the app supports (exclusive devices of third party partner apps or health and fitness sensors)	Pedometer (4), Heart rate monitor (3), Accelerometer (3)
Third party health and fitness trackers[a]	The third party health and fitness trackers the app connects to	Fitbit (19), UP® – Smart Coach for Health (10), Health Mate - Steps tracker & Life coach (10), Misfit (6), Garmin Connect™ Mobile (4), Record by Under Armour, connects with UA HealthBox (2), Samsung Gear (1)
Aggregators[a]	The third party data aggregators the app connects to	HealthKit (31), GoogleFit (17), Healthgraph (5), S Health (5), Human Api (3), Validic (2), Fitnesssyncer (2), HealthVault (1)

[a]Per characteristic multiple inputs were possible and hence the individual percentages do not add up to 100%

available information. The websites of 4 of the apps were not available in English. Except for information extracted from the app stores, no further information was extracted from these websites. In 11% of the cases, no Uniform Resource Locator (URL) was provided, and no app associated home page was found on Google Search (a support URL is required for publishing apps in the iTunes store). In 8% of the cases an URL was provided, but the website was unavailable, and in 3% of the cases the address referred to a social media landing page. In cases where no website was available for an app, no further information, other than the information published in the apps stores, was investigated.

Scientific relevance

Dietary assessment method

The most widely implemented method was a food diary ($n = 166$, 94%; see Table 1). Food diaries allowed for daily records of the foods and/or drinks people consumed at the individual level and at a certain moment in time (e.g., meals, snacks, date, time). Although in their feature descriptions 4% ($n = 8$) of the apps claimed to record food intake, no specifications could be obtained in the publicly available information regarding the specific method implemented to do so. A food image collection method for occasional photographic remembering and experience sharing purposes was implemented by 2 (1%) apps.

Dietary assessment inputs

Ninety-three (53%) apps allowed for inputs from pre-compiled food databases and 74 (42%) apps allowed for custom user compiled inputs. Links to verified sources of the precompiled database (e.g., Composition of foods integrated dataset; CoFID) were available for 7 (4%) apps. Food diaries allowed for various types of inputs. Generic food items could be logged in 91 (52%) apps. Labeled or packaged food products have been identified as possible input type in 44 (25%) apps and 39 (22%) apps implemented a barcode scanner for identification and logging of these labeled products. Food images have been allowed as input in 21 (12%) of the cases and recipes in 20 (11%). Some apps allowed for specific types of customizable or user-documented data inputs such as favorites (29; 16%), frequently consumed foods (14; 8%) or recently consumed foods (15; 8%).

Nutrient estimation

Based on the foods eaten, energy (94; 53%), macronutrients (78; 44%), and micronutrients (25; 14%) were estimated. In 8 (5%) of the apps, food images were used to estimate energy and nutrient intakes or provide a normative evaluation of the foods depicted in the images. These estimations or evaluations were provided by either diet coaches or users themselves. Three tools claiming to use an image recognition software were identified.

Portion size estimations

Portion size estimations were reported to be supported by standard household measures such as cups, spoons, slices (59; 34%), weight and volume (35; 20%), or visual aids in the form of images or graphics (1 app). No information on portion size estimation was provided for the remaining 46% of apps.

Interventional influences

One-hundred (57%) apps included some form of intended interventional influence on users' food consumption behaviour, including nutrition advice (53; 30%), reminders and recommendations (54; 30%) in the form of eating and drinking reminders, notifications, badges or rewards for coming close to and reaching predefined weight or nutrition goals. Sources of social support and motivation including connected users following each other's progress and posts (23; 13%), personal coaching for the achievement of user-specific diet or weight goals (19; 11%) and the option for inviting other users to compete or take part in weight loss or exercise challenges (17; 10%), were also identified.

Contextual data

One-hundred and seven (61%) of the dietary assessment tools collected some form of data related to motivation, including users' goals related to their desired intake of energy, nutrients, or water (59; 34%) or desired body weights (32; 18%) and states of physical fitness (10; 6%). Users' preferences such as preferred foods were identified in 29 (16%) of the apps, and 9 (5%) apps allowed users to record their mood or emotions.

Health and physical fitness indicators were identified in 108 (61%) apps. These indicators included body weight (76; 43%), body mass index (22; 13%), or body composition (11; 6%). Symptoms, in the form of subjective evidence of current diseases, were found in 12 (6%) apps and records of drugs or other substances used to treat diseases or injuries in 11 (7%). Some apps allowed for monitoring of blood sugar (8; 5%), blood pressure (8; 5%) or blood oxygen saturation (2; 1%).

Contextual data related to users' physical activity have been identified in 90 (51%) apps. This includes various types of activities (29; 16%; e.g., swimming, cycling, running) and number of steps taken (19; 11%). Sleep and sleeping patterns have been identified in 13 (7%) apps. Twenty-seven (12%) of the apps offered social media platform features for exchanging data and information with other connected users. Thirteen (7%) of the apps allowed their users to share their data and progress updates with popular social media networks. Eleven percent of the tools in the sample were identified as allowing for inputs of dishes from restaurant menus. This implies that food consumption data collected by these tools might contain information regarding the location where the food was purchased. Geo-coordinates provided by a GPS unit were identified in one of the apps.

Data management

In 55 (31%) apps the possibility for exporting user-documented food consumption data (from the app infrastructure, e.g., website) was identified (see Table 2). The most frequently implemented data export method was file download (40; 23%), which allowed users to download the collected data, in the form of a data file, directly from the apps' websites. Some apps allowed for email export from within the app (9; 5%), whereby the exported data file is sent as an attachment to an email address specified by the user. Exported data was found to be in various standard formats including portable document format (PDF; 18; 10%), and comma-separated values (CSV; 18; 10%). Only a few app vendors allowed data export through a public API (Application Programming Interface; 5; 3%). APIs enable a more seamless distribution of data, in comparison to manual data file export. By allowing the sharing of data between authorized organizations and their IT systems (e.g., apps), processes can be automated without the need for manual intervention. All implemented APIs stated their ability to respond in the JavaScript Object Notation (JSON), which is a lightweight and widely recognized and supported open-standard data format [38].

Although only a few app vendors stated that they utilized a public API, about a quarter (40; 23%) of the apps exchanged data with at least one other dietary assessment tool included in the sample. Apps with the greatest number of connections with other dietary assessment apps in our sample were apps which implemented an API for data exchange such as Fitbit, connecting with 19 (11%) of the sampled apps, followed by Jawbone Up, and MyFitnessPal connecting with 10 (6%) and 3 (2%) of the sampled apps respectively. Twenty-four (14%) of the investigated dietary assessment apps connected to at least one popular health and fitness tracker (e.g., Garmin, Misfit, Withings), all which implemented an API for data access.

About a quarter (44; 25%) of the apps were exchanging data with at least one data aggregator or central data collection hub. Aggregators are designed to allow health and fitness apps to work together and collate their data. These various streams of data from apps and devices such as data on body weight, exercises, activities or dietary consumption can then be accessed and visualized on a single dashboard. We found in total twelve data aggregators which integrated with at least one of the diet apps in our sample. The aggregators which integrated with most apps in our sample were Apple's HealthKit (31; 18%) and Google Fit (17; 10%). Other aggregators connecting to various diet apps in our sample were S-Health (5; 3%) HealthGraph (5; 3%) Human API (3; 2%) and Validic (2; 1%). All aggregators implement a documented API for data access.

Table 2 Investigated characteristics of user documented food consumption data related to data management and extracted information (n = 176)

Characteristic	Description	Extracted information (n)
Data export	Whether the data collected by the app is exportable directly via the apps infrastructure (not via integrated aggregators)	No information (117), Yes (55), No (4)
Access method[a]	The type of data export	File download (40), Email export (9), API (5), SDK (3), No information (3), Dropbox[b] (3), AirDrop[c] (1), Google Account[d] (1), Google Drive[e] (1)
Data format[a]	The format the data can be exported	PDF (18), CSV (18), Excel (9), No information (8), JSON (4), HTML (3), SQLite[f] data file (2)
External data sources[a]	What type of third parties systems does the app exchange data with	Aggregators (44), Partner apps (40), Health and fitness trackers (24)

[a]Per characteristic multiple inputs were possible and hence the individual percentages do not add up to 100%
[b]cloud storage provider or online backup service that is also used as a file-sharing platform
[c]lets Mac and iOS devices share files wirelessly
[d]required for access to certain Google online services and supports app data storage
[e]personal cloud storage service that lets users store and synchronize digital content across computers, laptops and mobile devices
[f]SQLite is a relational database management system
API Application Programming Interface, *SDK*, Software Development Kit, *PDF* Portable Document Format, *CSV* Comma Separated Values, *JSON* JavaScript Object Notation, *HTML* Hypertext Markup Language

Legal and ethical governance

Sixty-nine (39%) apps in our sample provided a terms and conditions document, and eighty (45%) provided a privacy statement (see Table 3). In fifty (28%) apps the user was described as the owner of the data and in forty-three (24%) of the apps users were required to grant the app vendor an irrevocable, worldwide, and royalty-free license to commercially exploit the collected user-documented data including reproduction, adaptation, distribution, and publication. More specific data usage and exploitation purposes were not further described. Seventy-four (42%) apps were described as collecting personally identifiable information (PII) including name, email address, phone number or date of birth. Thirty-eight (22%) apps created a public profile of the collected data, and twenty-one (12%) stated that they offer privacy settings in order to restrict data publishing of those public user profiles. Fifty-one (29%) apps stated that vendors would share collected PII with other affiliated parties without written consent. These affiliated third parties are required to comply with the privacy policies of the app vendors. Sharing PII with unaffiliated parties, which are not bound by the privacy policies of the app vendors was described in twenty-nine (16%) of the cases. In those cases, vendors claimed to ask for written consent prior to data sharing.

Discussion

We identified several potentials and challenges associated with the use of food consumption data collected by

Table 3 Investigated characteristics of user documented food consumption data related to legal governance and extracted information (n = 176)

Characteristic	Description	Extracted information (n)
Website	Whether the app can be associated with a working home/support page	Yes (140), No (36)
Contact information	Whether the app vendor provides contact information	Yes (117), No (59)
Terms & conditions	Whether the app provides a terms of use document	Yes (69), No (107)
Privacy statement	Whether the app provides a privacy policy document	Yes (80), No (96)
Ownership[a]	The parties who hold the ownership of the user generated data (User content)	User (50), Vendor (1), No information (125)
Usage license vendor	Whether the app vendor retains the right to access and exploit the user generated data (publish, distribute, publicly display)	Yes (43), No (9), No Information (124)
Personally identifiable information collection	Whether the app collects personal identifiable information (e.g., during registration)	Yes (74), No (5), No Information (97)
Type personally identifiable information[a]	The types of personal identifiable information does the app collect	Email address (44), Name (37), Username and or password (28), Date of birth (18), Phone number (16), Registration (16), Health data (15), Address (14), Financial information (11), Gender (10), Additional data (8), Optional registration (8), Physical characteristics (7), Demographics (7), Mandatory registration (7), Image (5), Postcode (4), Location (3), No information (3), Interactions (1), Home address (1), Personal video (1), Social network handle (1), Ethnicity (1)
Public profile	Whether the app creates a public profile of the users personal data	Yes (38), No (5), No Information (133)
Privacy settings public profile	Whether the is user able to configure the privacy settings for his or her public profile	Yes (21), No (1), No Information (16)
Cookies	Whether the homepage/ website of the app stores cookies on a user's computer	Yes (61), No Information (115)
Web Beacons	Whether the homepage/ website of the app stores web beacons on a user's computer	Yes (25), No (2), No Information (149)
PII data sharing affiliates	Whether the collected personal identifiable data will be shared with affiliated third parties (confidentiality agreements)	Yes (51), No (8), With consent (4), No information (113)
PII data sharing non affiliates	Whether the collected personal identifiable data will be shared with unaffiliated third parties (without confidentiality agreements)	Yes (4), No (11), With consent (29), No information (132)
Usage Analytics	Whether the homepage/ website of the app uses third-parties for advertising and usage analytics	Yes (41), No (1), No Information (134)
Data Storage[a]	The location where the system stores the data it collects	Device storage (78), Server storage (48), No information (81)
Data encryption	Whether the collected data is stored or transmitted in encrypted form	Storage: No information (176) Transfer: Yes (15), No information (161)
Data deletion	Whether the user is able to delete or ask for deletion of his or her personal identifiable information (e.g., after account termination)	Yes (33), No (1), No Information (142)

[a]Per characteristic multiple inputs were possible and hence the individual percentages do not add up to 100%

users of publicly available nutrition apps. Our findings have important implications for the scientific, technical, legal and ethical aspects associated with user-documented data and ultimately for developing strategies and policies aimed at the collection, integration, and sharing of this type of data.

Scientific implications

In our app sample, for the most part, food diaries were used for assessing people's diets, which is in line with previous findings [1, 2]. In addition to recording the time of consumption, food diaries have several advantages over other dietary assessment methods such as allowing for the collection of detailed actual intake data and being less prone to memory bias due to the focus on current food intake. Important challenges related to food diaries, however, are underreporting due to the large respondent burden and reactivity, meaning that keeping the diary affects habitual consumption behaviour. Hence, the completeness and quality of the user-documented food consumption data may decline over time [7]. Technical advances to support food logging might lower the user burden. Food diaries in our sample often allowed for precompiled food databases, which has been suggested to enable a more efficient and user-friendly data collection process [1, 2, 7, 8]. Barcode scanners which were also commonly described in our sample have been claimed to reduce the burden of food recording [14, 39] and have been evaluated as comprehensive, easy to use and non-intrusive data collection tools [40]. Similarly, food image processing technology, which has been characterized in some of the apps, aims at further increasing the accuracy of self-reported dietary recordings by increasing user adherence, automation, and standardization [41]. Although technical advances in dietary self-monitoring can make dietary assessment more efficient, they might not be sufficient for increasing users' adherence to diet apps. Self-regulation techniques such as goal-setting and intention formation features were also identified in a large number of apps. These features might be needed to promote user engagement and sustained use of apps [17]. Finally, since a large number of apps allowed users to add new foods to the underlying databases for current and future references, a more complete and representative insight into the prevalence and day-to-day variability of individual preferences and dietary patterns might be supported.

Technical advances, however, come with challenges. The clear challenge for database-driven food logging approaches is the quality of the databases [39]. References to verified database compilation standards were only available for a small number of apps and tests of the quality of food databases underlying food consumption apps including estimated nutrients are nearly absent [6, 42]. In addition, the investigated apps provided a limited set of nutrients for the foods eaten, with the vast majority of apps focusing on intake of energy and macronutrients. Since very limited information was provided on the content of the food composition databases underlying the apps, their quality and the availability of data for specific nutrients and also the degree of missing data for the nutrients included is not known. This might be a barrier for research interested in the associations between specific nutrients and health outcomes. The investigated apps might be useful for assessing intake on the food level. Product brand names and recipes can provide valuable information for researchers interested in users' food preferences and choices. Nutrient values for the consumed foods could be estimated post hoc by matching the identified foods to food entries in a quality controlled food composition database.

In addition, there is a clear scientific challenge to better understand the effects of the various app features on changes in food consumption behaviours [4, 10]. Food diaries are prone to changes in food consumption behaviours [43] and the presence of behaviour change features might often be non-evidence based [15, 44, 45]. This is problematic for generating unbiased insights into habitual food intake and its behavioural determinants and it complicates validation of apps against a reference standard [6].

Goal setting and intention formation features might not only increase user engagement but at the same time provide motivational and situational context to the collected food consumption data. Psychological factors such as users' goals, preferences and habits were the most prominent in the apps and provide potentially relevant determinants of people's food consumption behaviours [46]. Because energy expenditure drives food consumption [47], the collected data on body size and physical activity, including peoples' routines, might additionally provide relevant physical and physiological context. Overall, though, the emphasis of contextual data was on parameters relevant for weight management including weight goals, energy expenditure, body weight or BMI. There are potential gaps in relevant determinants of food consumption such as data related to users' emotional states, or the physical location of food consumption. Since the primary focus of the investigated tools was collecting data about the individual, relevant determinants of food consumption within the social and cultural context might have been lacking.

There seems to be a clear tendency towards integrating and enriching user-documented data with data from third-party apps or data aggregators [48, 49]. Food consumption episodes can be enriched with GPS locations, social media interactions or various kinds of health and activity related data through their connections with partner apps or aggregators. The strive towards integration and interconnectedness with other services and apps has the potential to provide a more complete overall summary about the user [44] and ultimately a more thorough understanding of the determinants of food consumption behaviours.

Data management implications

The lack of procedures for exporting collected food consumption data in the investigated apps poses a barrier towards data sharing and analysis [50–52] and is considered an important criterion of data quality [27]. A significant challenge for self-tracking technologies is fragmented data scattered across multiple platforms [53, 54]. This is not only challenging for researchers interested in investigating this type of data but also forms an important barrier for motivating users to adopt and use self-tracking technologies. Since the majority of popular health apps do not seem to allow individuals access to their data beyond what is presented through the commercial interfaces, the evolving data integration and sharing platforms might also have important implications for data management practices. The emerging network of apps and data aggregators might provide an alternative and more efficient opportunity for data access. All sampled data aggregators implemented APIs for requesting and digesting food and related health data from various systems. In order to support processing and visualization of collected data irrespective of the source, these data platforms might provide some degree of initial harmonization of the data. Due to the potential lack of portability of data from one system to another [55, 56], accessing data entities already integrated from multiple data sources could be a very effective strategy from a data management perspective. Since data generated by external sources remains difficult to harmonize, however, imposing post-hoc standardizations and controls might render data inconsistent with its original source and hence provides data portability at the expense of data quality [57].

Legal and ethical implications

The lack of formal documentation regarding terms of usage, ownership, and privacy identified in the apps we investigated, increases the risk of compromising data integrity and forms an important challenge for legal and ethical governance of user-documented food consumption data. There is a requirement for apps to cover data ownership and data privacy in their licensing agreement, which the consumer accepts at the time of first use [30–32]. Users express a clear interest in being in control over their generated data [51] and compromises to data integrity can occur when researchers are not aware of existing data ownership policies and consequently fail to adhere to the rights, obligations, and expectations regarding data usage [24]. In addition, a key principle of research ethics is that participants must have all of the information that might reasonably influence their willingness to participate in a study, including its purpose, implications, risks, and measures taken to protect appropriate levels of anonymity, confidentiality, or de-identification [58]. Vendors were often granted an irrevocable and royalty-free license to commercially exploit the user-documented data, however, without specifying its usage and purpose. The overall lack of documentation regarding these core elements of informed consent poses a clear challenge to maintaining the ethical and legal integrity of the data.

The new General Data Protection Regulation (GDPR) aims to standardize privacy rules and the protection of personal data across the European Union [59]. Considering the vast amounts of lifestyle and health parameters collected by the sampled apps and exchanged in a rapidly increasing network of integrated systems, distinguishing personal data from non-personal or non-identifiable data might become challenging. Food consumption behaviour is deeply rooted in people's personal and social identities [60, 61] and might make reference to locations, diseases, ethnical origins, or ethical and religious convictions. Hence in the context of the privacy standards set by the GDPR, it is prudent to argue that user-documented food consumption data could be categorized as personal data (or at least certain elements of it). This would have strong legal and ethical implications for future privacy policies regarding informed consent and sharing of these data, as well as important technical implication for data access and integration due to the "right of data portability" and the "right to be forgotten" associated with personal data. Legal and ethical government issues to some extent apply to all kinds of digital apps collecting personal identifying information. Since secondary data, however, varies in terms of the amount of identifying information it contains [19], the complex and dynamically increasing network of diet apps and its implications regarding personal data requires a more thorough investigation on a case by case basis.

Limitations and future research

The extent to which information about the apps was publicly available was critical for collecting the relevant data about the apps in our sample. For a large number of apps, however, the relevant public sources of information such as homepages or privacy and terms of use statements were unavailable. The availability of information is considered an important indication of the quality of online products and services [62], and hence the lack of available information can be interpreted as a potential limitation to their utilization. We are aware that due to our chosen method of investigating publicly available information of apps, our sample might lack important information that has not been publicly provided or might even contain false or biased information based on misinterpretations by the authors or misleading publication and marketing strategies by app vendors. Since we did not download a random subset of apps in order to validate our interpretations, we are unable to provide estimations regarding the extend of these potential errors.

Considering the sheer number of potentially relevant apps that collect user-documented food consumption data, the fundamental challenge was to provide a selection of apps which was able to capture the variety of data collection apps available on the market. The app selection procedure was dependent on the order of the apps retrieved from the app stores. This strategy might be biased based on the estimated app relevance assigned by the app stores at that moment of time. In addition, the present selection of apps was limited to apps available in the UK storefronts. Although a large number of apps in our sample were also available in other countries, a selection of apps searched in app stores of different countries might have revealed a somewhat different set of apps. Finally, the present research did not aim to create an inventory of food consumption apps, since that would require a continuous research effort. Rather, we aimed to gather information from a representative sample of apps and learn from this highly dynamic market. Since the content in the apps stores is changing at a fast pace, the selection of apps for the present sample should be considered a snapshot of apps at a certain moment in time.

The present research did not aim to provide a general quality framework nor recommendations for researchers who seek to identify the scientific relevance of diet apps in general. The selection of characteristics indicative of scientific relevance needs to be tailored to the needs, quality criteria and protocols, specific to a particular research objective. That is, objectives on the assessment of dietary intake and health behaviour, effectiveness in weight or diabetes management, or understanding consumer behaviour at the individual or group level, emphasize different sets of quality characteristics which do or do not qualify an app as 'fit for purpose'.

Our aim was not to evaluate the quality of user-documented data collected by individual apps or to provide informed recommendations for choosing one app over the other. In order to get app specific quality evaluations and informed comparisons of apps, we believe it is important to further examine and validate a smaller selection of apps more closely. In particular, the evaluation and validation of food databases are warranted. In a recent study, Maringer et al., investigated the quality of labelled food product databases underlying popular diet apps with barcode scanners [63]. The authors concluded that, due to the variations in availability and accuracy of nutrient information contained in these databases, they lack the necessary consistency and accuracy for assessing dietary intake on the nutrient level. In addition, Maringer et al., reported that for some apps, food consumption data were not available for individual foods or meals, but was aggregated over certain periods of time. Hence in order to get more app specific evaluations regarding the availability and accuracy of user-documented data, those apps which allow for the export of collected data in a standardized format needs closer inspection. In addition, data aggregators might help to overcome some of the fundamental challenges related to user documented food consumption data from apps, including data linkages to contextual data, seamless data access, data harmonization and standardization. Further research is needed, however, in order to better understand the types and quality of data they exchange.

Conclusion

Considering the dynamically changing domain of publicly available food consumption apps and their increasing use of technical innovations, determining whether the data collected by users of these apps are "fit for purpose" involves a continuous research effort. User-documented food consumption data has the potential of providing scientifically relevant insights into the prevalence and variability of individual preferences and dietary patterns. The collection of lifestyle data and strive towards integration and interconnectedness of data might help to better understand the determinants of food consumption behaviours. An important challenge for an efficient data management strategy, however, seems to be the lack of available or documented data access. The identified interconnectedness of apps and their data provides new opportunities for data management (efficient data access, standardized formats, data linkage). The overall lack of documentation regarding terms of usage and data privacy poses a clear challenge for legal and ethical data integrity. The strive towards integration and interconnectedness of user-documented data makes this task even more challenging.

Endnotes

[1]iTunes-search module version 1.0.1. Nodejs module to search app data on the iTunes search api. Url: https://github.com/connor/itunes-node

[2]Google-play-scraper module version 0.2.1. Nodejs module to search app data on the Google Play store. Url: https://github.com/facundoolano/google-play-scraper

Abbreviations

API: Application Programming Interface; CSV: Comma Separated Values; EU: European Union; GDPR: General Data Protection Regulation; GPS: Global Positioning System; JSON: JavaScript Object Notation; PDF: Portable Document Format; PII: Personally Identifiable Information; RI: Research Infrastructure; UK: United Kingdom; URL: Uniform Resource Locator

Acknowledgements

We thank Prof. Dr. Indira Carr for her advice and input regarding legal and ethical issues related to user-documented food consumption data. Indira Carr is a Professor of Law at the Faculty of Business, Economics and Law, University of Surrey, Guilford, Surrey, United Kingdom. We thank Dr. Barbara Korousic Seljak, for her advice and input on technical issues related to access and integration of user-documented food consumption data. Barbara Korousic Seljak is a senior researcher at the Computer Systems Department, Jožef Stefan Institute, Ljubljana, Slovenia.

Funding

The research leading to these results received funding from the European Union's Horizon 2020 research and innovation program (Call: INFRADEV-1-2014-Design Studies) under Grant Agreement No 654280 (RICHFIELDS).

Authors' contributions

MM Made substantial contributions to conception and design, acquisition of data, analysis and interpretation of data; Made substantial contributions to the manuscript draft. Given final approval of the manuscript to be published. PV Was involved in revising the manuscript critically for important intellectual content; Given final approval of the manuscript to be published. NK Contributed to the research design and was involved in critical revisions of the manuscript. Given final approval of the manuscript to be published. MV Was involved in conception and design of the work and provided critical revisions of the manuscript. Given final approval of the manuscript to be published. AN Contributed to the research design and provided critical revisions of the manuscript. Given final approval of the manuscript to be published. SE Contributed to the research design and provided critical revisions of the manuscript. Given final approval of the manuscript to be published. LT Contributed to the research design and provided critical revisions of the manuscript. Given final approval of the manuscript to be published. MR Made substantial contributions to conception and design, and interpretation of data; Was involved in critical revisions of the manuscript. Given final approval of the manuscript to be published. AG Made substantial contributions to conception and design, analysis and interpretation of data; Was involved in revising the manuscript critically for important intellectual content; Given final approval of the manuscript to be published.

Competing interests

The authors certify that they have NO affiliations with or involvement in any organization or entity with any financial interest (such as honoraria; educational grants; participation in speakers' bureaus; membership, employment, consultancies, stock ownership, or other equity interest; and expert testimony or patent-licensing arrangements), or non- financial interest (such as personal or professional relationships, affiliations, knowledge or beliefs) in the subject matter or materials discussed in this manuscript.

Author details

[1]Division of Human Nutrition, Wageningen University & Research, Wageningen, The Netherlands. [2]Food, Consumer Behaviour and Health Research Centre, University of Surrey, Guildford, Surrey, United Kingdom. [3]Wageningen Economic Research, Wageningen University & Research, Wageningen, The Netherlands. [4]Division of Bioscience and Materials, Agrifood and Bioscience, RISE Research Institutes of Sweden, Gothenburg, Sweden.

References

1. Franco RZ, et al. Popular nutrition-related mobile apps: a feature assessment. JMIR Mhealth Uhealth. 2016;4(3):e85. https://doi.org/10.2196/mhealth.5846.
2. Chen J, Cade JE, Allman-Farinelli M. The most popular smartphone apps for weight loss: a quality assessment. JMIR Mhealth Uhealth. 2015;3(4):e104. https://doi.org/10.2196/mhealth.4334.
3. Carter MC, Burley VJ, Cade JE. Weight loss associated with different patterns of self-monitoring using the mobile phone app my meal mate. JMIR Mhealth Uhealth. 2017;5(2):e8. https://doi.org/10.2196/mhealth.4520.
4. DiFilippo KN, et al. The use of mobile apps to improve nutrition outcomes: a systematic literature review. J Telemed Telecare. 2015;21(5):243–53. https://doi.org/10.1177/1357633x15572203.
5. Thompson FE, et al. Need for technological innovation in dietary assessment. J Am Diet Assoc. 2010;110(1):48–51. https://doi.org/10.1016/j.jada.2009.10.008.
6. Carter MC, et al. Adherence to a smartphone application for weight loss compared to website and paper diary: pilot randomized controlled trial. J Med Internet Res. 2013;15(4):e32. https://doi.org/10.2196/jmir.2283.
7. Shim JS, Oh K, Kim HC. Dietary assessment methods in epidemiologic studies. Epidemiol Health. 2014;36:e2014009. https://doi.org/10.4178/epih/e2014009.
8. Rusin M, Arsand E, Hartvigsen G. Functionalities and input methods for recording food intake: a systematic review. Int J Med Inform. 2013;82(8):653–64. https://doi.org/10.1016/j.ijmedinf.2013.01.007.
9. Wharton CM, et al. Dietary self-monitoring, but not dietary quality, improves with use of smartphone app technology in an 8-week weight loss trial. J Nutr Educ Behav. 2014;46(5):440–4. https://doi.org/10.1016/j.jneb.2014.04.291.
10. Thompson-Felty C, Johnston CS. Adherence to diet applications using a smartphone was associated with weight loss in healthy overweight adults irrespective of the application. J Diabetes Sci Technol. 2017;11(1):184–5. https://doi.org/10.1177/1932296816656209.
11. Laing BY, et al. Effectiveness of a smartphone application for weight loss compared with usual care in overweight primary care patients: a randomized, controlled trial. Ann Intern Med. 2014;161(10):S5–12. https://doi.org/10.7326/M13-3005.
12. Bardus M, et al. A review and content analysis of engagement, functionality, aesthetics, information quality, and change techniques in the most popular commercial apps for weight management. Int J Behav Nutr Phys Act. 2016; 13:35. https://doi.org/10.1186/s12966-016-0359-9.
13. Breton ER, Fuemmeler BF, Abroms LC. Weight loss-there is an app for that! But does it adhere to evidence-informed practices? Transl Behav Med. 2011; 1(4):523–9. https://doi.org/10.1007/s13142-011-0076-5.
14. Pagoto S, et al. Evidence-based strategies in weight-loss mobile apps. Am J Prev Med. 2013;45(5):576–82. https://doi.org/10.1016/j.amepre.2013.04.025.
15. Hales S, et al. Is a picture worth a thousand words? Few evidence-based features of dietary interventions included in photo diet tracking mobile apps for weight loss. J Diabetes Sci Technol. 2016; https://doi.org/10.1177/1932296816651451.
16. Azar KM, et al. Mobile applications for weight management: theory-based content analysis. Am J Prev Med. 2013;45(5):583–9. https://doi.org/10.1016/j.amepre.2013.07.005.
17. Helander E, et al. Factors related to sustained use of a free mobile app for dietary self-monitoring with photography and peer feedback: retrospective cohort study. J Med Internet Res. 2014;16(4):e109. https://doi.org/10.2196/jmir.3084.
18. Zaidan S, Roehrer E. Popular mobile phone apps for diet and weight loss: a content analysis. JMIR Mhealth Uhealth. 2016;4(3):e80. https://doi.org/10.2196/mhealth.5406.
19. Tripathy JP. Secondary data analysis: ethical issues and challenges. Iran J Public Health. 2013;42(12):1478–9.
20. Morrow V, Boddy J, Lamb R. The ethics of secondary data analysis. Novella: NCRM Working Paper; 2014.
21. van den Puttelaar J, Verain MCD, Onwezen MC, et al. The Potential of Enriching Food Consumption Data by use of Consumer Generated Data: a case from RICHFIELDS, in Measuring Behavior: 10th International Conference on Methods and Techniques in Behavioral Research. Dublin: A. Spink; 2016.
22. Lupton D. Cooking, Eating, Uploading: digital food cultures. In: LeBesco K, Naccarato P, editors. The Handbook of Food and Popular. London Forthcoming: Bloomsbury; 2016.
23. Hox JJ, Boeije HR. Data Collection, Primary Versus secondary. In: Kempf-Leonard K, editor. Encyclopedia of Social Measurement. San Diego, CA: Academic Press; 2005.
24. Loshin, D., Knowledge Integrity: Data Ownership, in Data Warehouse magazine (Online) June 8, 2004. 2002.
25. Apple Inc. Search API. [Accessed 17 July 2016]; Available from: https://affiliate.itunes.apple.com/resources/documentation/itunes-store-web-service-search-api/.
26. Xu W, Liu Y. mHealthApps: a repository and database of mobile health apps. JMIR Mhealth Uhealth. 2015;3(1):e28. https://doi.org/10.2196/mhealth.4026.
27. Dufty D, et al. A suggested framework for the quality of big data. In: UNECE big data quality task team; 2014.
28. Rutishauser IHE, Black AE. Introduction to human nutrition. In: Gibney M, Vorster H, Kok FJ, editors. The Nutrition Society Textbook Series. Oxford: Blackwell Publishing; 2002. p. 225–48.
29. Stok FM, et al. The DONE framework: creation, evaluation, and updating of an interdisciplinary, dynamic framework 2.0 of determinants of nutrition and eating. PLoS One. 2017;12(2):e0171077. https://doi.org/10.1371/journal.pone.0171077.
30. Adhikari R, Richards D, Scott K. Security and privacy issues related to the use of mobile health apps. in 25th Australasian Conference on Information Systems. 2014;
31. Cummings E, Borycki EM, Roehrer E. Issues and considerations for healthcare consumers using mobile applications. Stud Health Technol Inform. 2013;183:227–31.
32. Blenner SR, et al. Privacy policies of android diabetes apps and sharing of health information. Jama. 2016;315(10):1051–2. https://doi.org/10.1001/jama.2015.19426.
33. Sunyaev A, et al. Availability and quality of mobile health app privacy policies. J Am Med Inform Assoc. 2015;22(e1):e28–33. https://doi.org/10.1136/amiajnl-2013-002605.

34. Sharp M, O'Sullivan D. Mobile medical apps and mHealth devices: a framework to build medical apps and mHealth devices in an ethical manner to promote safer use - a literature review. Stud Health Technol Inform. 2017;235:363–7.
35. Mobile Health and Fitness Apps: What Are the Privacy Risks? http://www.privacyrights.org/mobile-medical-apps-privacy-technologist-research-report.pdf.
36. Vayena E, et al. Ethical challenges of big data in public health. PLoS Comput Biol. 2015;11(2):e1003904. https://doi.org/10.1371/journal.pcbi.1003904.
37. FDA. (2015). Mobile Medical Applications: Guidance for Industry and Food and Drug Administration Staff. http://www.fda.gov/downloads/MedicalDevices/.../UCM263366.pdf
38. ECMA. (2013). Standard: ECMA 404. The JSON data interchange format. Ecma international. http://www.ecma-international.org/publications/files/ECMA-ST/ECMA-404.pdf
39. Arens-Volland AG, Spassova L, Bohn T. Promising approaches of computer-supported dietary assessment and management-current research status and available applications. Int J Med Inform. 2015;84(12):997–1008. https://doi.org/10.1016/j.ijmedinf.2015.08.006.
40. Byrd-Bredbenner C, Bredbenner CA. Assessing the home food environment nutrient supply using mobile barcode (universal product code) scanning technology. Nutrition Food Sci. 2010;40(3):305–13. https://doi.org/10.1108/00346651011044005.
41. Probst Y, et al. Dietary assessment on a mobile phone using image processing and pattern recognition techniques: algorithm design and system prototyping. Nutrients. 2015;7(8):6128–38. https://doi.org/10.3390/nu7085274.
42. Goodman S, et al. Vitamin D intake among young Canadian adults: validation of a mobile vitamin D calculator app. J Nutr Educ Behav. 2015;47(3):242–7. https://doi.org/10.1016/j.jneb.2014.11.006.
43. Rebro SM, et al. The effect of keeping food records on eating patterns. J Am Diet Assoc. 1998;98(10):1163–5. https://doi.org/10.1016/s0002-8223(98)00269-7.
44. Higgins JP. Smartphone applications for Patients' health and fitness. Am J Med. 2016;129(1):11–9. https://doi.org/10.1016/j.amjmed.2015.05.038.
45. Davis SF, et al. Health behavior theory in popular calorie counting apps: a content analysis. JMIR Mhealth Uhealth. 2016;4(1):e19. https://doi.org/10.2196/mhealth.4177.
46. Symmank C, et al. Predictors of food decision making: a systematic interdisciplinary mapping (SIM) review. Appetite. 2017;110:25–35. https://doi.org/10.1016/j.appet.2016.11.023.
47. Hopkins M, King NA, Blundell JE. Acute and long-term effects of exercise on appetite control: is there any benefit for weight control? Curr Opin Clin Nutr Metab Care. 2010;13(6):635–40. https://doi.org/10.1097/MCO.0b013e32833e343b.
48. Mandl KD, Mandel JC, Kohane IS. Driving innovation in health systems through an apps-based information economy. Cell Syst. 2015;1(1):8–13. https://doi.org/10.1016/j.cels.2015.05.001.
49. Research2Guidance. (2016). mHealth App Developer Economics 2016. The current status and trends of the mHealth app market. 6th annual study on mHealth app publishing based on 2,600 plus respondents.
50. IMS Institute for Healthcare Informatics, Patient Adoption of mHealth. Use, Evidence and Remaining Barriers to Mainstream Acceptance. 2015.
51. Chen J, Bauman A, Allman-Farinelli M. A study to determine the most popular lifestyle smartphone applications and willingness of the public to share their personal data for Health Research. Telemed J E Health. 2016;22(8):655–65. https://doi.org/10.1089/tmj.2015.0159.
52. Chen J, et al. Designing health apps to support dietetic professional practice and their patients: qualitative results from an international survey. JMIR Mhealth Uhealth. 2017;5(3):e40. https://doi.org/10.2196/mhealth.6945.
53. Choe EK, et al. Understanding quantified-selfers' practices in collecting and exploring personal data; 2014. p. 1143–52.
54. Li I, Dey A, Forlizzi JA. A stage - based model of personal informatics systems. In: Chi '10; 2010.
55. Estrin D, Sim I. Health care delivery. Open mHealth architecture: an engine for health care innovation. Science. 2010;330(6005):759–60. https://doi.org/10.1126/science.1196187.
56. Open mHealth 3 painful lessons learned building with HealthKit. 2015 [Accessed 12 July 2016]; Available from: http://www.openmhealth.org/3-painful-lessons-learned-building-with-healthkit/.
57. Loshin, D., Understanding big data quality for maximum information usability (white paper). 2014. https://www.sas.com/en_us/offers/sem/2317617-understanding-big-data-quality.html?gclid=CMLGhND17NQCFSIM0wody5oJXg Accessed 3 July 2017.
58. European Union, Ethics for researchers: facilitating research excellence in FP7. 2013.
59. European Union. General Data Protection Regulation 2016 9 May 2017].
60. Hauck-Lawson A. Introduction to special issue on the food voice. Food, Culture Society. 2004 7(1):24–5.
61. Kittler PG, Sucher KP, Nelms MN. Food and culture. 6th ed. Belmont, CA: Wadsworth; 2012.
62. Aladwani AM, Palvia PC. Developing and validating an instrument for measuring user-perceived web quality. Information Management. 2002;39(6):467–76. https://doi.org/10.1016/S0378-7206(01)00113-6.
63. Maringer M, et al. Food identification by barcode scanning in the Netherlands: a quality assessment of labelled food product databases underlying popular nutrition apps. Public Health Nutrition (in press). 2018.

4

Correlates of metabolic syndrome among young Brazilian adolescents population

Michel Coutinho dos Santos[1*], Ana Paula Cicci de Castro Coutinho[1], Mônica de Souza Dantas[1], Letícia Ayran Medina Yabunaka[1], Dartagnan Pinto Guedes[2] and Silvia Aparecida Oesterreich[3]

Abstract

Background: Findings available in literature indicate that metabolic syndrome (*MetS*) diagnosed in young ages tends to remain in adulthood. The aim of the study was to identify demographic, nutritional, anthropometric and behavioral correlates of *MetS* in a sample of adolescents from Dourados, Mato Grosso do Sul, Brazil.

Methodology: This is a cross-sectional school-based study involving 274 participants aged 12–18 years (186 girls and 88 boys). Anthropometric measurements were performed and a questionnaire with structured questions was applied for data collection. *MetS* was identified according to criteria proposed by the *International Diabetes Federation*. Data were statistically treated using bivariate analysis and hierarchical multiple regression.

Results: The proportion of adolescents identified with *MetS* was equivalent to 4.7% [95% CI (3.6–6.0)]. Multivariate analysis showed that older age (OR = 1.22 [1.04–1.73]) and higher economic class (OR = 1.25 [1.07–1.96]) were significantly associated with *MetS*. Among behavioral factors, longer recreational screen time (OR = 1.26 [1.05–1.94]) and low fruits/vegetables intake (OR = 1.49 [1.23–2.41]) were independently associated with *MetS*. Likewise, excess body weight (OR = 1.52 [1.24–2.41]) was significantly associated with the outcome.

Conclusion: The high proportion of adolescents with *MetS* and the identification of their correlates reinforce the need for early life style intervention and awareness programs in this population group.

Keywords: Cardiometabolic risk, Metabolic syndrome, Lifestyle, Health promotion, Youth

Background

Currently, regardless of sex, age, economic class and geographic region, overweight and obesity have become a global epidemic [1], which decisively contributes to the onset and development of metabolic syndrome (*MetS*) [2]. Findings available in literature indicate that *MetS* diagnosed in childhood and adolescence tends to remain in adulthood [3]. Therefore, the diagnosis of the possible presence of *MetS* at early ages, accompanied by control interventions, should have a favorable impact on the health of young people and the prevention of adverse outcomes in the future.

MetS refers to a set of cardiometabolic components that, when altered, favor the occurrence of cardiovascular events and diabetes. These components include excess abdominal fat, high blood pressure, and altered triglyceride, lipoprotein, and blood glucose levels [4]. Currently, for the adult population, there is consensus regarding the cutoff points used to define the *MetS* components. However, it is not the case of adolescents, where the diagnostic criterion varies considerably among the different available proposals, with repercussion in clinical practice, making it difficult the comparison among studies [5].

Even considering this limitation and due to the importance and the need to diagnose the presence of *MetS* and correlates as early as possible, a number of studies have been carried out involving adolescents [6–12]. This is necessary because the adult prevalence is on the rise [13], and in the young population, evidence has pointed to similar phenomenon [9–11]. In addition, several attributes linked to health risk behaviors have been increasingly frequent in adolescents [14].

Therefore, the aim of the present study was to identify demographic, nutritional, anthropometric and behavioral

* Correspondence: michelsantos@ufgd.edu.br
[1]University Hospital of the Federal University of Grande Dourados, Dourados, MS, Brazil
Full list of author information is available at the end of the article

correlates of *MetS* in a sample of adolescents from Dourados, Mato Grosso do Sul, Brazil.

Methods

In order to carry out the study, information from the database of a larger project with longitudinal characteristics (*Health Education Program through Dietary and Physical Activity Interventions*) was used, which includes adolescents enrolled in the 2nd cycle of elementary school (6th to 9th grades) and high-school (from 1st to 3rd grades) of four public schools randomly selected in the city of Dourados, Mato Grosso do Sul, Brazil. In this case, data were collected at the initial moment of the project. The intervention protocols were approved by the Research Ethics Committee of the Federal University of Grande Dourados (Protocol No. 1.434.947).

The inclusion of adolescents in the study was due to their desire to participate in the experiment. To that end, all students enrolled in the 2016 school year of the four selected schools, along with their parents/guardians, were contacted and informed of the nature and aims of the study. The criteria adopted to exclude some adolescents interested in participating in the study were: (a) any health problem that temporarily or permanently prevented participation in the study; (b) using any type of medication that could induce changes in the study variables; (c) undergoing any type of specific diet; and (d) pregnancy. Of the 1200 students contacted, 274 adolescents (186 girls and 88 boys) aged 12–18 years confirmed participation in the project and signed the Free and Informed Consent Form.

The study performed anthropometric measures and components related to the identification of *MetS*, and a questionnaire consisting of items distributed in four sections: demographic aspects, eating habits, physical activity and sedentary behavior, was applied. The questionnaire was applied in a single moment, individually for each adolescent and in the place and time of classes. Data were collected between June and July/2016 and were carried out by a team of four researchers.

Regarding demographic aspects, in addition to sex and age, information related to ethnicity, economic class, schooling of parents/guardians, family structure and eventual work activity were collected. The family economic class was identified according to guidelines proposed by the National Association of Research Companies [15]. Information related to eating habits was obtained using semi-quantitative food frequency questionnaire from the Youth Risk Behavior Survey (YRBS) module, which was translated, adapted and validated for use in the Brazilian young population [16]. In this case, adolescents answered how often they consumed fruits/vegetables and sweetened products/soft drinks, taking as reference the week before data collection. From the intake frequency reported, the following indicators were considered: no intake; intake 1–4 days/week; intake ≥5 days/week.

For the physical activity, the Physical Activity Questionnaire for Adolescents - PAQ-A was used, which was translated and validated for use in young Brazilians [17]. The PAQ-A consists of eight structured questions aimed at sizing different aspects of physical activity in the last seven days. The response options are coded using an increasing scale from 1 to 5 points, and the physical activity score was computed using the mean of scores assigned to each question. For the categorization of physical activity scores, specific cutoff points for sex and age based on the distribution of tertiles was used. Thus, the group of less active adolescents was stratified with PAQ-A scores ≤1st tertile. The group of moderately active adolescents had scores between the 1st and 2nd tertiles, and the group of the most active adolescents had scores ≥2nd tertile.

Sedentary behavior was evaluated by exposure to excessive screen time through structured issues about watching TV and using computer, video game, tablet, and smartphone in a typical week. A predefined time scale was provided for response, in which the adolescent indicated his option among four categories, ranging from "none" to "> 4 hours/day". The questions considered separately screen time equivalent to watching TV and using computer, video game, tablet and smartphone on weekdays and on weekends (Saturday and Sunday). Weighted average involving data of weekdays and weekends was used to identify screen time per day reported by students. Excessive screen time was defined by the combined use of TV and other screen devices for time > 2 h/day [18].

In the anthropometric field, height, body weight and waist circumference measurements were performed according to methodology described by the World Health Organization [19]. Body mass index (BMI) was calculated using the ratio between body mass expressed in kilograms and height expressed in meters squared (kg/m^2). With BMI values, the anthropometric nutritional status of students was classified into four categories based on sex and age cutoff points proposed by the International Obesity Task Force (IOFT): low body weight, eutrophic, overweight and obese [20].

MetS was identified by analyzing the blood content of plasma lipids (triglycerides and HDL-C) and blood glucose, resting blood pressure (systolic and diastolic) and abdominal fat accumulation (waist circumference), according to criteria proposed by the International Diabetes Federation [21]. In this case, *MetS* was defined by the presence of high waist circumference (< 16 years: both sexes ≥ Percentile 90, ≥ 16 years: boys ≥90 cm and girls ≥80 cm) and at least two other compromised components: increased triglycerides (≥ 150 mg/dL), low HDL-C (< 16 years: both sexes < 40 mg/dL, ≥ 16 years: boys < 40 mg/dL and girls < 50 mg/dL), high fasting blood

Table 1 Descriptive information of the sample selected in the study

	n (%)
Demographic Indicators	
Sex	
Girls	186 (67.9)
Boys	88 (32.1)
Age	
12–15 years	159 (58.0)
16–18 years	115 (42.0)
Ethnicity	
Caucasian	199 (72.6)
Non-Caucasian	75 (27.4)
Economic class	
Class D-E (Low)	99 (36.1)
Class C	107 (39.1)
Class B-A (High)	68 (24.8)
Schooling of Parents/Guardians	
≤ 4 years	82 (29.9)
5–8 years	59 (21.5)
9–11 years	55 (20.1)
≥ 12 years	78 (28.5)
Family structure	
Father and mother	182 (66.4)
Separated Parents	64 (23.4)
Relatives	28 (10.2)
Labor Activity	
None	209 (76.3)
Eventual	20 (7.3)
≥ 20 h/week	45 (16.4)
Nutritional status Anthropometric	
Body mass index	
Low weight	18 (6.6)
Normal weight	185 (67.5)
Overweight	42 (15.3)
Obesity	29 (10.6)
Behavioral indicators	
Physical activity	
Less active	136 (49.7)
Moderately Active	76 (27.7)
More active	62 (22.6)
Screen Time	
≤ 2 h/day	66 (24.1)
> 2 h/day	208 (75.9)
Fruits/vegetables intake	
No intake	44 (16.1)
Intake 1–4 days/week	156 (56.9)
Intake ≥5 days/week	74 (27.0)
Sweetened products/soft drinks	
No intake	18 (6.6)
Intake 1–4 days/week	126 (46.0)
Intake ≥5 days/week	130 (47.4)
Metabolic Syndrome Components	
High Waist Circumference	42 (15.3)
Increased Triglyceride	18 (6.6)
Decreased HDL-cholesterol	69 (25.2)
Elevated fasting blood glucose	14 (5.1)
Altered Blood Pressure	24 (8.8)

glucose (≥100 mg/dL) and altered blood pressure (systolic ≥130 mmHg or diastolic ≥85 mmHg).

Data were statistically treated using the Statistical Package for Social Science (SPSS), version 22. The observed proportions (%) in the outcome of Interest (*MetS*) according to demographic, anthropometric, behavioral and nutritional correlates were presented with respective 95% confidence intervals (95% CI). To analyze the linearity of associations between *MetS* and potential correlates, prevalence ratio calculations were used. Statistical differences among strata under investigation were treated by the chi-square test (χ^2). In the sequence, correlates that indicated at least marginally significant associations ($p \leq 0.20$) in the bivariate analysis were selected to be included in hierarchical multiple regression procedures. In this case, correlates were included in blocks, and demographic aspects (level one) were the first to be included the model, followed by the anthropometric nutritional indicator (level two) and, finally, the behavioral components were included (level three). All correlates that presented statistical significance remained in the multivariate model, $p < 0.05$.

Results

Descriptive information characterizing the sample selected for the study is provided in Table 1. Approximately 1/3 of the sample is composed of boys (32.1%) and the highest concentration of adolescents is aged 12–15 years (58%). Most adolescents in the study were Caucasian (72.6%), live with parents (66.4%) and did not work (76.3%). Regarding the economic class and schooling of parents/guardians, the adolescents were proportionally distributed in the strata considered. In addition, 25.9% of adolescents were overweight (overweight + obesity), almost half were classified as minimally physically active (49.7%), and in each group of ten adolescents, seven reported remaining over 2 h in screen devices. Daily fruit/vegetable intake was reported by 27% of adolescents and 93.4% of them assumed

Table 2 Prevalence (95% CI) and prevalence ratio (95% CI) of metabolic syndrome with stratification for demographic, nutritional and behavioral correlates of adolescents from Dourados, Mato Grosso do Sul, Brazil, 2016

		Prevalence (95% CI)	Prevalence Ratio	*p*-value
	Overall	4.7 (3.6–6.0)		
Demographic Indicators				
Sex				0.217
	Girls	4.4 (3.5–5.4)	Reference	
	Boys	5.0 (3.8–6.4)	1.10 (0.95–1.41)	
Age				0.173
	12–15 years	4.2 (3.2–5.3)	Reference	
	16–18 years	5.2 (4.0–6.6)	1.21 (1.03–1.63)	
Ethnicity				0.341
	Caucasian	4.9 (3.8–6.1)	1.04 (0.92–1.29)	
	Non-Caucasian	4.6 (3.5–5.8)	Reference	
Economic class				0.139
	Class D-E (Low)	4.3 (3.3–5.4)	Reference	
	Class C	4.6 (3.6–5.8)	1.05 (0.93–1.39)	
	Class B-A (High)	5.4 (4.2–6.8)	1.23 (1.04–1.68)	
Schooling of Parents/Guardians				0.166
	≤ 4 years	4.2 (3.3–5.1)	Reference	
	5–8 years	4.6 (3.5–5.9)	1.07 (0.94–1.34)	
	9–11 years	4.9 (3.7–6.4)	1.14 (0.98–1.46)	
	≥ 12 years	5.2 (3.9–6.7)	1.21 (1.01–1.67)	
Family structure				0.367
	Father and mother	4.9 (3.8–6.1)	1.04 (0.93–1.30)	
	Separated Parents	4.6 (3.5–5.8)	Reference	
	Relatives	4.7 (3.7–5.8)	1.00 (0.89–1.36)	
Labor Activity				0.274
	None	4.9 (3.8–6.1)	1.03 (0.94–1.30)	
	Eventual	4.6 (3.4–5.9)	Reference	
	≥ 20 h/week	5.1 (3.9–6.5)	1.08 (0.95–1.35)	
Nutritional Anthropometric status				
Body mass index				< 0.001
	Low weight	4.0 (3.4–4.7)	Reference	
	Normal weight	4.4 (3.5–5.5)	1.08 (0.96–1.33)	
	Overweight	4.9 (3.8–6.1)	1.21 (1.02–1.69)	
	Obesity	5.6 (4.4–6.8)	1.38 (1.15–1.90)	
Behavioral indicators				
Physical activity				0.181
	Less active	5.1 (4.0–6.3)	1.19 (1.01–1.67)	
	Moderately Active	4.8 (3.8–5.9)	1.12 (0.96–1.45)	
	More active	4.2 (3.4–5.2)	Reference	
Screen Time				0.119
	≤ 2 h/day	4.2 (3.3–5.3)	Reference	
	> 2 h/day	5.3 (4.1–6.7)	1.24 (1.02–1.69)	

Table 2 Prevalence (95% CI) and prevalence ratio (95% CI) of metabolic syndrome with stratification for demographic, nutritional and behavioral correlates of adolescents from Dourados, Mato Grosso do Sul, Brazil, 2016 *(Continued)*

		Prevalence (95% CI)	Prevalence Ratio	*p*-value
Fruits/vegetables intake				0.002
	No consumption	5.4 (4.2–6.8)	1.35 (1.13–1.91)	
	Intake 1–4 days/week	4.9 (4.8–6.1)	1.22 (1.03–1.73)	
	Intake ≥5 days/week	3.9 (3.2–4.8)	Reference	
Sweetened products/soft drinks intake				0.159
	No intake	4.3 (3.3–5.4)	Reference	
	Intake 1–4 days/week	4.6 (3.5–5.9)	1.04 (0.94–1.34)	
	Intake ≥5 days/week	5.2 (4.0–6.5)	1.20 (1.01–1.69)	

to consume sweetened products/soft drinks at least once a week. Regarding the individual components of *MetS*, decreased HDL-cholesterol was predominant (25.2%), while increased triglyceride (6.6%) and high fasting blood glucose (5.1%) were the least prevalent.

The presence of *MetS* with stratification for demographic, nutritional status and behavioral correlates are presented in Table 2. Overall prevalence was equivalent to 4.7% [95% CI (3.6–6.0)]. Results from bivariate analyses showed that, from the list of potential correlates considered, sex, ethnicity, family structure and labor activity were not statistically indicated ($p < 0.20$).

Results of the hierarchical multiple regression are available in Table 3. In the case of demographic correlates, the final model pointed to significant associations between *MetS*, age and economic class. Likewise, the anthropometric correlate related to nutritional status (BMI) remained significantly associated with *MetS*. Among behavioral components, of the four correlates considered, two of them (screen time and fruits/vegetables intake) remained associated with the outcome.

Discussion

The aim of the study was to provide up-to-date information on demographic, anthropometric and behavioral nutritional correlates of *MetS* in a sample of adolescents from Dourados, Mato Grosso do Sul, Brazil. The main findings were that, using the same diagnostic criteria (IDF), the proportion of adolescents with *MetS* was higher than that found in the young Brazilian population [4.5% vs. 2.6%] [12]. When compared with international data, the proportion observed in the present study is lower than that reported in North American and European adolescents; however, higher than that found in adolescents from Asian countries [9–11]. Also, in addition to being older and belonging to higher economic class, adolescents identified with *MetS* were those who reported excessive screen time, lower fruits/vegetables intake and greater body weight accumulation.

In general, correlates of *MetS* identified in the present study are consistent with current literature [6–8]. However, it is noteworthy that, unlike the findings of some studies [9, 10]; but consistent with others [11, 12], sex had no significant association with the presence of *MetS*. In this case, possibly the differences observed among studies can be attributed to the several criteria used to identify *MetS* in children and adolescents, since to date, there is no consensus regarding the use of a single criterion [5]. Another hypothesis to be considered may be related to the known differences between sexes related to the prevalence of abdominal obesity, hypertension and dyslipidemia found in different young populations [9]. in more advanced ages.

Corroborating previous findings [6–12], age was a significant correlate for the presence of *MetS* among adolescents in this study. In this regard, the expected increase in blood pressure, triglyceride and fasting blood glucose levels, and visceral fat deposits in more advanced ages [22] may explain the higher proportion of *MetS* among older adolescents. Regarding the economic class, the presence of *MetS* was positively associated with the higher strata. Other studies have identified significant associations in the same direction [6, 8]; however, we also find information in literature pointing to an inverse relationship between economic class and presence of MetS [12]. Perhaps the different indicators used to classify the economic class and the interactions between family income and attributes of the socio-cultural context in which it is inserted can contribute to understand these differences.

Regarding sedentary behavior, in a certain way, the results found here coincides with results found in other studies and suggest that the possibility of the presence of *MetS* is progressively higher according to the increase in screen time reported by adolescents [8, 23, 24]. However, a fact that should be considered refers to the cutoff point used to define excessive screen time, typically recommended by current international guidelines and used in the present study (> 2 h/day). In this sense, in a study involving meta-analysis resources, primary and sensitivity

Table 3 Hierarchical multiple logistic regression for demographic (level 1), nutritional (level 2) and behavioral (level 3) correlates of metabolic syndrome of adolescents from Dourados, Mato Grosso do Sul, Brazil, 2016

Correlates	OR $_{Crude}$ (95% CI)[a]	OR $_{Adjusted}$ (95% CI)[b]
Level 1 – Demographic Indicators		
Age		
12–15 years	Reference	Reference
16–18 years	1.26 (1.03–1.88)	1.22 (1.04–1.73)
Economic class		
Class D-E (Low)	Reference	Reference
Class C	1.17 (0.98–1.73)	1.15 (0.97–1.61)
Class B-A (High)	1.29 (1.03–2.13)	1.25 (1.07–1.96)
Schooling of Parents/Guardians		
≤ 4 years	Reference	Reference
5–8 years	1.14 (0.95–1.77)	1.11 (0.93–1.71)
9–11 years	1.18 (0.97–1.95)	1.14 (0.96–1.82)
≥ 12 years	1.24 (1.01–2.06)	1.19 (0.98–1.89)
Level 2 – Nutritional Anthropometric status		
Body mass index		
Low weight	Reference	Reference
Normal weight	1.16 (0.97–1.77)	1.10 (0.95–1.69)
Overweight	1.25 (1.02–2.17)	1.18 (0.98–1.99)
Obesity	1.67 (1.29–2.78)	1.52 (1.24–2.41)
Level 3 – Behavioral indicators		
Physical activity		
Less active	1.23 (1.02–2.04)	1.18 (0.98–1.87)
Moderately Active	1.19 (0.99–1.83)	1.13 (0.96–1.69)
More active	Reference	Reference
Screen Time		
≤ 2 h/day	Reference	Reference
> 2 h/day	1.29 (1.05–2.11)	1.26 (1.05–1.94)
Fruits/vegetables intake		
No intake	1.59 (1.24–2.65)	1.49 (1.23–2.41)
Intake 1–4 days/week	1.29 (1.08–2.27)	1.24 (1.06–2.03)
Intake ≥5 days/week	Reference	Reference
Sweetened products/soft drinks intake		
No intake	Reference	Reference
Intake 1–4 days/week	1.15 (0.94–1.98)	1.09 (0.93–1.76)
Intake ≥5 days/week	1.21 (1.01–2.17)	1.14 (0.97–1.96)

[a]Unadjusted odds ratio
[b]Odds ratio adjusted by the other variables included in the model

analyses performed based on this cutoff point did not reveal significant associations between screen time and *MetS*. In this case, individual studies included in the meta-analysis that indicated significant associations adopted cutoff points close to 4 h/day [25].

Regarding physical activity, no significant associations between scores equivalent to PAQ-A and *MetS* were found. To our knowledge, this was the first study that used PAQ-A to address possible associations between physical activity and *MetS*. However, according to current literature, it was verified that studies involving other types of questionnaires also found no significant differences in the physical activity of adolescents identified and not with *MetS* [26, 27]. On the other hand, studies that identified significant association between low levels of physical activity and greater chance of identifying *MetS* used the accelerometry technique [28] as a measure of physical activity. These findings are confirmed through meta-analysis resources, which demonstrated the reliance on the use of accelerometers to identify significant associations between physical activity practice and *MetS* in young populations [25].

Another finding from the present study was the significant association detected between fruits/vegetables intake and *MetS*. It is important to highlight that this food habit remained significantly associated even through adjustments to potential confounding variables. In this case, the protection attributed to higher fruits/vegetables intake is consistent with evidence presented by other studies involving different experimental designs and statistical treatments [6–8, 26]. Dietary pattern exerts influence on *MetS* through a specific effect on the plasma lipid-lipoprotein profile, blood pressure and body fat. Unlike diets in which fat-rich foods predominate, diets with higher fruits/vegetables intake tend to have lower intake of simple carbohydrates and saturated fat, while higher amounts of complex carbohydrates and fibers are inversely related to altered blood glucose and triglycerides, increased accumulation of abdominal fat and high blood pressure, and positively with more favorable HDL-C, all known components of *MetS* [29].

Based on the findings of the present study, the higher the excess body weight, the higher the proportion of *MetS*, with an abrupt increase in obesity cases. Similar findings are found in literature [6–9, 12], which corroborates the hypothesis that anthropometric nutritional status is strongly associated with *MetS*. In this sense, studies have detected important associations between obesity and *MetS* from early ages. Using a longitudinal design, among a set of biological and behavioral variables, it was found that childhood obesity is the strongest predictor of *MetS* and other risk factors for cardiovascular diseases in early adulthood [30].

The research method used to identify behavioral indicators involved a self-report questionnaire, thus allowing possible memory bias or even tendentious statements towards the desirable, being among the study limitations. However, the reporting of these indicators by adolescents themselves is a current procedure in studies with these characteristics, being the most feasible form of school-based or population-based surveys. In addition, the small sample size may somehow potentiate possible inaccuracy of the calculated estimates. The cross-sectional approach of data does not allow making inferences of causality in the association between the identification of *MetS* and the investigated correlates, because the outcome and the other variables have been identified at the same time.

Conclusions

In conclusion, the results of the study are considered as a preliminary observation among the young Brazilian adults population as a high risk group for *MetS*. In approximately 5% of adolescents selected in this study the presence of *MetS* was identified, with emphasis on older individuals and those of higher economic class. Significant inverse associations between *MetS* and fruits/vegetables intake, coupled with the direct association with higher screen time and greater body weight accumulation, suggest that policies and interventions aimed at health education programs targeting school and family contexts should include actions focusing on the attempt to reduce the incidence of *MetS*.

Abbreviations

BMI: Body mass index; HDLc: High density lipoproteins; IC95%: 95% Confidence intervals; IDF: International diabetes federation; IOFT: International obesity task force; MetS: Metabolic syndrome; PAQ-A: Physical activity questionnaire for adolescents; SPSS: Statistical package for the social science; YRBS: Youth risk behavior survey; χ2: Chi-square test

Acknowledgments

We thank all of the data collection: José Botelho Sena Neto, Nerilda Ribeira Veiga, Adriana Favero de Lima, Mara Lourenço Vermeiro, Mi Ye Marcaida Olimpio, Luis Henrique Almeida Castro and the clinical analysis team: Viviane Regina Noro and Andessa Leite Ferraz de Melo.

Funding

The study was partially funded by the Federal University of Grande Dourados and the University Hospital of Grande Dourados.

Authors' contributions

MCS acquisition of data and been involved in drafting the manuscript, APCCC acquisition of data, revising it critical, MSD acquisition of data, and been involved in drafting the manuscript, LAMY acquisition of data and involved in the laboratory analysis of biological samples, DPG contributions to conception and design, statistical analysis and corrected the manuscript, SAO contributions to conception and design, analysis and interpretation of data, general supervision of the research. All authors read and approved the final manuscript.

Competing interests

The authors declare that they have no competing interests in this section.

Author details

[1]University Hospital of the Federal University of Grande Dourados, Dourados, MS, Brazil. [2]Northern University of Paraná, Londrina, PR, Brazil. [3]Faculty of Health Sciences, Federal University of Grande Dourados, Dourados, MS, Brazil.

References

1. Ng M, Fleming T, Robinson M, Thonsom B, Graetz N. Margono, et al. global, regional, and national prevalence of overweight and obesity in children and adults during 1980-2013: a systematic analysis for the global burden of disease study 2013. Lancet. 2014;384(9945):766–81.
2. Zimmet P, Alberti G, Kaufman F, Tajima N, Silink M, Arslanian S, et al. The metabolic syndrome in children and adolescents. Lancet. 2007;369(9579): 2059–61.
3. Magnussen CG, Koskinen J, Chen W, Thomson R, Schmidt MD, Srinivasan SR, et al. Pediatric metabolic syndrome predicts adulthood metabolic syndrome, subclinical atherosclerosis, and type 2 diabetes mellitus but is no better than body mass index alone: the Bogalusa heart study and the cardiovascular risk in young Finns study. Circulation. 2010;122(16):1604–11.
4. Alberti KG, Eckel RH, Grundy SM, Zimmet PZ, Cleeman JI, Donato KA, et al. Harmonizing the metabolic syndrome: a joint interim statement of the international diabetes federation task force on epidemiology and prevention; National Heart, Lung, and Blood Institute; American Heart Association; world heart federation; international atherosclerosis society; and International Association for the Study of obesity. Circulation. 2009;120(16):1640–5.
5. Agudelo GM, Bedoya G, Estrada A, Patiño FA, Muñoz AM, Velásquez CM. Variations in the prevalence of metabolic syndrome in adolescents according to different criteria used for diagnosis: which definition should be chosen for this age group? Metab Syndr Relat Disord. 2014;12(4):202–9.
6. Ekelund U, Anderssen S, Andersen LB, Riddoch CJ, Sardinha LB, Luan J, et al. Prevalence and correlates of the metabolic syndrome in a population-based sample of European youth. Am J Clin Nutr. 2009;89(1):90–6.
7. You MA, Son YJ. Prevalence of metabolic syndrome and associated risk factors among Korean adolescents: analysis from the Korean national survey. Asia Pac J Public Health. 2012;24(3):464–71.
8. Mehairi AE, Khouri AA, Naqbi MM, Muhairi SJ, Maskari FA, Nagelkerke N, et al. Metabolic syndrome among Emirati adolescents: a school-based study. PLoS One. 2013;8(2):e56159.
9. Friend A, Craig L, Turner S. The prevalence of metabolic syndrome in children: a systematic review of the literature. Metab Syndr Relat Disord. 2013;11(2):71–80.
10. Tailor AM, Peeters PH, Norat T, Vineis P, Romaquera D. An update on the prevalence of the metabolic syndrome in children and adolescents. Int J Pediatr Obes. 2010;5(3):202–13.
11. Poyrazoglu S, Bas F, Darendeliler F. Metabolic syndrome in young people. Curr Opin Endocrinol Diabetes Obes. 2014;21(1):56–63.
12. Kuschnir MC, Bloch KV, Szklo M, Klein CH, Barufaldi LA, Abreu GA, et al. ERICA: prevalence of metabolic syndrome in Brazilian adolescents. Rev Saúde Pública. 2016;50(supl 1):11s.
13. Grundy SM. Metabolic syndrome pandemic. Arterioscler Thromb Vasc Biol. 2008;28(4):629–36.
14. Nunes HEG, Gonçalves ECA, Vieira JAJ, Silva DAS. Clustering of risk factors for non-communicable diseases among adolescents from southern Brazil. PLoS One. 2016;11(7):e0159037.
15. Associação Brasileira de Empresas de Pesquisa – ABEP. Critério de Classificação Econômica Brasil. São Paulo: Associação Brasileira de Empresas de Pesquisa; 2014.
16. Guedes DP, Lopes CC. Validation of the Brazilian version of the 2007 youth risk behavior survey. Rev Saude Publica. 2010;44(5):840–50.
17. Guedes DP. Measuring physical activity in Brazilian youth: reproducibility and validity of the PAQ-C and PAQ-A. Rev Bras Med Esporte. 2015;21(6):425–32.
18. American Academy of Pediatrics; Council on Communications and Media. Children, adolescents, obesity, and the media. Pedriatrics. 2011;128(1):201–8.
19. WHO. World Health Organization. Physical status: the use and interpretation of anthropometry. Report of a WHO expert committee. [technical report series n° 854]. Geneva: WHO; 1995.
20. Cole TJ, Lobstein T. Extended international (IOTF) body mass index cut-offs for thinness, overweight and obesity. Pediatr Obes. 2012;7(4):284–94.

21. Zimmet P, Alberti KG, Kaufman F, Tajima N, Silink M, Arslanian S, et al. The metabolic syndrome in children and adolescents - an IDF consensus report. Pediatr Diabetes. 2007;8(5):299–306.
22. Werneck AO, Silva DR, Collings PJ, Fernandes RA, Ronque ERV, Barbosa DS, et al. Biological maturation, central adiposity, and metabolic risk in adolescents: a mediation analysis. Child Obes. 2016;12(5):377–83.
23. Kang HT, Lee HR, Shim JY, Shin YH, Park BJ, Lee YJ. Association between screen time and metabolic syndrome in children and adolescents in Korea: the 2005 Korean National Health and nutrition examination survey. Diabetes Res Clin Pract. 2010;89(1):72–8.
24. Mark AE, Janssen I. Relationship between screen time and metabolic syndrome in adolescents. J Public Health. 2008;30(2):153–60.
25. Oliveira RG, Guedes DP. Physical activity, sedentary behavior, cardiorespiratory fitness and metabolic syndrome in adolescents: systematic review and meta-analysis of observational evidence. PLoS One. 2016;11(12):e0168503.
26. Pan Y, Pratt CA. Metabolic syndrome and its association with diet and physical activity in US adolescents. J Am Diet Assoc. 2008;108(2):276–86.
27. Budak N, Oztürk A, Mazicioglu M, Yazici C, Bayram F, Kurtoglu S. Decreased high-density lipoprotein cholesterol and insulin resistance were the most common criteria in 12- to 19-year-old adolescents. Eur J Nutr. 2010;49(4): 219–25.
28. Nguyen TH, Tang HK, Kelly P, Van d PHP, Dibley MJ. Association between physical activity and metabolic syndrome: a cross sectional survey in adolescents in ho chi Minh City, Vietnam. BMC Public Health. 2010;10:141.
29. Calton EK, James AP, Pannu PK, Soares MJ. Certain dietary patterns are beneficial for the metabolic syndrome: reviewing the evidence. Nutr Res. 2014;34(7):559–68.
30. Srinivasan SR, Myers L, Berenson GS. Predictability of childhood adiposity and insulin for developing insulin resistance syndrome (syndrome X) in young adulthood: the Bogalusa heart study. Diabetes. 2002;51(1):204–9.

5

Five year trends in the serve size, energy, and sodium contents of New Zealand fast foods: 2012 to 2016

Helen Eyles[1*], Yannan Jiang[1], Tony Blakely[2], Bruce Neal[3], Jennifer Crowley[1], Christine Cleghorn[2] and Cliona Ni Mhurchu[1]

Abstract

Background: The nutritional composition of foods and beverages consumed away from the home has important implications for population health. Our objective was to determine if the serve size, energy, and sodium contents of fast foods sold at chain restaurants in New Zealand (NZ) changed between 2012 and 2016.

Methods: Serve size and nutrient data were collected in annual cross-sectional surveys of all products sold at 10 major fast food chains. Changes over time may occur due to alterations in product availability or individual product reformulation. Linear regression adjusting for food group and chain was used to estimate overall changes in serve size and nutrients. Random effects mixed models were used to estimate reformulation changes on same products available for two or more years.

Results: Across all products ($n = 5468$) increases were observed in mean serve size (+ 9 (3, 15) g, + 5%), energy density (+ 54 (27, 81) kJ/100 g, + 6%), energy per serve (+ 178 (125, 231) kJ, + 14%), and sodium per serve (+ 55 (24, 87) mg, + 12%). Sodium density did not change significantly. Four of 12 food groups (Desserts, Pizza, Sandwiches, and Salads) and four of 10 fast food chains (Domino's, Hell Pizza, Pizza Hut, and Subway) displayed large, undesirable changes for three or more (of five) outcomes (≥10%; $p < 0.05$). One food group (Asian) and one chain (St Pierre's) displayed large, desirable changes for two or more outcomes. The only significant reformulation change was a drop in sodium density (− 22 (− 36, − 8) mg/100 g, − 7%).

Conclusions: The serve size and energy density of NZ fast food products has increased significantly over the past 5 years. Lower sodium concentration in new and reformulated products has been offset by overall increases in serve size. Continued monitoring and development and implementation of Government-led targets for serve size and nutrient content of new and existing fast food products are required.

Keywords: Fast foods, Portion size, Sodium, Energy intake

Background

Consumption of food prepared away from the home is increasing globally, and is an important contributor to population diets in many countries [1]. In the United States (US), food away from home as a share of household food expenditure has risen from ~ 26% in 1970 [2] to >50% in 2014 [3], with children consuming one quarter of their dietary energy from restaurant foods and beverages [4]. A similar trend is emerging in New Zealand (NZ) with food away from home contributing 25% in 2016 [5]. No recent data are available on the contribution food away from home makes to the energy intakes of New Zealanders, but in the most recent adult nutrition survey (2008/09) 14% reported consuming restaurant food and 28% reported consuming fast food over the past 24 h, with the highest rates observed for young adults (19 to 30 yrs.; 15 and 42%, respectively) [6]. Moreover, a recent (2017) market research panel survey reported 80% of NZ adults have consumed fast food in the

* Correspondence: h.eyles@auckland.ac.nz
[1]National Institute for Health Innovation, School of Population Health, The University of Auckland, Private Bag 92019, Auckland Mail Centre, Auckland 1142, New Zealand
Full list of author information is available at the end of the article

past month, and 27% consumed fast food more than five times in that month [7].

Fast food can be defined as food which is generally cheap, requires minimal preparation and where no table service is provided [8]. The contribution that fast food makes to food away from home in NZ is currently unknown. However, fast food is of particular concern for population health because it is an independent predictor of body size [9]. Furthermore, compared with foods prepared at home, fast foods are generally more processed, higher in adverse nutrients such as sodium and saturated fat, and lower in positive nutrients such as fibre [9]. Serving sizes of foods and beverages available at fast food restaurants in the US have also increased steadily over time [10].

There is a clear mandate from the World Health Organization (WHO) to reduce serving sizes and population consumption of sugar and sodium [11–13]. As such, there is pressure for fast food companies to provide healthier options. Several countries have responded by implementing national sodium reduction strategies [14] and taxing foods and beverages high in sugar and sodium [15–17], and recently Public Health England outlined a series of actions to reduce children's energy intakes, including portion size reduction [18]. However, the focus to date has been on packaged foods, and although existing nutrient profiling models exist which could be modified fast foods [19], there are currently no agreed serve size or nutrient guidelines for fast food companies to work towards. Moreover, the availability and composition of products available at popular global fast food chains varies markedly by country [20].

In NZ, there is currently no Government-led national sodium strategy or any food or beverage taxes aimed at improving health. However, there is a Government-led (voluntary) front-of-pack labelling system for packaged foods [21], and a national childhood obesity plan [22]; the obesity plan includes 'The Healthy Kids Industry Pledge' [23] where food companies have been encouraged (since 2015) to make voluntary pledges to improve their products and help reduce obesity rates for children. However, there are no product guidelines for industry; McDonalds is the only fast food chain to have made a pledge to date, and there are no specific, measureable goals to improve the serve size or nutrient content of their products. This is despite evidence that there is plenty of opportunity to improve the healthiness of NZ fast foods; a 2013 survey found burger combo meals sold at NZ fast food chains contribute up to 68% of the adult recommended dietary intake for sodium, and more than 94% of the WHO maximum recommended ideal free sugars intake [24].

The first objective of this project was to determine if the overall serving size, energy and sodium contents of fast foods sold by major NZ chain restaurants changed between 2012 and 2016, and whether any observed changes differed by food group or chain. This objective was assessed for all fast food products available for sale, where changes over time could arise due to new products having a different nutrient profile to discontinued products, and/or reformulation of products available for sale over time. The second objective more specifically examined reformulation within products available for sale in two or more years.

Methods

Data source

Annual cross-sectional surveys were undertaken between 2012 and 2016 of all food and beverage products available for sale at major fast food chains in NZ (≥20 stores nationwide). Fast food chains were defined as per Fleischhacker et al. [8] and described in the Background. The following data were collected by trained fieldworkers between February and March each year: product name, serving size, and nutrient information. It is not mandatory for any of this information to be available or displayed under the Australian and NZ Food Standards Code [25], and thus serving size and nutrient data were missing for some products. Data were recorded directly from company websites. Visits to one large store representing each fast food chain were also completed to capture any information not available on-line. Stores selected for visits were in Auckland, New Zealand's largest city, and chosen based on size and location to provide the largest product range possible.

Data management

Food and beverage data were entered into an Excel spreadsheet and classified using a three-tiered food classification system based on that developed by The Global Food Monitoring Group [26]. Identical products available for sale across years were matched manually using product name. Once matched, a unique code was allocated to each product to enable it to be tracked over time for reformulation analyses.

Outcomes

There were five main outcomes of interest: serve size (g), energy density (per 100 g), sodium density (per 100 g), energy content per serve (kJ), and sodium content per serve (mg). Serve size was defined as the amount intended to be consumed in one sitting. For the majority of products the serve size was the same as the product unit or package size. However, for pizza and chicken products intended to be shared by a group, the serve size was as recommended by the manufacturer ($n = 1539$ and 115 total products, respectively).

Preparation of the dataset for analysis

Additional file 1: Appendix 1 shows the preparation of the dataset for analysis. The initial dataset included 14,840 products. Three phases of data cleaning were completed: In phase 1 products with no recorded information on any outcome of interest were removed ($n = 7281$). In phase 2, duplicate products with different serving sizes were removed. For example, sides such as barbeque ribs were available in two sizes and thus only the largest serving size was retained ($n = 137$). Finally, in phase 3 all food groups and fast food chains with <100 products available for sale across all 5 years, and/or with data missing for one or more years were removed ($n = 2091$ products).

Statistical analysis

The total number of product records included in each year were first summarised overall and by fast food group and chain separately. Descriptive information on serving size, energy, and sodium contents were presented for each year including the number of products with available information, mean, standard deviation, median and range. The sample was considered sufficiently large for the central limit theorem to apply, where the mean of the sample was considered approximately equal to the mean of the population [27].

For Objective 1, linear regression models were used to estimate the change in serve size, energy, and sodium contents with adjustment for fast food chain and food group to account for variation in the types of products sold during the study period. Overall analyses therefore estimated the change in nutrients over time, averaged across all food groups and fast food chains. Year was included as a continuous variable in the model (coded as 2012 = 0, 2013 = 0.25, 2014 = 0.5, 2015 = 0.75, and 2016 = 1) such that the coefficient gave an estimated change over 5 years. The interaction between year and fast food chain was tested in the main model to see if the observed change on nutrients was different between fast food chains. The same interaction was tested between year and food group. Where significant interaction was present, subgroup analyses were carried out for individual food groups and chains separately. However, results for sub-groups must be interpreted with caution due to multiple comparisons and diminishing statistical power. Average percentage change over the 5 years was calculated by dividing the adjusted mean change by an estimated mean for 2012 i.e. the overall mean minus half of the adjusted mean change. For completeness, all regression models were also run with year as a categorical variable to estimate the change between individual years e.g. 2012 to 2013, 2013 to 2014 etc.; these analyses are not included in the main results but are available in Additional file 1: Appendices 4 and 5.

For Objective 2 on reformulation analyses, random effects mixed models were used to estimate the 5-year change on serve size, energy and sodium contents for

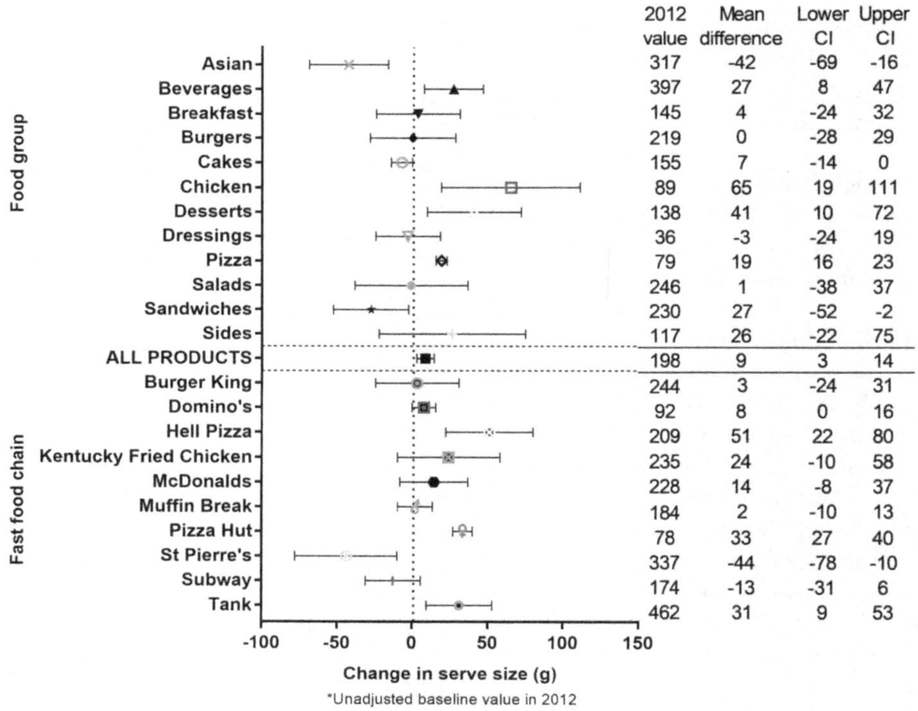

Fig. 1 Five year changes in the serve size of fast food products from major NZ chains (2012 to 2016). * Unadjusted baseline value in 2012

same products that are available for sale in two or more years. A random product effect was included in the regression model to account for within product change. Same covariates were considered in the fixed effects model as for Objective 1. Due to the limited number of products available for sale in two or more years, analyses by food group were only completed for outcomes where a significant change was observed over time.

All statistical analyses were performed using SAS version 9.4 (SAS Institute Inc., Cary, NC, USA). All statistical tests were two-sided at 5% significance level, with no adjustment for multiple testing.

Results

Characteristics of the data set

The total number of product records included for Objective 1 analysis was $N = 5468$ across 12 food groups and 10 major fast food chains (Additional file 1: Appendix 2). Overall product availability was relatively consistent across years (1359 in 2012, 1803 in 2013, 1211 in 2014, 1460 in 2015 and 1589 in 2016) but varied by food group and chain, ranging from $n = 130$ for Desserts to 1626 for Pizza, and from $n = 173$ for St Pierre's (Sushi) to 1098 for McDonalds. The total number of unique products available for sale in two or more years and included in Objective 2 analysis was $N = 1025$ (Additional file 1: Appendix 3), including 632 products available in 2 years, 194 in 3 years, 107 in 4 years, and 92 available across all 5 years (a total of 2734 product records).

Objective 1: change over 5 years for all products, and by food group and fast food chain

Serve size

The unadjusted mean (SD) serve size across all products in all years was 186.2 (135.8) g (Additional file 1: Appendix 2). The model-adjusted mean difference (95% CI) estimated over the 5 year period was + 8.8 (3.1 to 14.8) g, or equivalently an increase of 4.8% (Fig. 1). Significant interaction was found between year and food group, and between year and fast food chain ($p < 0.0001$). Large (≥10%), significant increases in serve size were observed for 3/11 food groups (Chicken (+ 70%), Desserts (+ 36%), and Pizza (+ 25%)), and 3/10 fast food chains (Domino's (+ 10%), Hell Pizza (+ 34%) and Pizza Hut (+ 44%)). Large, significant decreases in serve size were observed for two food groups (Asian (Chinese food and Sushi; – 13%) and Sandwiches (– 11%)) and one fast food chain (St Pierre's; – 14%) (Fig. 1).

Energy density

The mean (SD) energy density of all products over the 5 year period was 893.5 (484.6) kJ/100 g. There was a significant increase of + 54 (27 to 81) kJ/100 g

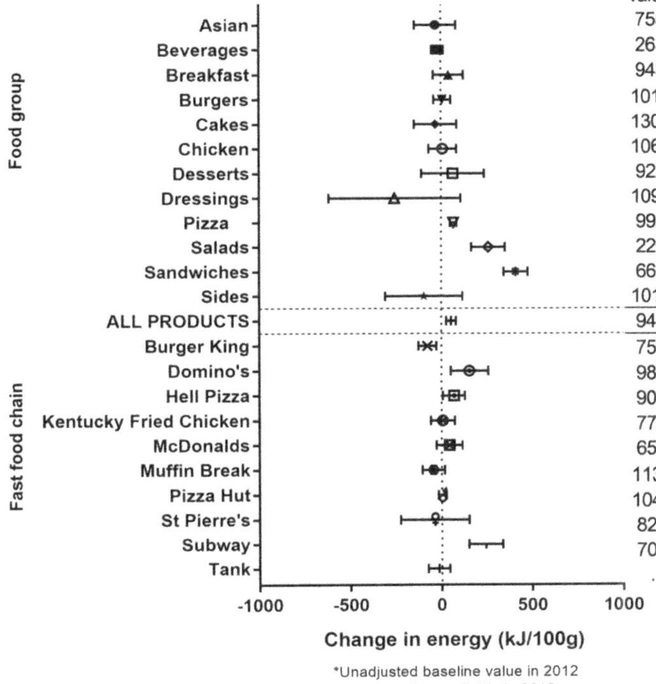

	2012 value	Mean difference	Lower CI	Upper CI
Asian	755	-30	-144	83
Beverages	263	-18	-50	14
Breakfast	943	42	-42	125
Burgers	1014	7	-40	54
Cakes	1300	-30	-147	86
Chicken	1060	9	-67	85
Desserts	922	65	-107	237
Dressings	1093	-255	-618	108
Pizza	992	67	49	85
Salads	220	259	168	350
Sandwiches	662	411	344	477
Sides	1010	-95	-306	117
ALL PRODUCTS	946	54	27	81
Burger King	752	-76	-125	-27
Domino's	980	155	52	258
Hell Pizza	907	69	7	130
Kentucky Fried Chicken	778	7	-58	73
McDonalds	651	44	-27	115
Muffin Break	1139	-44	-105	17
Pizza Hut	1042	5	-17	27
St Pierre's	823	-36	-224	152
Subway	701	244	152	337
Tank	.	-15	-74	44

Fig. 2 Five year changes in the energy density of fast food products from major NZ chains (2012 to 2016). * Unadjusted baseline value in 2012. - No value available in 2012

predicted by the linear regression over the 5 years, or + 6% (Fig. 2). Significant interaction was found between year and food group, and between year and fast food chain ($p < 0.0001$). One food group (Sandwiches) showed a large, significant increase in energy density (+ 78%), but no food groups showed large (i.e. 10% or more) significant decreases. Across fast food chains one showed a large, significant increase in energy density (Domino's Pizza; + 15%), and none showed large, significant decreases (Fig. 2).

Sodium density

The mean (SD) sodium density across all products over the 5 years was 352.6 (316.6) mg/100 g. Overall, there was no significant change observed over the 5 year period (– 3.2 (– 20.4 to 14.1) mg/100 g; Fig. 3). However, significant interaction was found between year and food group, between year and fast food chain ($p < 0.0001$). Large, significant increases in sodium density were observed for Salads and Sandwiches (+ 102% and + 39%, respectively), and for Subway (27%). Large, significant decreases in sodium density were also observed for three fast food chains (Burger King (– 23%), Hell Pizza (– 12%) and Pizza Hut (– 13%), but no food groups.

Energy per serve

The mean (SD) energy per serve across all products over the 5 years was 1346 (803) kJ, and there was a significant increase over the 5 years of 178 (125 to 231) kJ or + 13% (Fig. 4). Significant interaction was found between year and food group, and between year and fast food chain ($p < 0.0001$). Large, significant increases in energy per serve were observed for four food groups (Desserts, Pizza, Salads, and Sandwiches; + 65, 34, 240, and 61%, respectively) and five fast food chains (Domino's Pizza, Hell Pizza, Kentucky Fried Chicken, Pizza Hut, and Subway; + 16, 80, 23, 43, and 101%, respectively), and large, significant decreases were observed for one food group (Asian; – 16%), and one fast food chain (St Pierres; – 16%) (Fig. 4).

Sodium per serve

The mean (SD) sodium content per serve across all products over the 5 years was 454.0 (458.8) mg, and there was a significant increase over time of + 55.3 (23.9 to 86.7) mg, or + 11% (Fig. 5). Significant interaction was found between year and food group, and between year and fast food chain ($p < 0.0001$). Large, significant increases in sodium per serve were seen for 4/11 food groups (Desserts (+ 92%), Pizza (+ 16%), Salads (+ 176%), and Sandwiches (+ 32%)) and 4/10 fast food chains (Hell Pizza (+ 38%), Kentucky Fried Chicken (+ 24%), Pizza

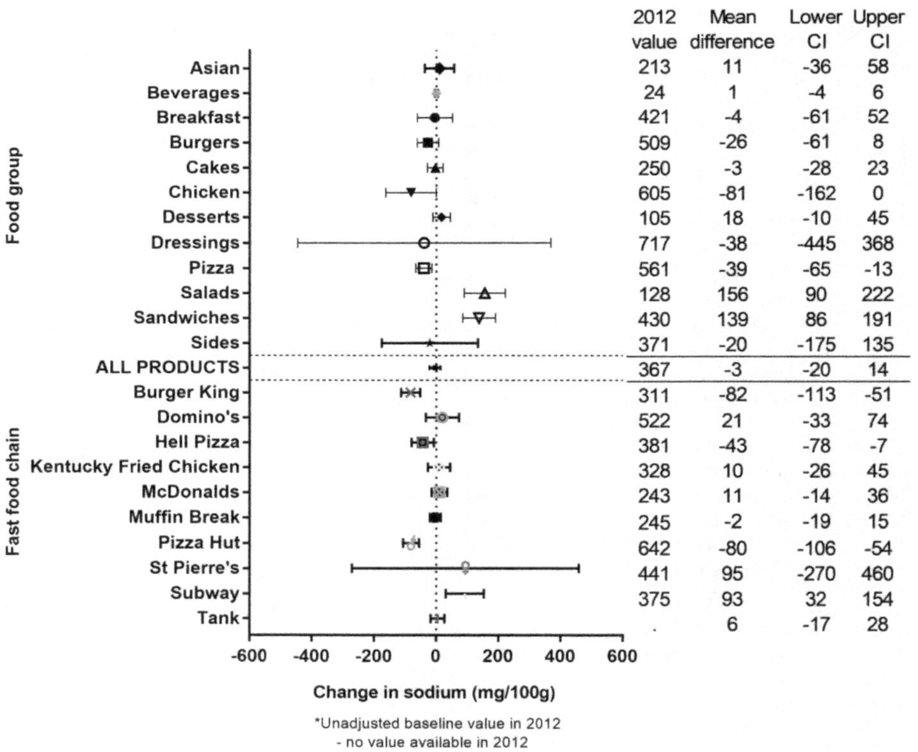

Fig. 3 Five year changes in the sodium density of fast food products from major NZ chains (2012 to 2016). * Unadjusted baseline value in 2012. - No value available in 2012

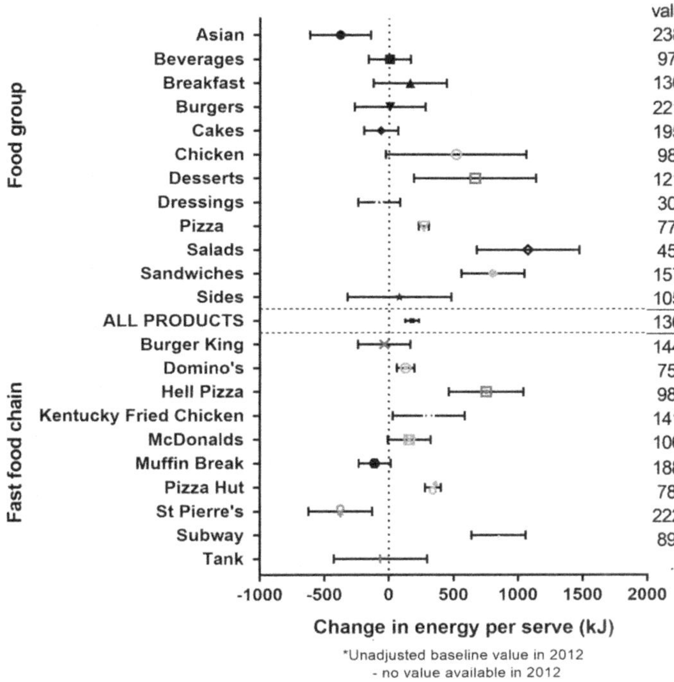

	2012 value	Mean difference	Lower CI	Upper CI
Asian	2381	-377	-614	-141
Beverages	970	5	-158	167
Breakfast	1309	162	-121	444
Burgers	2216	7	-267	280
Cakes	1956	-62	-194	69
Chicken	984	517	-26	1061
Desserts	1218	663	192	1135
Dressings	308	-77	-239	85
Pizza	774	268	228	307
Salads	459	1074	677	1471
Sandwiches	1574	802	558	1047
Sides	1059	79	-323	480
ALL PRODUCTS	1367	178	125	231
Burger King	1446	-37	-240	166
Domino's	755	128	61	196
Hell Pizza	982	751	462	1041
Kentucky Fried Chicken	1412	308	29	586
McDonalds	1068	157	-9	322
Muffin Break	1889	-110	-234	14
Pizza Hut	782	340	279	400
St Pierre's	2224	-376	-624	-129
Subway	893	848	638	1058
Tank	.	-67	-429	296

Fig. 4 Five year changes in energy per serve of fast food products from major NZ chains (2012 to 2016). * Unadjusted baseline value in 2012. - No value available in 2012

Hut (+ 28%), and Subway (+ 77%)). However, there were no large, significant decreases in sodium per serve for any food group or chain (Fig. 5).

Overall findings by food group and fast food chain

Table 1 summarises the overall findings by food group and fast food chain; this table should be interpreted with caution given energy per serve is a function of serve size and energy density, and sodium per serve is a function of serve size and sodium density. Four of 12 food groups displayed large, undesirable changes for the majority of outcomes assessed (≥10%, $p < 0.05$, three or more of five outcomes) i.e. Desserts and Pizza (serve size, energy per serve, and sodium per serve); Sandwiches (energy density, sodium density, energy per serve and sodium per serve); and Salads (sodium density, energy per serve, and sodium per serve). Similarly, four fast food chains displayed large, undesirable changes for the majority of outcomes i.e. Domino's (serve size, energy density, and energy per serve); Hell Pizza and Pizza Hut (serve size, energy per serve and sodium per serve); and Subway (sodium density, energy per serve, and sodium per serve). Only one food group and one fast food chain displayed large, desirable changes for two or more outcomes i.e. Asian and Subway, where both displayed large significant decreases in serve size and energy per serve.

Objective 2: reformulation of products for sale in two or more years

Reformulation analysis on products available for sale in two or more years suggested a moderate and significant reduction over time for sodium density of − 21.8 mg (− 35.7 to − 7.9), or equivalently a 7% reduction. Across the food groups, the largest absolute reduction was seen for Burgers (− 59.7 (− 74.2 to − 45.1) mg/100 g), and across fast food chains the largest absolute reductions were seen for Burger King and Hell Pizza (− 57.5 (− 70.3 to − 44.8) and − 46.2 (− 72.1 to − 20.31) mg/100 g, respectively) (Fig. 6). No reformulation changes were observed for the remaining four outcomes (Additional file 1: Appendix 5).

Discussion

Overall, we found moderate to large increases in the serve size, energy content (per 100 g and per serve), and sodium content (per serve) of foods and beverages sold at major NZ fast food chains from 2012 to 2016. Of the 12 food groups included, four displayed large (≥10% increase; $p < 0.05$), nutritionally undesirable changes for the majority of (at least three of five) outcomes we assessed i.e. Desserts, Pizza, Sandwiches, and Salads. Similarly, products sold at four of the 10 fast food chains displayed undesirable changes for the majority of outcomes i.e. Domino's, Hell Pizza, Pizza Hut, and Subway. There were two exceptions, with one food group and

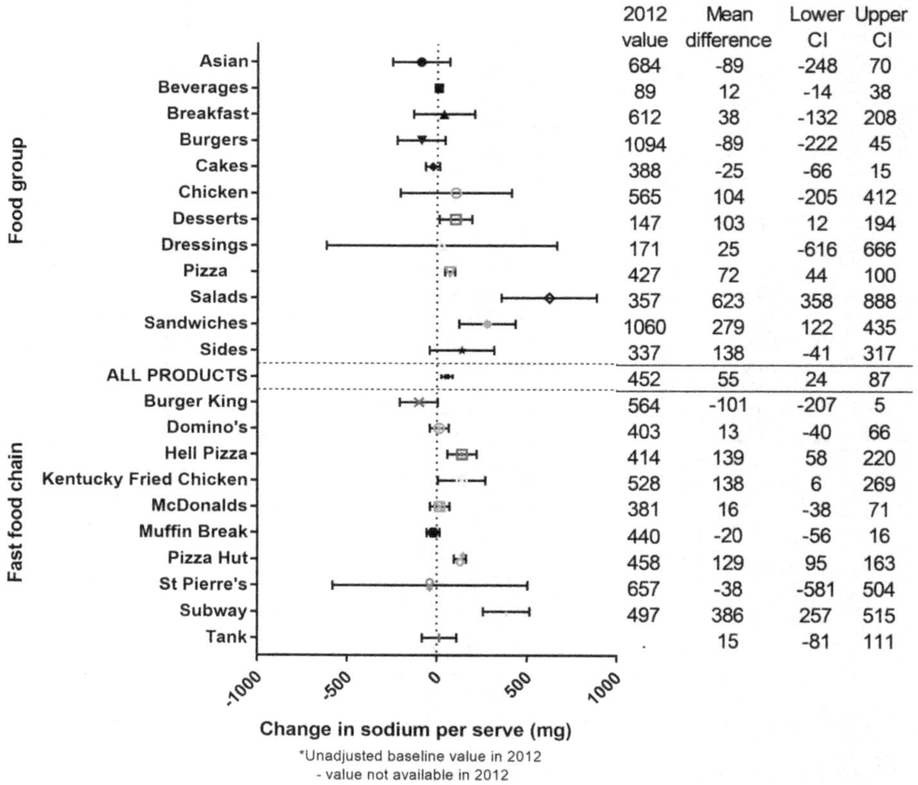

Fig. 5 Five year changes in the sodium per serve of fast food products from major NZ chains (2012 to 2016). * Unadjusted baseline value in 2012. - No value available in 2012

one fast food chain making large desirable changes for two or more outcomes i.e. Asian and St Pierre's (reduced serve size and energy per serve in both cases; Table 1). We found minimal evidence of reformulation of individual products, with no changes in the serve size, energy density, energy per serve, or sodium per serve of products sold in two or more years. The one exception was sodium density where a significant overall reduction of − 7% was observed, largely driven by the Burgers food group, and Burger King and Hell Pizza fast food chains.

A particular strength of this analyses was the comprehensive dataset ($n = 5468$), which means our findings should be broadly generalizable to all fast foods in NZ. However, the limitations include that smaller numbers of products were available for reformulation analyses ($n = 1025$), and matches of same products over time may have been incomplete due to the manual process used and lack of a common identifier. Nonetheless, our findings are robust given we only completed reformulation analyses for sub-groups with >100 products. We also took a cautious approach to reporting sub-group findings by focussing on those food groups with large effect sizes (>10%) and statistical significance ($p < 0.05$). Should the representativeness of products have varied over time e.g. with unhealthy products having a greater probability of being included in later years, then this would generate a selection bias and false trends in our outcome data. However, this is unlikely given we only included food groups and chains with data available each year, and companies are more likely to provide serve size and nutrition information for their full range of products rather than a changing selection. Further, information about fast food purchases are not publicly available in NZ, and thus our data were not sales weighted. However, if there were any bias created we do not think it varied over time, so would not distort trends. Finally, retention of only the largest serve size for duplicate products may have slightly inflated the mean increase in serve size observed over the 5 years. However, this was the case for only 137 products, and retaining the largest serve size in each year means our results reflect the actual, relative increase in all serve sizes available from the included companies.

Trends in the overall nutritional quality of fast foods have also been assessed in Australia and the US. In Australia, the energy density of all fast foods sold at five major chains in New South Wales was assessed over a 7 year period (2009 to 2015) [28]. In contrast to the significant increase we observed across all products over a similar time frame, no change was found in the overall

Table 1 Summary of 5-year changes in the serve size, energy, and sodium content of fast food products sold at major New Zealand chains (2012 to 2016)**

	Serve size	Energy density	Sodium density	Energy per serve	Sodium per serve
All products	*	*		*	*
Food group					
Asian	*	*		*	
Beverages	*	*			
Breakfast					
Burgers					
Cakes					
Chicken	*	*			
Desserts	*	*		*	*
Dressings					
Pizza	*	*	*	*	*
Salads			*	*	*
Sandwiches	*	*	*	*	*
Sides					
Fast food chain					
Burger King			*		
Domino's	*	*		*	
Hell Pizza	*	*	*	*	*
Kentucky Fried Chicken				*	*
McDonalds					
Muffin Break					
Pizza Hut	*	*	*	*	*
St Pierre's	*	*		*	
Subway			*	*	*
Tank	*	*			

**Dark green indicates ≥10% decrease, light green 9 to 5% decrease, no colour 4% decrease to 4% increase, light red 5 to 9% increase, and dark red ≥10% increase. * Indicates statistically significant change ($p < 0.05$). Interactions of year with food group and fast food chain with year all had p values of <0.001. Table should be interpreted with caution given energy per serve is a function of serve size and energy density, and sodium per serve is a function of serve size and sodium density

energy content of Australian products, either per 100 g or per serve. However, items on sale for a limited time did increase by 74 kJ per 100 g, which is similar to our finding that the increase in energy density was likely due to new products. In the US Urban and colleagues [29] undertook reformulation analyses and found the energy content per serve of 56% of french fries, cheeseburgers, grilled chicken sandwiches and regular cola ($n = 27$) on sale at three fast food chains increased between 1996 and 2013. Sodium per serve of matched products also increased in 33% of items, despite some reduction in sodium per serve for a small proportion (18%) of products. Our time period was shorter than this previous study (5 years compared with 17), and our data did not include information for all 5 years for all products. However, for 187 products where we had similar, matched outcome data available for 2012 and 2016, we found energy content per serve had increased for 24% of products (and remained unchanged for 46%), and sodium per serve had increased for 24% of products (unchanged for 47%). In another US study, Rudelt et al. [30] examined changes in the sodium density (per 100 g) within 695 lunch and dinner items sold at eight major fast food chains over 14 years (1997/98 to 2009/10), reporting an overall increase of 23% (+ 146 mg/100 g), but with reductions in the sodium content of some side dishes for some chains. We also found a decrease within NZ fast food products due to reformulation of sodium per 100 g; although our drop was smaller (– 7%), we assessed the trend over a shorter (5 years) and more recent (2012 to 2016) time frame.

The overall increases in energy and sodium we observed per serve were attributable to the overall increase in serve size, rather than large increases in energy and sodium concentration per se. For sodium, there were significant reductions per 100 g for Pizza and at Burger King, Hell Pizza, and Pizza Hut, and evidence of reformulation in products available for sale in two or more years. However, these reductions per 100 g did not translate to a drop in sodium per serve, due to the increase in serve size; this is an important finding given larger serve sizes for products such as Beverages and

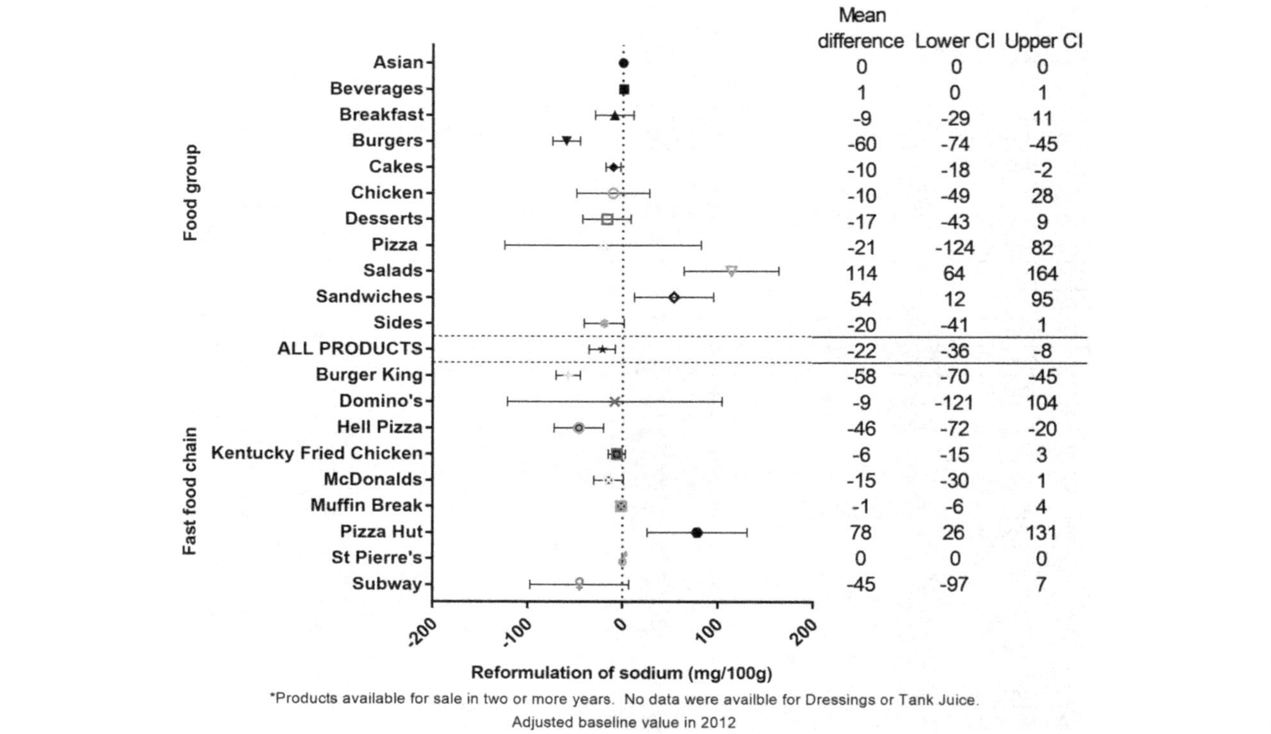

Fig. 6 Five year reformulation changes in sodium content of fast food products from major NZ chains (2012 to 2016)*. * Products available for sale in two or more years. No data were available for Dressings or Tank Juice. Adjusted baseline value in 2012

Desserts would result in an increase in total sugar per serve, and for chains such as Domino's, Hell Pizza, and Pizza Hut, higher saturated fat per serve.

The increases observed in the overall energy and sodium contents of Salads and Sandwiches and Wraps, and across products at Subway and Tank Juice is particularly concerning, as consumers are likely to view these foods and fast food chains as healthier options. Substantial increases in the numbers of products available in these food groups (salads increased from 20 in 2012 to 67 in 2016), and changes in the types of options available (there was a 600% increase in salads including heavy root vegetables and legumes and grains) may account for some of the increase in energy observed, despite no significant change in serve size.

An important consideration of our analyses is that it excluded fish and chips, which are an iconic part of the NZ fast food culture; in 2017 42% of NZ adults consumed fish and chips in the past month [7]. However, fish and chip outlets are independently owned and operated, and while there are important opportunities to improve the type of fat [31] and amount of added salt, the operating structure of fast food restaurants within chains provides substantial and widespread opportunities for reformulation. Further, the consumption of products from fast food companies in NZ is likely to be much larger overall than that of fish and chips, with McDonalds and Kentucky Fried Chicken alone being consumed by 38 and 23% of NZ adults respectively, in the last month [7]. Growth over the past 2 years was also higher for many fast food chains (39% for Domino's Pizza, 30% for Sushi, and 20% for Indian) compared with fish and chips (11%).

Another important consideration is the impact our findings might have on children and young people, the highest consumers of fast foods [32]. Products on sale at McDonalds, the one fast food chain which made a 'Healthy Kids Industry Pledge' [23] displayed no overall changes in serve size or nutrient content. A separate analysis of products included in children's Happy Meals was similar with no overall changes in product profiles or evidence of reformulation [33].

Conclusions

In conclusion, NZ fast foods have become larger and more energy dense over the past 5 years. Lower sodium concentration in new and reformulated products has been offset by overall increases in serve size. Systematic monitoring and implementation of Government-led targets for serve size, energy and nutrient content of fast food products could improve the composition of NZ fast foods and population diets; if improvements are not observed then regulation should be considered. Products marketed to and favoured by children and young people should also be carefully considered, because they are the most frequent consumers of fast food. Finally, in NZ, fast food chains should be encouraged to make 'Healthy Kids Industry' pledges [23] outlining measurable improvements to the serve size, energy, and nutrient content of their products.

Additional file

Additional file 1: Appendix 1. Preparation of fast food data for analysis. **Appendix 2.** Total products and unadjusted mean (SD) values included in main analyses by year, food group, fast food chain, and outcome*. **Appendix 3.** Summary of products included in reformulation analyses sold in two or more years by year, food group, fast food chain, and outcome. **Appendix 4.** Model adjusted means, 95% CI's and *p*-values for all products in main analyses by year, food group, and outcome*. **Appendix 5.** Model adjusted means, 95% CI's and *p*-values for reformulation analyses including products available for sale in two or more years by year, fast food chain, and outcome*.

Acknowledgements
We would like to thank John Fa'atui for data management, Rita George and Rachel Sullivan for data cleaning, Yeun-Hyang (Catherine) Choi for her contribution to early iterations as a data analyst, and the following fieldworkers for data collection: Ashmita Chand, Emma Shields, and Chantel Vinet.

Funding
This work was supported by a Health Research Council of New Zealand programme grant (13/724).

Authors' contributions
HE conceived the study, supervised collection of data, completed data cleaning, contributed to the study design and interpretation of the data, created all graphs and tables, and drafted the manuscript. YJ contributed to study design, completed statistical analyses, and contributed to interpretation of the data. TB contributed to study design, statistical analyses, and interpretation of data. BN contributed to study design and interpretation of data. JC and CC contributed to an early version of the draft paper and interpretation of data. CNM contributed to study design, statistical analysis and interpretation of data, and provided overall advice. All authors provided comments on the draft manuscript and approved the final version.

Competing interests
The authors declare that they have no competing interests.

Author details
[1]National Institute for Health Innovation, School of Population Health, The University of Auckland, Private Bag 92019, Auckland Mail Centre, Auckland 1142, New Zealand. [2]Department of Public Health, University of Otago, Wellington, New Zealand. [3]The George Institute for Global Health, The University of Sydney, Sydney, Australia.

References
1. Lachat C, Nago E, Verstraeten R, Roberfroid D, Van Camp J, Kolsteren P. Eating out of home and its assocation with dietary intake: a systmatic review of the evidence. Obes Rev. 2011; https://doi.org/10.1111/j.1467-1789X.2011.00953.x.
2. Food away from home. Available: https://www.ers.usda.gov/topics/food-choices-health/food-consumption-demand/food-away-from-home.aspx#nutrition. Accessed 25 Sept 2017.
3. US food-away-from-home sales topped food-at-home sales in 2014. Available: https://www.ers.usda.gov/data-products/chart-gallery/gallery/chart-detail/?chartId=58364. Accessed 25 Sept 2017.
4. Food and nutrient intake data: Taking a look at the nutritional quality of foods eaten at home and away from home. Available: https://www.ers.usda.gov/amber-waves/2012/june/data-feature-food-and-nutrient-intake-data/. Accessed 25 Sept 2017.
5. Statistics New Zealand. Household expenditure statistics: Year ended June 2016. 2016. Available: http://www.stats.govt.nz/browse_for_stats/people_and_communities/Households/HouseholdExpenditureStatistics_HOTPYeJun16.aspx. Accessed 25 Sept 2017.
6. Smith C, Gray AR, Fleming EA, Parnel WR. Characteristics of fast-food/takeaway-food and restaurant/cafe-food among New Zealand adults. Public Health Nutr. 2013;17:23668–2377.
7. Fish and chips are still top dog in New Zealand. Available: http://www.nielsen.com/nz/en/insights/news/2017/fish-and-chips-are-still-top-dog-in-new-zealand.html. Accessed 25 Sept 2017.
8. Fleischhacker SE, Evenson KR, Rodriguez DA, Ammerman AS. A systematic review of fast food access studies. Obes Rev. 2011;12:e460–71. https://doi.org/10.1111/j.1467-789X.2010.00715.x.
9. De Vogli R, Kouvonen A, Gimeno D. The influence of market deregulation on fast food consumption and body mass index: a cross-national time series analysis. Bull World Health Organ. 2014;92:99–107A. https://doi.org/10.2471/BLT.13.120287.
10. Young L, Nestle M. Portion sizes and obesity: response of fast-food companies. J Public Health Policy. 2007;28:238–48.
11. World Health Organization. Guideline: Sodium intake for adults and children. 2012. Available: http://www.who.int/nutrition/publications/guidelines/sodium_intake_printversion.pdf. Accessed: 18 Feb 2013.
12. World Health Organization. Sugars intake for adults and children. (World health Organization ed. Geneva: World Health Organization; 2015. Available: http://www.who.int/nutrition/publications/guidelines/sugars_intake/en/. Accessed 10 Aug 2015
13. Limiting portion sizes to reduce the risk of childhood overweight and obesity. Available: http://www.who. nt/elena/titles/portion_childhood_obesity/en/. Accessed 25 May 18.
14. Webster JL, Dunford EK, Hawkes C, Neal BC. Salt reduction initiatives around the world. J Hypertens. 2011;29:1043–50.
15. Colchero MA, Popkin BM, Rivera JA, Ng SW. Beverage purchases from stores in Mexico under the excise tax on sugar sweetened beverages: observational study. Br Med J. 2016; https://doi.org/10.1136/bmj.h6704.
16. Caro JC, Ng SW, Smith Taillie L, Popkin BM. Designing a tax to discourage unhealthy food and beverage purchases the case of Chile. Food Policy. 2017;71:86–100. https://doi.org/10.1016/j.foodpol.2017.08.001.
17. Hagenaars LL, Theo PP, Klazinga NS. The taxation of unhealthy energy-dense foods (EDFs) and sugar-sweetened beverages (SSBs): an overview of patterns observed in the policy content and policy context of 13 case studies. Health Policy. 2017;121:887–94. https://doi.org/10.1016/j.healthpol.2017.06.011.
18. Public Health England. Calorie reduction: the scope and ambition for action. London: Public Health England; 2018. Available: https://www.gov.uk/government/publications/calorie-reduction-the-scope-and-ambition-for-action. Accessed 25 May 2018
19. Drewnowski A. Uses of nutrient profiling to address public health needs: from regulation to reformulation. Proc Nutr Soc. 2017;76:220–9. https://doi.org/10.1017/S0029665117000416.
20. Dunford EK, Webster JL, Woodward M, Czernichow S, Yuan WL, Jenner K, Ni Mhhurchu C, Jacobson M, Campbell NRC, Neal BC. The variability of reported salt levels in fast foods across six countries: opportunities for salt reduction. 2012; https://doi.org/10.1503/cmaj.111895.
21. Health star ratings. Health star ratings are a quick and easy way for you to choose healthier packaged foods. Available: http://www.mpi.govt.nz/food-safety/food-safety-for-consumers/food-labelling/health-star-ratings/. Accessed 18 Jan 2018.
22. Childhood obesity plan. Available: https://www.health.govt.nz/our-work/diseases-and-conditions/obesity/childhood-obesity-plan. Accessed 23 Nov 2017.
23. Healthy kids industry pledge. Available: https://www.health.govt.nz/our-

work/diseases-and-conditions/obesity/childhood-obesity-plan/healthy-kids-industry-pledge. Accessed 23 Nov 2017.

24. Waterlander WE, Eyles H, Whitworth L. Healthiness of popular fast food items in New Zealand: plenty of room for improvement. N Z Med J. 2014; 127:102–5.
25. Food Standards Australia New Zealand. Nutrition Information User Guide to Standard 1.2.8 Nutrition Information Requirements. Available: http://www.foodstandards.govt.nz/code/userguide/Documents/Userguide_Prescribed%20Nutrition%20Information%20Nov%2013%20Dec%202013.pdf. Accessed 27 Feb 15.
26. The Food Monitoring Group. International collaborative project to compare and track the nutritional composition of fast foods. BMC Public Health. 2012;12 https://doi.org/10.1186/1471-2458-1112-1559.
27. Lumley T, Diehr P, Emerson S, Chen L. The importance of the normality assumption in large public health data sets. Annu Rev Public Health. 2002; 23:151–69.
28. Wellard-Cole L, Goldsbury D, Havill M, Hughes C, Watson WL, Dunford EK, Chapman K. Monitoring the changes to the nutrient composition of fast foods following the introduction of menu labelling in new South Wales, Australia: an observational study. Public Health Nutr. 2017; https://doi.org/10.1017/S1368980017003706.
29. Urban LE, Roberts SB, Fierstein JL, Gary CE, Lichtenstein AH. Temporal trends in fast food restaurant energy, sodium, saturated fat, and trans fat content, United States, 1996-2013. Prev Chronic Dis. 2014;11:140202. http://dx.doi.org/10.5888/pcd11.140202.
30. Rudelt A, French S, Harnack L. Fourteen-year trends in sodium content of menu offerings at eight leading fast-food restaurants in the USA. Public Health Nutr. 2013;17:1682–8.
31. Skeaff CM. Feasibility of recommending certain replacement or alternative fats. Eur J Clin Nutr. 2009;63:S34–49. https://doi.org/10.1038/sj.ejcn.1602974.
32. Ministry of Health, University of Otago. A focus on nutrition: Key findings of the 2008/09 New Zealand adult nutrition survey. Wellington: Ministry of Health; 2011. Available: http://www.health.govt.nz/publication/focus-nutrition-key-findings-2008-09-nz-adult-nutrition-survey. Accessed 11 Nov 2015
33. Happy meal. Kids love a treat. So it's good to know there's a menu just for them. Available: https://mcdonalds.co.nz/menu/happy-meal. Accessed 19 Jan 2018.

6

Evaluation of the online Beverage Frequency Questionnaire (BFQ)

Lana Vanderlee[1,2], Jessica L. Reid[2], Christine M. White[2], Erin P. Hobin[1,3,4], Rachel B. Acton[2], Amanda C. Jones[2], Meghan O'Neill[2,4], Sharon I. Kirkpatrick[2] and David Hammond[2*]

Abstract

Background: The contribution of beverages to overall diet is of increasing interest to researchers and policymakers, particularly in terms of consumption of drinks high in added sugars; however, few tools to assess beverage intake have been developed and evaluated. This study aimed to evaluate the relative validity of a new online Beverage Frequency Questionnaire (BFQ) among young adults in Canada.

Methods: A cross-sectional relative validation study was conducted among young adults aged 16–30 years ($n = 50$). Participants completed a 17-item BFQ, a 7-day food record (7dFR), and a single-item measure of sugary drink intake. Pearson correlations and paired t-tests were used to evaluate correlation and agreement between the measures for 17 individual beverage categories, total drink consumption, total alcoholic beverage consumption, and two definitions of drinks with excess sugars. Cognitive interviews were conducted to examine participant interpretation and comprehensiveness of the BFQ.

Results: Estimates of beverage intake based on the BFQ and the 7dFR were highly correlated, specifically for the total number and volume of beverages consumed, total alcoholic beverage consumption, sugary drink intake, and each of the 17 beverage categories with 3 exceptions: coffee or tea with sugar or cream, specialty coffees, and hard alcohol with caloric mix. Paired t-tests between the BFQ and the 7dFR indicated that the average reported volume was significantly different only for sweetened fruit drinks. The single-item measure of sugary beverage intake was not significantly correlated with the 7dFR. Cognitive interviewing demonstrated high comprehension levels, and confirmed the appropriateness of the BFQ beverage categories and sizes.

Conclusions: Overall, the results suggest that the BFQ performed well relative to a 7dFR and had high usability among this study population, indicating its promise for collecting population-level data on beverage intake, including sugar-sweetened beverages, which are known indicators of diet and health.

Keywords: Relative validity, Sugary drinks, Sugar sweetened beverages, Dietary assessment, Food frequency screener

Background

Beverages, especially those high in free sugar, are of particular and growing interest among researchers and policymakers. A well-established body of evidence has demonstrated the link between high consumption of sugar-sweetened beverages (SSBs), which are beverages containing added sugars, and diseases such as type 2 diabetes, metabolic syndrome, cardiovascular disease, dental caries, and several cancers [1–11]. Sugar-sweetened beverages have been associated with these diseases primarily through their contribution to excess weight gain, [12, 13] and contribute substantial caloric energy, have low nutrient density, are associated with poorer quality diets, and offer low satiety in comparison to foods [14, 15]. Additionally, there is growing evidence suggesting that 100% juice, which contains free sugars, has similar impact as SSBs in terms of dietary compensation and the effects of sugars in juice on diabetes and other health conditions [5, 13, 16, 17].

Sugary drinks, which include SSBs and 100% juice, are the single leading source of sugar in Canadians' diets. In 2004, Canadians reported consuming an average of 371

* Correspondence: dhammond@uwaterloo.ca
[2]School of Public Health and Health Systems, University of Waterloo, 200 University Ave W, Waterloo, ON, Canada
Full list of author information is available at the end of the article

g of sugary drinks per day [18–20]. Canadian youth (14 to 18 years) and young adults (19 to 30 years) were the largest consumers of sugary drinks, consuming an average of 643 mL and 500 mL per day, respectively. Regular carbonated soft drinks have long dominated the Canadian sugary beverage market. However, an increasing number of novel beverage categories are being introduced, which have partially offset declines in sales of traditional sugary drinks, such as carbonated soft drinks, fruit drinks and 100% fruit juice [21]. Between 2004 and 2015, sales of flavoured water, flavoured milk, drinkable yogurt, and energy drinks grew from negligible proportions to accounting for approximately 12% of all sugary drink sales volume in Canada [21].

Given the unique contribution of sugary drinks to key metabolic diseases, and their prominent role in Canadians' diets, it is important to accurately monitor beverage consumption at a population level. Beverage intake has historically been measured using a variety of tools. Both 24-h recalls and dietary records (or 'food diaries') provide comprehensive data on foods and beverages consumed by participants in the previous day or over a specified period of time, and have been used to derive beverage intake data [22, 23]. However, such tools can be resource intensive to administer, and place a high burden on participants' time and effort. Online versions of 24-h recalls and records, such as the Automated Self-Administered 24-h Dietary Assessment Tool (ASA24), have been developed to reduce the cost and enhance the feasibility of collecting such comprehensive dietary intake data, from which beverage intake information can be obtained [24]; however, the time required to complete such tools may be prohibitive for some studies. To further enhance the feasibility of collecting beverage intake data from large samples, smaller multi- or single-item beverage frequency questionnaires have been developed to examine changes in beverage intake over time [25, 26].

Frequency-based screeners can play an important role in population-based research. Although frequency-based measures have the limitation of requiring respondents to 'average' intake, which imposes cognitive challenges and contributes bias, depending on the number of items included, they can be considerably shorter and thus may be more feasible than 24-h recalls to administer in some situations. Further, screeners can be used to assess 'typical patterns' of intake, which are of interest in most population-level research [27–29]. However, the existing beverage frequency measures have several important limitations. For example, tools may include general beverage categories without breaking out sub-categories of interest, such as sugary drinks. Existing tools may also have inadequate coverage of new or emerging beverage categories, such as vitamin waters or non-caloric drinks [30–32]. Additionally, most beverage frequency tools use paper-based methods and have not been adapted or tested for online administration. A large majority have been evaluated only in US populations, using US-based beverage container sizes and measurements. Most existing beverage frequency tools do not utilise visual cues for indication of beverage sizes, instead relying on participants to recall numeric sizes, such as "355 mL", or do not inquire about container or portion size [30–32]. In addition, beverage measures have historically failed to include alcoholic beverages, which are a major contributor to intake of both energy and sugars, particularly among those more likely to engage in binge drinking behaviours, such as adolescent and young adult populations [33–36]. Finally, it is challenging to accurately capture intake of episodically-consumed beverages, such as alcohol and energy drinks, as well as sugary drinks, among occasional consumers using 24-h recalls or food records collected for one or a few days.

Given the increasing political and public health focus on sugary drinks, it is important that effective and efficient measures are available with which to characterize beverage consumption at a population level. The objectives of the current study were to compare a newly developed Beverage Frequency Questionnaire (BFQ) to a 7-day dietary record, to examine the ability of the tool to capture the frequency of consumption of drinks with added and free sugar, and to examine whether the BFQ performed better than a single-item measure that has been used in population-level surveys to assess intake of SSBs. It was hypothesized that there would be good agreement between the BFQ and the 7-day food record, and that the BFQ would provide more accurate estimates of beverage intake relative to the 7-day record than the single-item measure that has been widely used in population-based surveys to date.

Methods

Participants

This study was conducted in April and May 2016 with a convenience sample of 50 young adults from a university campus and its surrounding community in southwestern Ontario, Canada. Participants were eligible if they were between 16 and 30 years old, and could read and speak English. Quotas were set to ensure an even proportion of males and females. Participants were recruited until the target sample size was reached, and were remunerated with $40 CAD. This study received ethics clearance through a University of Waterloo Research Ethics Committee (#21304).

Study design

Eligible participants attended two group sessions. During Visit 1, participants provided written consent and completed a brief socio-demographic survey and the BFQ. At this session, participants were provided with verbal and written instructions for completing a food record, and were asked to complete the food record for the next 7 days. Participants returned for Visit 2 eight days after the initial visit to submit their food record, complete a single-item measure of SSB intake and a second BFQ, and participate in cognitive interviewing. All surveys were self-administered using a provided laptop with the pre-loaded online tools.

Measures

Beverage Frequency Questionnaire (BFQ)

The BFQ is an online beverage frequency screener that examines consumption of 17 categories of beverages, including alcoholic beverages (see Additional file 1: Figure S1 for the full list of categories and examples provided in the BFQ). Categories were modelled after previous existing questionnaires for beverage consumption, [30–32] with substantial adaptations to ensure that categories could adequately discern between sweetened and unsweetened beverages, caloric and non-caloric beverages, and individual beverage categories. Within caloric and non-caloric drinks, distinctions were made to distinguish between key beverage attributes (e.g., carbonated vs. non-carbonated, heavily caffeinated products).

First, the survey asked participants, "During the PAST 7 DAYS, how many times did you drink each of the following beverages?" for each drink category. Next, for each of the categories that the participant consumed, the participant was asked, "On average, how much did you usually drink each time?" and was shown a series of images, adapted from ASA24, of commonly-used containers with the volume in millilitres below the container [24]. Response options for 'Less' than the smallest image amount and 'More' than the largest image amount were also available. Figure 1 provides an example of container sizes for the "regular soda or pop" beverage category. Additional information regarding the online format is available from the corresponding author.

Seven-day food record (7dFR)

Participants were provided with a standard food record booklet with spaces for a description of the specific food or beverage item consumed (including brand information, when possible), the location at which it was prepared, and the number and portion size or amount that was consumed. Participants completed the food record for 7 days, beginning the day after Visit 1. Participants were instructed to record all meals, beverages and snacks consumed each day, ideally in real-time as foods and beverages were consumed, and were asked to provide as much detail as possible.

Single-item measure of sugar-sweetened beverage intake

Prior to completing the BFQ at Visit 2, participants were asked, "During the PAST 7 DAYS, how many drinks with added sugar did you have, such as pop, fruit drinks, sports drinks, vitamin waters, energy drinks and specialty coffees? Do NOT count diet or sugar-free drinks. Do NOT include today." This measure did not specifically include 100% fruit juice, and was meant to capture SSBs.

Socio-demographic questionnaire

Participants were queried about sex, age, education level, and race/ethnicity, as well as self-reported weight and height, which were used to calculate body mass index (BMI), according to World Health Organization (WHO) categories of underweight, normal weight, overweight and obese [37].

Cognitive interviewing

Cognitive interviewing was conducted with participants to assess the comprehensiveness of the BFQ, their comprehension of the BFQ and interpretation of the instructions, and to examine how participants used the tool. After completing the BFQ at Visit 2, participants were provided with paper copies of the screens they had seen on the computer when completing the tools. Cognitive interviewing was conducted in small groups of one to

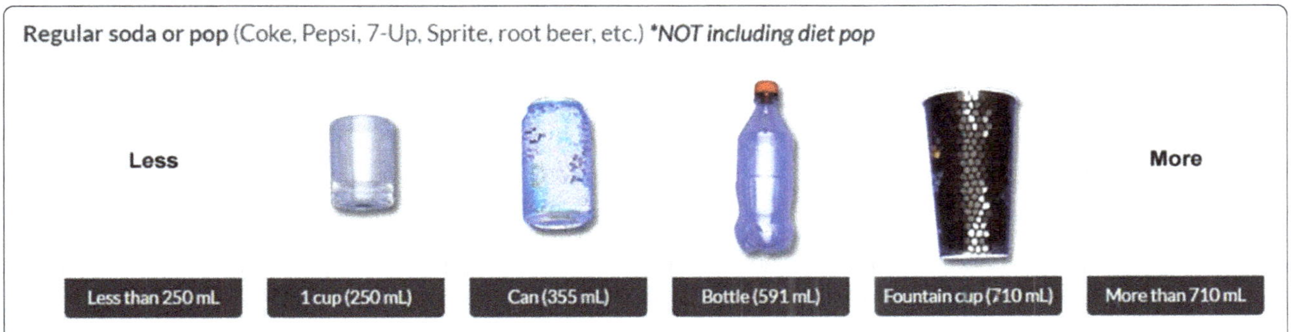

Fig. 1 Example of images used in the BFQ

four participants by a trained research assistant, who took notes on responses.

First, participants were asked if they had trouble recalling the number of drinks for any specific categories, if there were any drinks not on the current list that they felt should be added, and whether or not they were thinking about each of the 7 days individually or gave an estimated amount based on their usual patterns. Participants were also asked whether they recalled seeing images for serving sizes, and, if so, whether they used the shape of the container or the amount written under the container, or both, to identify their serving size. Lastly, they were asked if, over the course of the week, they had the same type of drink in different sizes of containers (e.g., a can of pop one day and a bottle the next day), and if so, how they chose which container/size to select.

Analysis

Food records

Data from the 7dFRs were coded by a trained research assistant to identify incidences of consumption and amounts consumed of beverages in the categories included in the BFQ, as well as other beverages not captured by the BFQ. Because the BFQ relates to a 7-day period, the volume consumed within each beverage category was summed over the 7-day period. When beverages were consumed in dining establishments outside of the home, restaurant websites were used to estimate the volume of beverage containers (e.g., for fountain drinks). When the frequency of consumption was not reported, it was assumed that the beverage category was consumed zero times. When size was not reported in the food record, the smallest size for the specific beverage category in the BFQ was used. Assumptions were required in at least one instance in 14 food records (4 instances for the frequency of consumption and 14 instances for the volume consumed).

Beverage Frequency Questionnaire (BFQ)

Data from the BFQ estimated of the number of times each drink category was consumed. This number was multiplied by the usual serving size selected (in mL) to estimate the total volume consumed over the past 7 days for each beverage category. When a participant reported consuming less than the smallest size provided, the amount was estimated as 50% of the smallest size option in that beverage category; when a participant reported consuming more than the largest size provided, the amount was estimated as 125% of the largest size. For example, if a participant reported consuming less than the smallest size of regular soda or pop (250 ml), it was assumed that they consumed 125 ml of regular pop or soda; if they reported consuming more than the largest size of regular soda or pop (710 ml), it was assumed they consumed 888 ml of regular soda or pop. Some questions were combined to create definitions for beverage categories, such as alcoholic drinks, which included: beer, cider or coolers; wine (red or white); hard alcohol with mix, cocktails that have calories; and hard alcohol with no mix or non-caloric mix.

Definitions of beverages with excess free and added sugars

Two definitions were used to classify beverages with excess sugar content. The first was a typical definition of *SSBs*, which included: regular soda or pop; sweetened fruit drinks; flavoured waters or vitamin waters with calories; sports drinks; energy drinks; and, specialty coffees. A more comprehensive definition of *sugary drinks* was also utilized, which included the aforementioned beverages, as well as: 100% fruit or vegetable juice; chocolate milk; regular coffee with cream or sugar; and hard alcohol with mix or cocktails that had calories. Analyses were conducted to examine the correlation between the food record and the BFQ for the two definitions of beverages with excess sugar content.

Statistical analysis

Pearson correlations were used to examine the relationship between the number of times (drinks) and total volume of beverages consumed per 7-day period, as reported in the food record and the BFQ for each drink category, for the *SSB* and *sugary drinks* definitions, for alcoholic drinks, and for all drinks combined. Analyses comparing the *SSB* and *sugary drinks* definitions were also conducted stratified by race/ethnicity. Agreement and correlations were also examined comparing the single-item measure to the 7dFR using paired samples t-tests and Pearson correlations. Cognitive interviewing notes were summarized by the interviewer, and suggestions for amendments to the BFQ were collated. Bland-Altman plots were generated to compare the measurements from the two tools.

Results

Participant characteristics

The final sample of 50 participants were primarily normal weight university students, with diverse racial/ethnic backgrounds (Table 1).

Beverage consumption

The number of BFQ beverage categories reported by participants ranged from 0 to 7, out of a possible 17 categories, with an average of 3.16 categories (s.d. = 1.74). Three participants reported not consuming any BFQ beverages (note: plain water was not included as a category).

Table 1 Sample characteristics

		(Frequency)
Mean Age (SD)	22 (2.99)	(50)
Gender		
Male	50.0%	(25)
Female	50.0%	(25)
Body Mass Index (BMI) category		
Underweight	6.0%	(3)
Normal weight	72.0%	(36)
Overweight	12.0%	(6)
Obese	8.0%	(4)
Not stated	2.0%	(1)
Race/ethnicity		
White	42.0%	(21)
Other	58.0%	(29)
Educational attainment		
High school or less	22.0%	(11)
Some university, no degree	42.0%	(21)
Completed university degree	30.0%	(15)
Postgraduate degree	6.0%	(3)

When the data from the BFQ and 7dFR were compared (Table 2), both the number of drinks and the volume of drinks were positively correlated between the BFQ and 7dFR for all 17 beverage categories, with three exceptions: coffee or tea with sugar or cream, specialty coffees, and hard alcohol with caloric mix. There were also positive correlations between the number and volume of drinks in the BFQ and food record for all drinks combined and all alcoholic drinks combined. Paired t-tests between the BFQ and the 7dFR indicated that the average volume was not significantly different for any category except sweetened fruit drinks. When qualitatively compared, food records from 16 participants included beverages that were not captured in the BFQ: 11 participants reported consuming smoothies and five reported consuming protein drinks, neither of which had dedicated categories on the BFQ.

Definitions of drinks with excess sugar content

Correlations between the BFQ and 7dFR for the total number of beverages and the total volume consumed were significant for both *sugar-sweetened beverages* (regular soda or pop; sweetened fruit drinks; flavoured waters or vitamin waters with calories; sports drinks; energy drinks; and specialty coffees) and *sugary drinks* (sugar-sweetened beverages plus 100% fruit or vegetable juice; chocolate milk; regular coffee with cream or sugar; and hard alcohol with mix or cocktails that had calories). When stratified by race/ethnicity, trends were similar and all findings remained significant within each category (results not shown). Bland-Altman plots suggested no proportional bias with the limited definition of SSBs ($t = 0.32$, $p = 0.75$) and for the sugary drinks definition ($t = 1.78$, $p = 0.08$). Figure 2 shows that 94% of the differences for both SSBs and sugary drinks, respectively, fell within the limits of agreement (2 standard deviations from the mean).

Comparison to single-item measure

The mean number of *SSBs* reported over 7 days was 3.66 (s.d. 4.39; range: 0–18) based on the single-item measure, compared to 2.70 (s.d. 3.59; range: 0–14) based on the 7dFR, and 2.14 (s.d. 2.85, range: 0–15) based on the BFQ. While there was no significant difference in the mean number of SSBs consumed based on the single-item measure and the 7dFR ($t = 1.36$, $p = 0.18$), there was not a significant correlation between the number of SSBs based on the single-item measure and the 7dFR (0.23, $p = 0.10$).

Cognitive interviewing

Overall, 32% of the participants ($n = 16$) reported that they had trouble reporting the number of drinks for the categories provided in the BFQ. When asked how they recalled the number of drinks they consumed in the last week, 54% ($n = 27$) of the participants reported that they considered each of the past 7 days, 22% ($n = 11$) gave an estimate based on their usual patterns, and 24% ($n = 12$) reported using a combination of considering each of the past 7 days and estimating based on their usual patterns. In addition, 20% ($n = 10$) of participants reported that they could not find a drink on the list and felt that it should be added to the BFQ ($n = 3$ suggested protein drinks and n = 3 suggested smoothies).

In total, 22% of the 49 participants who viewed images depicting typical container sizes for at least one beverage category had trouble selecting an image for the beverage category. Participants reported that the container or volume of beverages they consumed was not captured in the images and they had to guess the closest size. When participants were asked whether they tried to match the shape of the container or the amount written under the container when they selected an image, 27% indicated they tried to match the shape, 29% tried to match the amount, and 45% used both the shape and the amount written under it. Overall, 2 participants (4%) reported that alcohol was particularly hard to recall due to oddly shaped glasses that they were served in.

Across the sample, 42% ($n = 21$) reported that they consumed the same type of beverage in different sizes of containers over the course of the week. When selecting an image, 36% ($n = 18$) of participants reported that they selected the size that they consumed the most often, and 3 selected the larger container size.

Table 2 Average number of beverages and volume consumed, according to the Beverage Frequency Questionnaire (BFQ) and 7-day food record (7dFR)

Beverage category	Mean # of drinks (s. e.)		r_p # of drinks	*p*-value	Mean total volume in ml (s. e.)		Mean volume difference between BFQ and Record (s. e.)	r_p total volume	*p*-value	t-test for total volume	*p*-value
	7dFR	BFQ			7dFR	BFQ					
1. Regular soda or pop	0.78 (0.27)	0.86 (0.26)	0.58	< 0.001	277 (99)	388 (133)	+ 298 (112)	0.51	< 0.001	−0.93	0.36
2. Diet soda or pop	0.00	0.06 (0.0)	–	< 0.001	0 (0)	21 (21)	21 (21)	–		−1.00	0.32
3. 100% fruit/vegetable juice	2.00 (0.46)	1.88 (0.45)	0.56	< 0.001	506 (117)	494 (115)	387 (104)	0.48	< 0.001	0.10	0.92
4. Fruit drinks with added sugars	1.06 (0.34)	0.52 (0.18)	0.46	< 0.001	359 (94)	154 (57)	295 (72)	0.56	< 0.001	2.62	0.01
5. Flavoured water/vitamin water with calories	0.08 (0.48)	0.06 (0.04)	0.91	< 0.001	37 (23)	35 (26)	13 (8)	0.95	< 0.001	0.20	0.84
6. Sports drinks	0.12 (0.06)	0.22 (0.10)	0.60	< 0.001	82 (46)	124 (56)	63 (31)	0.82	< 0.001	−1.33	0.19
7. Energy drinks	0.12 (0.07)	0.12 (0.06)	0.91	< 0.001	51 (29)	57 (29)	23 (13)	0.89		−0.40	0.69
8. Calorie-free drinks	0.00	0.02 (0.02)	–	< 0.001	0 (0)	12 (12)	12 (12)	–		−1.00	0.32
9. Unsweetened milk or alternatives	1.60 (0.45)	2.08 (0.56)	0.47	< 0.001	478 (135)	640 (233)	469 (178)	0.59	< 0.001	−0.86	0.39
10. Chocolate or sweetened milk and alternatives	0.90 (0.27)	0.88 (0.37)	0.58	< 0.001	336 (109)	255 (112)	311 (103)	0.49	< 0.001	0.73	0.47
11. Coffee/tea with cream or sugar	2.32 (0.56)	2.06 (0.39)	0.20	0.1	833 (223)	517 (135)	747 (225)	0.13	0.37	1.29	0.20
12. Coffee/tea no cream or sugar	1.66 (0.48)	1.74 (0.61)	0.65	< 0.001	570 (197)	729 (282)	588 (165)	0.76	< 0.001	−0.87	0.39
13. Specialty coffee	0.54 (0.16)	0.36 (0.14)	0.23	0.11	211 (64)	116 (43)	208 (62)	0.26	0.07	1.41	0.16
14. Beer/cider/coolers	0.58 (0.21)	0.60 (0.20)	0.92	< 0.001	271 (106)	250 (78)	143 (50)	0.87	< 0.001	0.40	0.69
15. Wine	0.10 (0.06)	0.12 (0.07)	0.60	< 0.001	58 (42)	29 (18)	57 (36)	0.50	< 0.001	0.82	0.42
16. Hard alcohol with caloric mix	0.16 (0.09)	0.28 (0.13)	0.18	< 0.001	56 (33)	70 (31)	40 (21)	0.78	< 0.001	−0.64	0.53
17. Hard alcohol no mix or non-caloric mix	0.30 (0.19)	0.24 (0.14)	0.18	0.23	9 (11)	13 (8)	24 (12)	0.16	0.25	0.51	0.61
Sugar-sweetened beverages[a]	2.70 (0.51)	2.14 (0.40)	0.53	< 0.001	1017 (183)	875 (173)	634 (147)	0.54	< 0.001	0.82	0.41
Sugary drinks[b]	8.08 (1.18)	7.24 (0.94)	0.63	< 0.001	2749 (392)	2211 (316)	1368 (291)	0.55	< 0.001	1.57	0.12
All alcoholic drinks	1.14 (0.31)	1.24 (0.34)	0.58	< 0.001	405 (120)	361 (96)	44 (76)	0.78	< 0.001	0.58	0.57
All drinks	12.32 (1.40)	12.10 (1.20)	0.62	< 0.001	4145 (484)	3904 (463)	241 (428)	0.59	< 0.001	0.56	0.57

[a]Includes: regular soda or pop; sweetened fruit drinks; flavoured waters or vitamin waters with calories; sports drinks; energy drinks; and specialty coffees

[b]Includes: regular soda or pop; sweetened fruit drinks; flavoured waters or vitamin waters with calories; sports drinks; energy drinks; specialty coffees; 100% fruit or vegetable juice; chocolate milk; regular coffee with cream or sugar; and hard alcohol with mix or cocktails that had calorie

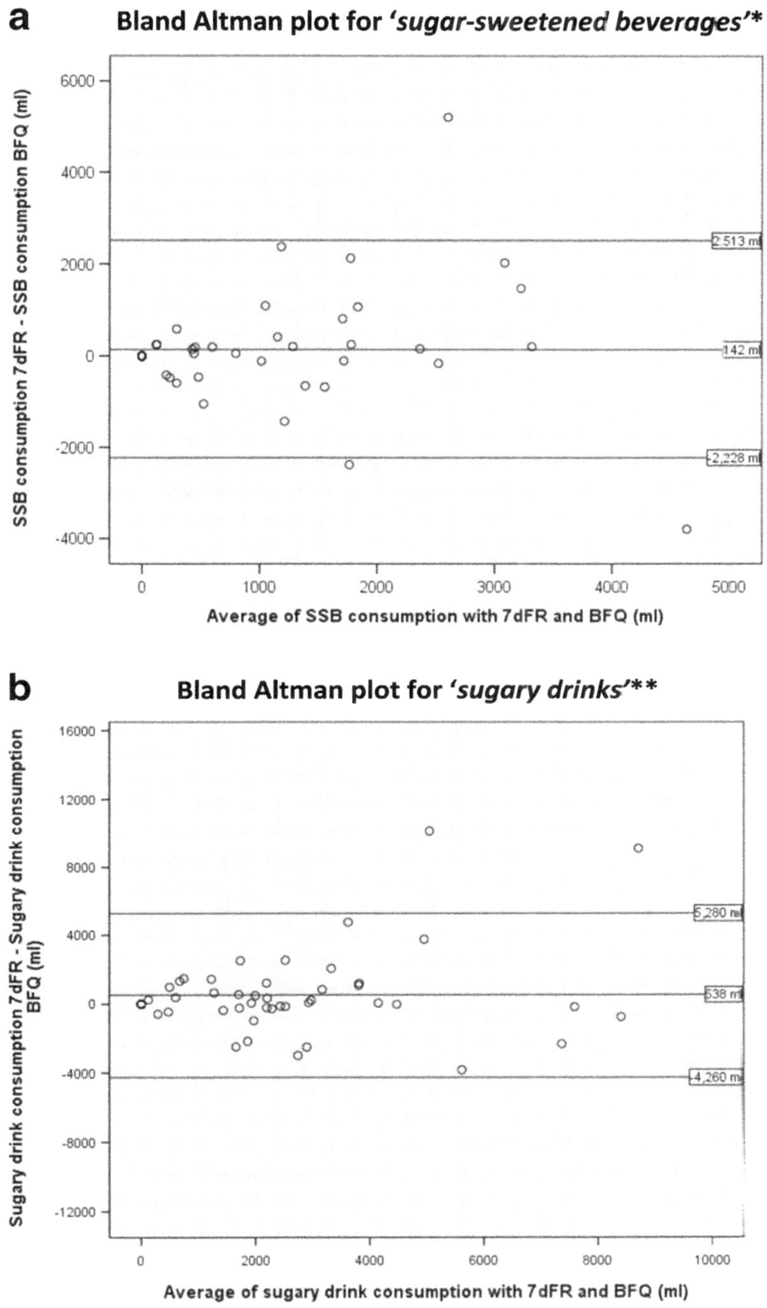

Fig. 2 a Bland Altman plot for *'sugar-sweetened beverages*'*. **b** Bland Altman plot for *'sugary drinks*'**

Discussion

The results indicate strong correlation and agreement between the BFQ and the 7dFR for the vast majority of beverage categories and for the overall definitions of *sugar-sweetened beverages* and *sugary drinks*. These results are very similar to a 2010 validation study of a paper-based beverage frequency questionnaire that also did not find significant correlations for hard alcohol, or coffee with cream or sugar when compared to a 4-day food record; however, the current study found higher correlations across all beverage categories [31]. Coffee with cream or sugar was among the most frequently consumed beverages, and was consumed in large volumes, which may contribute to poorer recall of instances of consumption and greater likelihood of having to select an average container size that may not precisely reflect all of the various container sizes consumed. Given that the overall contribution of added sugar or calories from this category are likely to be small, this is unlikely to influence estimates of energy or added sugar intake. The reasons for poor recollection of consumption of specialty coffees and caloric alcoholic drinks is unclear, although both were consumed relatively infrequently. The cognitive interview data suggest that this could be due to alcohol being served in unusual beverage containers, which may create challenges in completing a frequency-type questionnaire. Future iterations of the BFQ may consider additional container sizes and shapes for alcoholic beverages and additional prompts to improve recall of coffee and tea with cream or sugar, and coffee and tea with cream or sugar will be removed from the definition of *sugary drinks*.

The BFQ performed better relative to the 7dFR than the single-item measure in assessing SSB and sugary drink intake. While there are advantages to using an abbreviated measure, such as the single-item measure, in terms of time and respondent burden, the findings indicate a more comprehensive tool, such as the BFQ, can improve recall and estimation of the frequency and amount of beverages consumed, without creating the level of participant burden that might be associated with administering 24-h recalls or food records to capture the total diet. However, the BFQ obviously does not provide information on other aspects of the diet that may be of interest, for example, for considering how beverage intake patterns relate to other characteristics of eating patterns, which would be captured in a 24-h recall or food record.

Most participants did not report difficulty using the BFQ, and used the BFQ as intended by considering each of the previous 7 days when estimating intake, rather than basing estimates solely on usual patterns. Additionally, the participants typically selected the size consumed most often, rather than the largest or smallest size consumed, which should decrease any bias towards over- or under-reporting. The cognitive interviewing indicated that participants benefited from having the images to guide estimation of container size, as more than half of participants used both the container shape and the volume amount to guide their selection; however, this study did not explicitly test whether or not this improved volume estimations, and portion size estimation is known to be a challenging aspect of dietary assessment.

With regards to face validity, the results suggest that the BFQ reasonably captures most beverages that are consumed by this age group, with the exception of protein shakes and smoothies. During the cognitive interviewing, participants noted that these two drink categories were missing from the beverage questionnaire. These beverages' potentially high sugar contents and their reported frequent consumption position them as potentially meaningful sources of dietary sugar. A revised version of the BFQ for use in future research includes these categories. Few young adults in this sample consumed calorie-free drinks, consistent with national data based on dietary recalls indicating highest consumption among adults over 30 years of age [19, 20]. Consumption of these types of beverages may become more prevalent as efforts to reduce dietary sugar intake increase with age.

Study limitations and strengths

This study assessed relative validity of the BFQ by comparing intake estimates to another self-report measure. 7dFRs are one of the most widely used methods for capturing self-reported dietary intake, but may be subject to reactivity in addition to other sources of bias [38]. The correlations between the BFQ and 7dFR data may reflect agreement both in terms of true intake as well as biases that may be common to data collected using the two tools (e.g., underreporting of certain categories of beverages due to social desirability biases). An objective measure is needed to overcome these challenges; however, there is no biomarker for beverage intake and observation is not feasible for the 7-day period of study in this research, and can also lead to reactivity. Future research may make use of biomarkers of sugar intake to shed further light on the ability of tools such as the BFQ to capture intake of total, free, and added sugars [39, 40].

Further, the order of administration of tools may have affected responses. For example, the completion of the 7dFR may have led to increased accuracy on the BFQ completed at the 2nd visit, possibly inflating the correlations between the BFQ and the food record. Additionally, the sample size was relatively small and a small number of respondents reported consumption of beverages in some categories, lending uncertainty to the estimates for those categories. The relatively demanding task of recording dietary intake over 7 days may have resulted in sample selection bias in that those with knowledge and interest in nutrition were motivated to participate; however, this was potentially reduced by the remuneration provided as an incentive to participate. While the population under study was restricted primarily to university students, the study population included a large sample of non-White participants, and included those with high variation in beverage intake behaviours, increasing the generalizability to the young adult population in Canada.

Tool limitations and strengths

Given the challenge of recalling plain water consumption, this was not included in the BFQ; therefore, the BFQ cannot capture shifts from caloric beverages to plain water. Further, the BFQ does not provide data on the total diet, limiting its use for examining beverage intake in relation to other characteristics of eating patterns. Lastly, the tool was not developed to examine other characteristics of beverages, such as caffeine consumption or added components such as vitamins and minerals, which may be of interest to some researchers. Strengths of the BFQ include the inclusion of specific categories of beverages with attention to contributions to intake of energy and sugars, as well as categories frequently consumed in the current marketplace. The tool captures consumption of beverages that may be episodically consumed, such as energy drinks. Finally, this tool captures both alcoholic and non-alcoholic drinks. Given the high amounts of sugar in some alcoholic drinks and the contribution of alcohol to calorie intake, this is an important addition to the literature. Additionally, the revised version of the BFQ has been translated into French and Spanish (although it has only been evaluated in English to date), and has been adapted for use in other countries (United States, Mexico, United Kingdom and Australia) by changing brand names and portion/container sizes. Future work with the tool will include developing country-specific category averages of total sugar, free/added sugar, and calories, using branded food and beverage databases that can be applied to beverage categories to estimate added sugar and energy consumption from beverages.

Conclusions

Overall, this study showed that the online BFQ performs well relative to a more comprehensive measure of intake for capturing intake of regularly-consumed beverage categories, including the frequency and volume of beverages with excess sugars, and is a promising tool to measure population-level beverage intake. The unique features of this tool, including its online application, the use of images to improve reporting of serving sizes, and the reference period of 7 days to capture episodically-consumed beverages, make this a novel tool for researchers and practitioners seeking to gather data about beverage consumption patterns.

Funding

This project has been made possible through funding from the Public Health Agency of Canada (PHAC). The views expressed herein do not necessarily represent the view of the Public Health Agency of Canada. Additional funding for this project has been provided by a PHAC – Canadian Institutes of Health Research (CIHR) Chair in Applied Public Health, which supports Professor Hammond, staff, and students at the University of Waterloo. LV is a CIHR Banting Postdoctoral Fellow.

Authors' contributions

LV, JLR, CW, EPH and DH designed the BFQ; LV and DH designed the research study; LV, JLR, CW and MO conducted the research; LV and SIK designed the analysis; LV and MO analyzed data; LV, RBA, and ACJ wrote the paper; LV had primary responsibility for final content. All authors have read and approved the final manuscript.

Competing interests

Lana Vanderlee, Jessica L. Reid, Christine M. White, Erin P. Hobin, Rachel B. Acton, Amanda C. Jones, Meghan O'Neill, Sharon I. Kirkpatrick declare that they have no competing interests.

DH has provided paid expert testimony on behalf of public health authorities in response to legal challenges from the food and beverage industry.

Author details

[1]Department of Nutritional Sciences, University of Toronto, Toronto, Canada. [2]School of Public Health and Health Systems, University of Waterloo, 200 University Ave W, Waterloo, ON, Canada. [3]Public Health Ontario, Toronto, Canada. [4]Dalla Lana School of Public Health, University of Toronto, Toronto, Canada.

References

1. Forouzanfar MH, Alexander L, Anderson HR, Bachman VF, Biryukov S, Brauer M, Burnett R, Casey D, Coates MM, Cohen A, et al. Global, regional, and national comparative risk assessment of 79 behavioural, environmental and occupational, and metabolic risks or clusters of risks in 188 countries, 1990–2013: a systematic analysis for the global burden of disease study 2013. Lancet. 2015;386(10010):2287–323.
2. O'Connor TM, Yang SJ, Nicklas TA. Beverage intake among preschool children and its effect on weight status. Pediatrics. 2006;118(4):e1010.
3. Malik VS, Popkin BM, Bray GA, Després J-P, Willett WC, Hu FB. Sugar-sweetened beverages and risk of metabolic syndrome and type 2 diabetes. Diabetes Care. 2010;33(11):2477–83.
4. Xi B, Huang Y, Reilly KH, Li S, Zheng R, Barrio-Lopez MT, et al. Sugar-sweetened beverages and risk of hypertension and CVD: a dose–response meta-analysis. Br J Nutr. 2015;113(5):709–17.
5. Te Morenga LA, Howatson AJ, Jones RM, Mann J. Dietary sugars and cardiometabolic risk: systematic review and meta-analyses of randomized controlled trials of the effects on blood pressure and lipids. Am J Clin Nutr. 2014;100(1):65-79. https://doi.org/10.3945/ajcn.113.081521.
6. The Prospective Studies Collaboration. Body-mass index and cause-specific mortality in 900 000 adults: collaborative analyses of 57 prospective studies. Lancet. 2009;373(9669):1083–96.
7. The Global BMI MOrtality Collaboration. Body-mass index and all-cause mortality: individual-participant-data meta-analysis of 239 prospective studies in four continents. Lancet. 2016;388(10046):776–86.
8. Lauby-Secretan B, Scoccianti C, Loomis D, Grosse Y, Bianchini F, Straif K. Body fatness and cancer—viewpoint of the IARC working group. N Engl J Med. 2016;375(8):794–8.
9. Singh GM, Danaei G, Farzadfar F, Stevens GA, Woodward M, Wormser D, Kaptoge S, Whitlock G, Qiao Q, Lewington S, et al. The age-specific quantitative effects of metabolic risk factors on cardiovascular diseases and diabetes: a pooled analysis. PLoS One. 2013;8(7):e65174.
10. Kodama S, Horikawa C, Fujihara K, Yoshizawa S, Yachi Y, Tanaka S, Ohara N, Matsunaga S, Yamada T, Hanyu O, et al. Quantitative relationship between body weight gain in adulthood and incident type 2 diabetes: a meta-analysis. Obes Rev. 2014;15(3):202–14.
11. Lu Y, Hajifathalian K, Ezzati M, Woodward M, Rimm EB, Danaei G. Metabolic mediators of the effects of body-mass index, overweight, and obesity on coronary heart disease and stroke: a pooled analysis of 97 prospective cohorts with 1·8 million participants. Lancet. 2014;383:970–83.
12. Malik VS, Pan A, Willett WC, Hu FB. Sugar-sweetened beverages and weight gain in children and adults: a systematic review and meta-analysis. Am J Clin Nutr. 2013;98(4):1084–102
13. Te Morenga L, Mallard S, Mann J. Dietary sugars and body weight: systematic review and meta-analyses of randomised controlled trials and cohort studies. BMJ. 2013;346:e7492.

14. Malik VS, Schulze MB, Hu FB. Intake of sugar-sweetened beverages and weight gain: a systematic review. Am J Clin Nutr. 2006;84(2):274.
15. Malik VS, Popkin BM, Bray GA, Després J-P, Hu FB. Sugar-sweetened beverages, obesity, type 2 diabetes mellitus, and cardiovascular disease risk. Circulation. 2010;121(11):1356–64.
16. Popkin BM. Hyson's review ignores long-term research and recent global guidelines that recommend no more than 4 ounces of fruit juice a day due to adverse health effects. Adv Nutr. 2015;6(5):625–6.
17. Auerbach BJ, Wolf FM, Hikida A, Vallila-Buchman P, Littman A, Thompson D, et al. Fruit juice and change in BMI: a meta-analysis. Pediatrics. 2017;139(4):e20162454.
18. Langlois K, Garriguet D. Sugar consumption among Canadians of all ages. Health Rep. 2011 Sep;22(3):23–7.
19. Garriguet D. Beverage consumption of Canadian adults. Health Rep. 2008;19(4):23.
20. Garriguet D. Beverage consumption of children and teens. Health Rep. 2008;19(4):17.
21. Jones AC, Veerman JL, Hammond D. The health and economic impact of a tax on sugary drinks in Canada. 2017.
22. Han E, Powell LM. Consumption patterns of sugar-sweetened beverages in the United States. J Acad Nutr Diet. 2013;113(1):43–53.
23. Nissensohn M, Castro-Quezada I, Serra-Majem L. Beverage and water intake of healthy adults in some European countries. Int J Food Sci Nutr. 2013;64(7):801–5.
24. Subar AF, Kirkpatrick SI, Mittl B, Zimmerman TP, Thompson FE, Bingley C, et al. The automated self-administered 24-hour dietary recall (ASA24): a resource for researchers, clinicians and educators from the National Cancer Institute. J Acad Nutr Diet. 2012;112(8):1134.
25. Falbe J, Thompson HR, Becker CM, Rojas N, McCulloch CE, Madsen KA. Impact of the Berkeley excise tax on sugar-sweetened beverage consumption. Am J Public Health. 2016;106(10):1865–71.
26. Park S, Pan L, Sherry B, Blanck HM. Peer reviewed: consumption of sugar-sweetened beverages among US adults in 6 states: behavioral risk factor surveillance system, 2011. Prev Chronic Dis. 2014;11
27. Subar AF, Kipnis V, Troiano RP, Midthune D, Schoeller DA, Bingham S, et al. Using intake biomarkers to evaluate the extent of dietary misreporting in a large sample of adults: the OPEN study. Am J Epidemiol. 2003;158(1):1–13.
28. Kipnis V, Subar AF, Midthune D, Freedman LS, Ballard-Barbash R, Troiano RP, et al. Structure of dietary measurement error: results of the OPEN biomarker study. Am J Epidemiol. 2003;158(1):14.
29. Prentice RL, Mossavar-Rahmani Y, Huang Y, Van Horn L, Beresford SA, Caan B, et al. Evaluation and comparison of food records, recalls, and frequencies for energy and protein assessment by using recovery biomarkers. Am J Epidemiol. 2011;174(5):591–603.
30. Nelson MC, Lytle LA. Development and evaluation of a brief screener to estimate fast-food and beverage consumption among adolescents. J Am Diet Assoc. 2009;109(4):730–4.
31. Hedrick VE, Savla J, Comber DL, Flack KD, Estabrooks PA, Nsiah-Kumi PA, et al. Development of a brief questionnaire to assess habitual beverage intake (BEVQ-15): sugar-sweetened beverages and total beverage energy intake. J Acad Nutr Diet. 2012;112(6):840–9.
32. Hedrick VE, Comber DL, Estabrooks PA, Savla J, Davy BM. The beverage intake questionnaire: determining initial validity and reliability. J Am Diet Assoc. 2010;110(8):1227–32.
33. Battista K, Leatherdale ST. Estimating how extra calories from alcohol consumption are likely an overlooked contributor to youth obesity. Health Promot Chronic Dis Prev Can. 2017 Jun;37(6):194–200.
34. Traversy G, Chaput J-P. Alcohol consumption and obesity: an update. Current Obesity Rep. 2015;4(1):122–30.
35. Sayon-Orea C, Martinez-Gonzalez MA, Bes-Rastrollo M. Alcohol consumption and body weight: a systematic review. Nutr Rev. 2011;69(8):419–31.
36. Yeomans MR. Alcohol, appetite and energy balance: is alcohol intake a risk factor for obesity? Physiol Behav. 2010;100(1):82–9.
37. World Health Organization Regional Office for Europe. Body mass index - BMI. Available at http://www.euro.who.int/en/health-topics/disease-prevention/nutrition/a-healthy-lifestyle/body-mass-index-bmi. Accessed 23 July 2018.
38. Rebro SM, Patterson RE, Kristal AR, Cheney CL. The effect of keeping food records on eating patterns. J Am Diet Assoc. 1998;98(10):1163–5.
39. Beasley J, Jung M, Tasevska N, Wong W, Siega-Riz A, Sotres-Alvarez D, et al. Biomarker-predicted sugars intake compared with self-reported measures in US Hispanics/Latinos: results from the HCHS/SOL SOLNAS study. Public Health Nutr. 2016;19(18):3256–64.
40. Tasevska N. Urinary sugars—a biomarker of total sugars intake. Nutrients. 2015;7(7):5816–33.

7

Severely malnourished children with a low weight-for-height have a higher mortality than those with a low mid-upper-arm-circumference: I. Empirical data demonstrates Simpson's paradox

Emmanuel Grellety[1*] and Michael H. Golden[2]

Abstract

Background: According to WHO childhood severe acute malnutrition (SAM) is diagnosed when the weight-for-height Z-score (WHZ) is <−3Z of the WHO_{2006} standards, the mid-upper-arm circumference (MUAC) is < 115 mm, there is nutritional oedema or any combination of these parameters. Recently there has been a move to eliminate WHZ as a diagnostic criterion on the assertion that children meeting the WHZ criterion are healthy, that MUAC is universally a superior prognostic indicator of mortality and that adding WHZ to the assessment does not improve the prediction; these assertions have lead to a controversy concerning the role of WHZ in the diagnosis of SAM.

Methods: We examined the mortality experience of 76,887 6–60 month old severely malnourished children admitted for treatment to in-patient, out-patient or supplementary feeding facilities in 18 African countries, of whom 3588 died. They were divided into 7 different diagnostic categories for analysis of mortality rates by comparison of case fatality rates, relative risk of death and meta-analysis of the difference between children admitted using MUAC and WHZ criteria.

Results: The mortality rate was higher in those children fulfilling the WHO_{2006} WHZ criterion than the MUAC criterion. This was the case for younger as well as older children and in all regions except for marasmic children in East Africa. Those fulfilling both criteria had a higher mortality. Nutritional oedema increased the risk of death. Having oedema and a low WHZ dramatically increased the mortality rate whereas addition of the MUAC criterion to either oedema-alone or oedema plus a low WHZ did not further increase the mortality rate. The data were subject to extreme confounding giving Simpson's paradox, which reversed the apparent mortality rates when children fulfilling both WHZ and MUAC criteria were included in the estimation of the risk of death of those fulfilling either the WHZ or MUAC criteria alone.

Conclusions: Children with a low WHZ, but a MUAC above the SAM cut-off point are at high risk of death. Simpson's paradox due to confounding from oedema and mathematical coupling may make previous statistical analyses which failed to distinguish the diagnostic groups an unreliable guide to policy. WHZ needs to be retained as an independent criterion for diagnosis of SAM and methods found to identify those children with a low WHZ, but not a low MUAC, in the community.

(Continued on next page)

* Correspondence: Emmanuel.Grellety.Bosviel@ulb.ac.be
[1]Research Center Health Policy and Systems - International Health, School of Public Health, Université Libre de Bruxelles, Bruxelles, Belgium
Full list of author information is available at the end of the article

(Continued from previous page)
Keywords: Nutrition, Acute malnutrition, Severe acute malnutrition, SAM, Mid-upper-arm circumference, MUAC, Weight-for-height, WHZ, Mortality, Case fatality rate, Wasting, Oedema, Kwashiorkor, Diagnosis, Simpson's paradox, Mathematical coupling, Child, Human, Meta-analysis

Background

About 19 million children are estimated to have severe wasting, of whom about half to one million die each year [1]. These estimates were made from prevalence data using weight-for-height (WHZ) as the single criterion. As the deaths related to a low mid-upper-arm-circumference (MUAC) or nutritional oedema (kwashiorkor) were not included in these estimates the actual prevalence is much higher than this estimated burden. Furthermore, although the prevalence may have been overestimated with respect to WHZ [2], the incidence was not taken into account; this would increase the annual burden much more substantially [3]. Whatever the actual magnitude it is clear that severe acute malnutrition (SAM), with other nutritional insults, are major neglected conditions leading to death and poor development of children globally and as such constitute a critical public health priority. The criteria used to define SAM have a crucial effect upon all aspects of the condition.

Not only assessments of the numbers of children affected but also their individual eligibility for treatment is affected by the criteria used to define SAM. These criteria have changed repeatedly over the years so that different numbers and degrees of severity have characterised those designated as having SAM. These schemes initially included those based upon weight-for-age, introduced by Gomez [4] and adopted by The Wellcome Trust [5], as the basic parameter [6]. Later weight-for-height was suggested [7] and forms a classification by Waterlow [8] to differentiate underweight children (weight-for-age) into those that are light because they are wasted (weight-for-height, WHZ) from those that are small because they are stunted (height-for-age). Wasting and stunting are thought to represent acute and chronic malnutrition and to be appropriately treated, respectively, with an acute intervention to reverse the wasting and prevent death or long term support to the child and family to permit sustained improvement of growth and development. The normal references to which the malnourished children are compared have also been refined successively from the Baldwin-Wood [9], Harvard [10], NCHS [11], CDC_{2000} [12] and more recently to the WHO_{2006} references [13]. The WHO_{2006} references are now promulgated as being standards, rather than references, to which all children should aspire for optimal health [14]. They have rendered all other references obsolete.

Since Waterlow's classification [8], SAM has been defined as children having a low WHZ and/or nutritional oedema. More recently WHO has endorsed the additional criterion of a low absolute MUAC as an independent criterion to classify children with SAM [15]. Therefore the universal definitions of childhood SAM now mandated by WHO are a WHZ of <−3Z of the WHO_{2006} standards or an absolute MUAC of < 115 mm or nutritional oedema, or any combination of these three criteria.

Because of its simplicity, ease of use and relative cheapness as a diagnostic tool MUAC has been readily taken up to screen children for SAM in the community and elsewhere [16]. It can even be used by mothers themselves [17]. The development of a therapeutic food suitable and safe to give at home [18] has led to a revolution in the care of SAM children [19, 20], to scaling up of treatment programs (SUN movement) and "coverage" assessed by the proportion of SAM children diagnosed by MUAC in the community that are receiving treatment [21]. Thus, MUAC has been widely adopted by many agencies and some governments as the preferred criterion for diagnosis of SAM and is used to select children for treatment from the community and health facilities in accordance with WHO recommendations [22]; these agencies no longer assess WHZ and now run "MUAC only" programs. Children admitted by MUAC show as good a response to treatment in the community as those admitted by the WHZ criterion [23] particularly if they have a good appetite, are uncomplicated and are relatively close to the 115 mm threshold. Community programs prevent the milder forms of SAM from deteriorating further and developing complications and have enabled many children to access treatment at home who would otherwise have remained untreated.

Although the prevalence of SAM (and moderate acute malnutrition - MAM), is about the same in nutritional surveys when diagnosed by MUAC and WHZ, different children are identified by the two criteria with a considerable discordance in individual countries [24–41]. We previously collected data from representative community surveys of children from 47 countries to assess the degree of overlap for SAM and MAM by the two anthropometric criteria, to examine the external validity, the scale and direction of discordance and how it varied by country [42]. We found that the two criteria performed quite differently in the various countries and regions, with some diagnosing most SAM children with MUAC and others nearly all SAM children with WHZ. There was no satisfactory explanation for this phenomenon (see [42] for discussion). The mean overlap for SAM (children fulfilling both the WHZ and MUAC criteria) was 16.5%, so that more than 80% of children in the community had SAM by one or the other but not by both criteria. About 45% of the children fulfilled the WHZ definition for SAM but not the MUAC criterion; i.e. they were identified by WHZ alone because they had an absolute MUAC of over 115 mm. As the two diagnostic parameters select different children we proposed that both MUAC and WHZ should continue to be used routinely to identify those children who should receive treatment.

This suggestion led to a direct criticism from Briend et al. [43] who maintain that only MUAC should be used to identify severely malnourished children, that this is a public health priority and nothing should divert resources from universal use of MUAC as the only criterion for diagnosing and selecting children. The position taken by Briend et al. appears to have widespread approval shown by his numerous co-authors and support from humanitarian agencies and donors. However, Briend et al's proposal has led to a controversy among the humanitarian and nutritional community concerning whether WHZ should or should not be abandoned as a criterion for the diagnosis of SAM. A major assertion justifying their point of view is that children with a low WHZ are relatively healthy [44–50] and therefore are not in need of treatment. Briend et al. [43, 46] also contend 1) that WHZ can be abandoned on the grounds that MUAC has repeatedly been shown to be a better indicator of mortality than WHZ, based solely on comparison of receiver operating characteristic curves (ROC) to predict long-term, all-cause mortality risk, 2) that they only have a low WHZ because their legs are relatively long, 3) that the two criteria are proxies for each other and 4) that when children satisfy both criteria their mortality rate is not additive, but that MUAC mortality is always higher than that of WHZ [43, 46, 49–51], and 5) that the addition of WHZ to MUAC does not increase the prognostic sensitivity or specificity of death prediction [51]. These contentions have each been rebutted [52] (rebuttal follows after [43]). At stake is the fate of the 45% of children with SAM by WHZ but not by the MUAC; if they are indeed relatively healthy at a low risk of death then dropping the use of WHZ may have merit, however, if they are at a high risk of death such a policy would lead to a large proportion of SAM children being denied treatment.

The purpose of this study is to address the controversy by examining the relative mortality rates of children who have SAM by the three different WHO recommended criteria; a WHZ of <−3Z using the WHO_{2006} standards, a MUAC of < 115 mm, and nutritional oedema (kwashiorkor and marasmic-kwashiorkor), each separately as well as the various combinations of the three criteria.

Our a priori hypotheses were 1) that children with SAM by MUAC-only and WHZ-only both have a substantial mortality risk, 2) that the two conditions are additive so that children satisfying both criteria have an augmented mortality risk and 3) that nutritional oedema further augments the risk of death. We did not hypothesise that SAM by MUAC-only or WHZ-only would have a higher mortality rate in older or younger children. On one hand younger children are more likely to have a MUAC < 115 mm but also have an inherently higher mortality rate, on the other hand an older child who fulfils the MUAC criterion will be more severely malnourished. Thus, we a priori determined to examine relative mortality by age group.

Methods

We re-analysed data from in-patient treatment facilities (IPFs), out-patient treatment programs (OTPs) and supplementary feeding centres (SFCs) to determine the mortality rates associated with combinations of the different diagnostic criteria: MUAC, WHZ and oedema using the WHO_{2006} recommended criteria that now define marasmus, kwashiorkor and marasmic-kwashiorkor.

In order to have a sufficient number of deaths, admission weight, height, MUAC, oedema, age, sex and outcome data were collected from patients that had been treated for SAM from three sources: 1) Therapeutic feeding centres and hospitals in African countries; these children, with complicated SAM were all under intensive daily care and are collectively referred to as being treated in in-patient facilities (IPFs); 2) Children with uncomplicated SAM with a reasonable appetite were treated in out-patient therapeutic programs (OTPs), and followed weekly; and, 3) Children initially classified as having MAM who were given take-home supplementary food and followed either every 2 weeks or monthly at supplementary feeding centres (SFCs).

All the data were retrospective and involved only children that were being treated using standard WHO therapeutic protocols [53] for earlier studies and updated versions for later studies [54] and for those treated as outpatients [55]. Although the treatment given in each type of program was different, the treatment given in each mode of treatment was standardised according to WHO and updates, derivative National Guidelines on Integrated Management of Severe Malnutrition and derivate Non-Governmental Organisations' (NGO) guidelines. There were only minor differences between the documents. Most programs were carried out by International NGOs so that cross facility and country treatment was the same and the supervisory staff had had the same training at head-quarter level. A few were conducted under the auspices of UNICEF and again followed standard treatment guidelines.

Each child's individual data had been recorded on forms designed specifically for the management of the severely malnourished according to the guidelines (they are not designed for research purposes). During original data collection these were verified by checking with the centres' admission's registry.

The data from all the IPFs, OTPs and SFCs were combined to give three separate datasets of individual patients admitted for one of the three modes of treatment. This was because individual facilities did not contain sufficient deaths to allow for meaningful statistical analysis. Some of the IPF data has already been reported [56]; others were obtained personally for the purpose of program evaluation during visits by MHG and Dr. Yvonne Grellety for National Governments, UNICEF and NGOs; most were from ongoing therapeutic programs by various NGOs.

SFCs should not have recruited any SAM children as these are specifically designed for treatment of MAM children only. However, with the introduction of the WHO_{2006} standards some children who had been classified as moderately malnourished using the NCHS reference or a MUAC cut-off of < 110 mm now satisfied the criteria for SAM with the WHO_{2006} standards and the introduction of a higher MUAC cut-off point as admission criteria for SAM. The data for those children, re-classified as SAM, were abstracted from the SFC data and constitutes a separate dataset for the purpose of this study. As the difference between the NCHS and the WHO standards affect mainly children below about 72 cm in height when NCHS <–3Z was used and all children when < 70% of the NCHS median was used as the admission criterion, the reclassification mainly selected younger children. These children would all have milder forms of SAM as their WHZ fell into the "tram-lines" between the two references; those with more serious illness would have been treated in the OTP or IPF.

The individual datasets from each centre and program had been recorded by the authors or by the staff of the NGO running the program using either SPSS, Epi-info or Excel (various versions). They were all transferred to ENA-for-SMART software [57] and their WHZ computed using the WHO_{2006} gender specific standards.

All children that did not meet at least one of the criteria for SAM, were below 6 or above 60 months or the data for weight, height, MUAC or outcome was absent were excluded. The data were examined for gross errors of recording (such as a child with a height of 10 cm, a weight of 30 kg or a MUAC of 50 mm) which could not occur in children from 6 to 60 months; these records were also excluded. A flow-chat of the data handling and cleaning is given in Fig. 1. No records were excluded on the basis of either WHO or SMART flagging of extreme values; it was assumed that children who were below the cut-off points used during data-cleaning for survey analysis would still fall below the cut-off points for SAM and so were correctly categorised.

As no data were being analysed that depended upon accurate recording of age, where age was not recorded they were retained in the analysis if their heights were between 55 and 115 cm and assigned an age according to their height so that breakdown of the children's outcome into broad age groups would not be biased (71 children: less than 0.01% of all patients). Where oedema was not recorded they were assumed to be oedema free. Oedema status was not recorded for any of the children in SFC as the presence of oedema is a criterion for direct admission to SAM treatment programs; all these children were assumed to be oedema free. Where sex was not recorded they were assigned a sex at random (12 children).

In keeping with intention-to-treat practice, for each dataset, children that defaulted were retained in the analysis as they were at risk of death prior to their default and most deaths from malnutrition occur early after admission before most defaults occur and children in extremis are less likely to default (the numbers of defaulting children are given in Table 1. Children recorded as failing to respond to treatment were retained. The outcome of non-responders and defaulters after quitting the service is unknown; there was no recorded follow-up of such children in any of the programs. Some of the children in the OTP were recorded as "other"; these were children who moved out of the catchment area, were transferred to a different OTP or started their treatment in the IPF and continued treatment successfully in the OTP. They were retained in the analysis (they were not included in the IPF data).

Children from the SFC who were recorded as being transferred to an OTP or IPF were excluded if the data from the receiving treatment facility were available, otherwise they were included. Similarly, for the OTP, children that were transferred to the IPF were excluded from the analysis if the corresponding IPF data were available, otherwise they were included (i.e. no child was counted in both programs). Children that were transferred to other facilities from the IPF were included in the analysis and assumed to have survived; they were mostly children sent for surgery, tuberculosis or other specialised treatment after their initial severe malnutrition has been successfully managed.

The absolute numbers of children admitted in one of the following categories was determined for each data set divided by whether they left the program alive or dead. Children having:

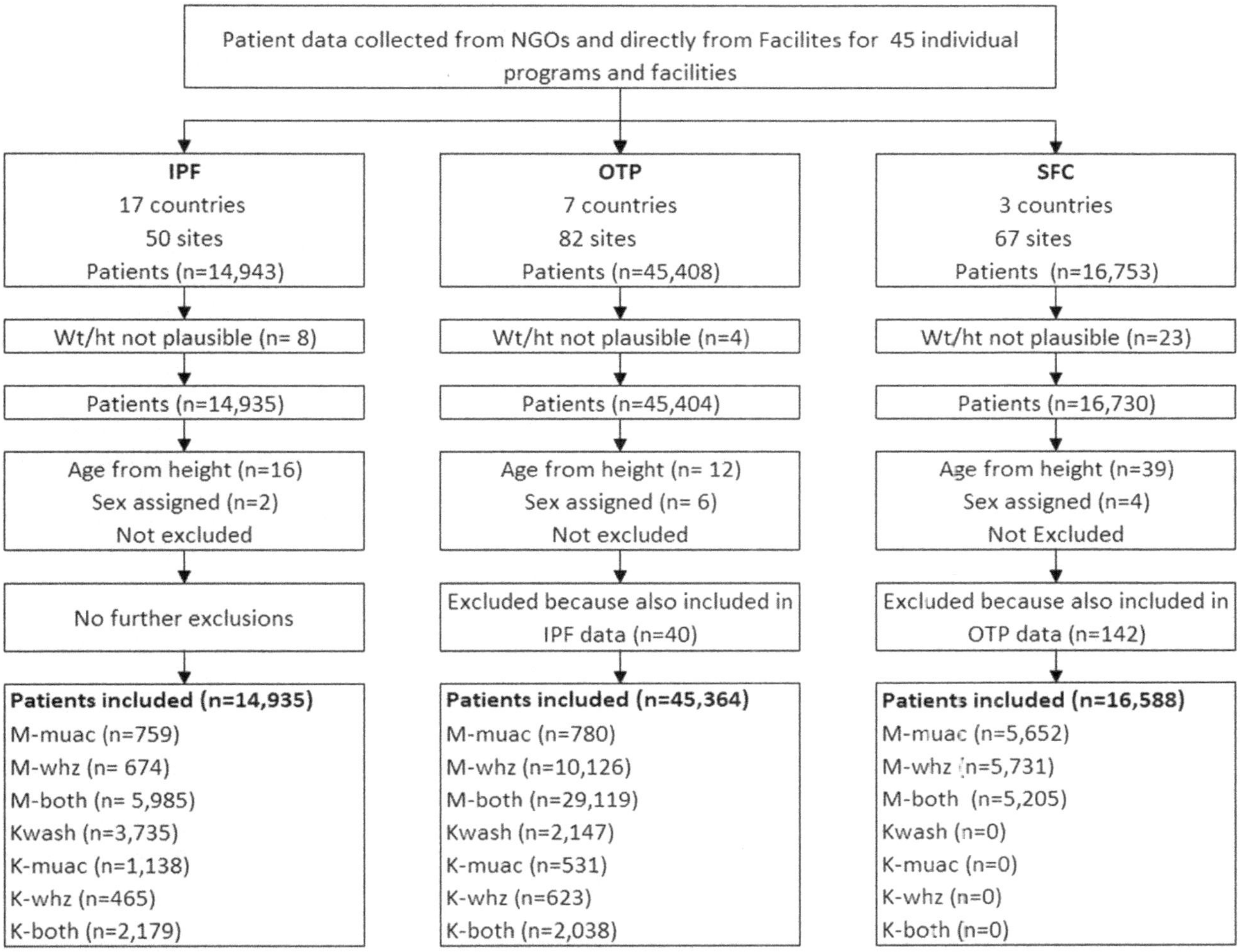

Fig. 1 Flow chart of analyses of admissions for treatment of Severe Acute Malnutrition in Africa. *NGO's* Non-Governmental Organizations; *IPF* In-patient Facility (Hospital. Therapeutic Feeding Center); *OTP* Out-patient Treatment Program (Home treatment); *SFC* Supplementary Feeding Center; *Wt/ht* Weight or height; *M-muac* MUAC < 115 mm with WHZ ≥ −3Z and no oedema (marasmus by MUAC only); *M-whz* WHZ < −3Z with MUAC ≥115 mm and no oedema (marasmus by WHZ only); *M-both* MUAC < 115 mm & WHZ < −3Z and no oedema (marasmus by both diagnostic criteria); *Kwash* nutritional oedema/Kwashiorkor without meeting either MUAC or WHZ criteria; *K-muac* oedema & MUAC < 115 mm with WHZ ≥ −3Z (marasmic kwashiorkor by MUAC only); *K-whz* oedema & WHZ < −3Z with MUAC ≥115 mm (marasmic kwashiorkor by WHZ only); *K-both* oedema & MUAC < 115 mm & WHZ < −3Z (marasmic kwashiorkor by both diagnostic criteria)

1. MUAC < 115 mm as the only criterion for admission (WHZ ≥ −3Z, no oedema) - (M-muac);
2. WHZ < −3Z as the only criterion for admission (MUAC ≥115 mm, no oedema) - (M-whz);
3. MUAC < 115 mm and WHZ < −3Z (no oedema) - (M-both);
4. oedema with MUAC ≥115 mm and WHZ ≥ −3Z - (Kwash);
5. oedema with MUAC < 115 mm and WHZ ≥ −3Z - (K-muac);
6. oedema with MUAC ≥115 mm and WHZ < −3Z - (K-whz);
7. oedema with MUAC < 115 mm and WHZ < −3Z - (K-both).

The abbreviations given in parenthesis are used where M- indicates marasmus, K- indicates kwashiorkor/ oedematous malnutrition, "muac" is used when the *only* anthropometric criterion is a MUAC of < 115 mm, "whz" when the *only* anthropometric criterion is a WHZ < −3Z WHO_{2006}, and the suffix "both" when the child has both a MUAC < 115 mm and a WHZ < −3Z.

The data for non-oedematous and oedematous children were analysed separately. Those children who were alive at exit from the program compared to those that had died were analysed by 2 × 3 and 2 × 4 Chi-squared analysis respectively. The post-hoc individual comparisons were made using the Marascuilo procedure [58, 59]. The complete data were also analysed using a 2 × 7 chi-squared analysis with post hoc Marascuilo comparisons to confirm the significance of comparisons of interest with increased degrees of freedom (data not presented as they include a number of comparisons that were not considered a priori).

The individual comparisons were then re-tested by grouping all the children with a low MUAC (i.e. M-muac + M-both) to give a count of all the children admitted who had a low MUAC – designated as "ALL-muac". Similarly all children with a low WHZ (M-whz + M-both) were combined to be analysed as "ALL-whz". This was repeated with the K-muac, K-whz and K-both groups and also with the grand total of oedematous and non-oedematous children combined. These additional analyses were made because most of the published literature on comparison of MUAC and WHZ criteria for diagnosis of SAM includes children that are oedematous and most do not distinguish those who have a single deficit from those that have both a low MUAC and a low WHZ (studies reviewed in the companion paper – [60]).

Because we anticipated that there would be a difference in the relative mortality in younger and older age groups all the analyses were repeated using children 6 to < 18, 18 to < 36 and 36 to 60 months of age.

To determine whether there were regional differences in case fatality rates (CFRs) of children who were admitted by MUAC-only or WHZ-only we combined the data from countries within each region of Africa (see Additional file 1: Table S1 for combinations of countries) by treatment program for comparison of the respective mortality risks. The data were analysed by binary meta-analysis using MetaXL version 5.3 [61]. The odds ratios comparing the case fatality rates for children admitted with M-muac v M-whz and also K-Muac v K-whz were compared using Peto's method [62] of weighting the groups. No adjustment for the quality of each set of data was made. We did not have sufficient access to any potential confounding data to adjust for confounding.

Ethical statement

This is a secondary analysis of existing anonymous data which had been collected and analysed for programmatic purposes: that is, to audit services, compare the performance with the Sphere standards [63], identify were performance needed improvement and assess case-loads for future staff and product requirement planning. As no individual, location or administrative district could be identified formal ethical clearance was not required.

Results

The children's countries of residence, mode of treatment and outcomes are shown in Table 1. The corresponding breakdown of the children by diagnostic criteria is given in Additional file 2: Table S2. There were 76,887 children with SAM in the three modes of treatment of which 3588 died. They are divided into the 7 different diagnostic categories of SAM depending upon the criteria present at the time of admission. Their mortality rates are presented by mode of treatment and age group in Table 2. The significances of the paired differences between the diagnostic groups are given Table 3. Figs. 2 and 3 show, respectively, the CFRs and the relative risks of death (RR) calculated against M-muac (the lowest RR) to show how the risks of death for each of the 7 categories of patient relate to one another. The data for the IPF and OTP combined (i.e. excluding those children reclassified as SAM from the SFC) are given in Additional file 3: Table S3.

Considering marasmus, overall the mortality is significantly higher in those with WHZ < –3Z than in those with MUAC < 115 mm. WHZ-only children also had a higher mortality in each of the age groups although this does not reach significance in the children 36 to 60 months. The children who had both anthropometric deficits had more than twice the mortality of either the WHZ-only or the MUAC-only groups. The children with complicated SAM (IPF) and those without complications (OTP) show the same pattern of mortality, but, as expected, it is higher in the complicated than uncomplicated cases. For both the complicated and un-complicated cases examined separately, the higher mortality with WHZ than with MUAC was present in each of the age groups. There was no indication that MUAC mortality dominated death in either the younger or older age groups. WHZ-only consistently had equivalent or higher mortality than MUAC-only across all age groups.

For the oedematous children, those without severe wasting (Kwash) had about the same mortality rate as the marasmic children with both anthropometric deficits (M-both), but higher than children with single deficits. It was significantly higher in the complicated than the uncomplicated cases; this is presumably because only children with mild or moderate oedema are admitted to the OTPs whereas those with severe oedema are always admitted to the IPF as well as those with complications. Table 2 also shows the RR of oedematous children calculated against those without an anthropometrical deficit (Kwash). The children with oedema and a low MUAC (K-muac) did not have a higher mortality than oedematous cases without a low MUAC (Kwash) in either the OTP or IPF so that the addition of the MUAC criterion to oedematous cases did not increase their mortality risk (K-muac). This is in marked contrast to the children with oedema and a WHZ below <–3Z (K-whz); these particular children in both the OTP and IPF experienced a very high CFR and a RR of between 2 and 3 times the risk for children with either Kwash or K-muac. Their mortality was, well above the Sphere standards. The fact that the severely oedematous cases (+++) were not included in the

Table 1 Outcome of patients admitted for treatment of SAM by treatment program and country

Data characteristics	Defaulter		Recovery		Death		Non-response		Other		Transfer		Total
	9893	12.9	58,097	75.6	3588	4.7	3490	4.5	1062	1.4	758	1.0	76,887
	n	%	n	%	n	%	n	%	n	%	n	%	n
IPFs by countries													
Angola	34	8.4	346	85.6	24	5.9	0	0.0	0	0.0	0	0.0	404
Burundi	202	13.2	1134	73.9	147	9.6	0	0.0	0	0.0	51	3.3	1534
Chad	59	12.2	364	75.5	26	5.4	0	0.0	0	0.0	33	6.8	482
Congo	21	7.6	236	85.5	19	6.9	0	0.0	0	0.0	0	0.0	276
DRC	249	8.9	2342	83.6	150	5.4	23	0.8	0	0.0	37	1.3	2801
Ethiopia	83	21.1	256	65.1	52	13.2	0	0.0	0	0.0	2	0.5	393
Guinea	18	3.7	417	85.5	44	9.0	0	0.0	0	0.0	9	1.8	488
Kenya	70	15.8	275	62.2	52	11.8	42	9.5	0	0.0	3	0.7	442
Liberia	76	11.3	528	78.5	44	6.5	2	0.3	0	0.0	23	3.4	673
Mali	23	10.4	171	77.4	27	12.2	0	0.0	0	0.0	0	0.0	221
Rwanda	150	9.2	1225	74.7	174	10.6	22	1.3	0	0.0	68	4.1	1639
Sierra Leon	18	16.4	71	64.5	8	7.3	0	0.0	0	0.0	13	11.8	110
Somalia	92	31.6	160	55.0	27	9.3	0	0.0	0	0.0	12	4.1	291
South Sudan	14	8.3	143	84.6	3	1.8	1	0.6	0	0.0	8	4.7	169
Sudan	366	30.3	684	56.7	74	6.1	5	0.4	0	0.0	77	6.4	1206
Tanzania	64	11.4	470	84.1	12	2.1	0	0.0	0	0.0	13	2.3	559
Uganda	550	16.9	2106	64.9	530	16.3	38	1.2	0	0.0	23	0.7	3247
Total	2089	14.0	10,928	73.2	1413	9.5	133	0.9	0	0.0	372	2.5	14,935
OTPs by countries													
Chad	61	29.5	106	51.2	7	3.4	20	9.7	0	0.0	13	6.3	207
DRC	73	2.6	2496	90.2	141	5.1	16	0.6	0	0.0	40	1.4	2766
Ethiopia	17	11.5	91	61.5	23	15.5	17	11.5	0	0.0	0	0.0	148
Kenya	4	8.2	33	67.3	4	8.2	8	16.3	0	0.0	0	0.0	49
Niger	4229	10.5	33,077	82.1	1848	4.6	138	0.3	789	2.0	191	0.5	40,271
South Sudan	76	9.8	665	85.9	20	2.6	12	1.6	1	0.1	0	0.0	774
Uganda	107	9.3	954	83.0	21	1.8	67	5.8	0	0.0	0	0.0	1149
Total	4567	10.1	37,422	82.5	2064	4.5	278	0.6	790	1.7	244	0.5	45,364
SFCs by countries													
DRC	185	7.3	1716	67.6	21	0.8	203	8.0	272	10.7	142	5.6	2539
Kenya	262	22.7	209	18.1	3	0.3	679	58.9	0	0.0	0	0.0	1153
Uganda	2790	21.6	7822	60.7	87	0.7	2197	17.0	0	0.0	0	0.0	12,896
Total	3237	19.5	9747	58.8	111	0.7	3079	18.6	272	1.5	142	0.9	16,588

IPF In-patient Facility (Hospital. Therapeutic Feeding Center), *OTP* Out-patient treatment program (Home treatment), *SFC* Supplementary Feeding Centre, *DRC* Democratic Republic of Congo

OTP group did not seem to ameliorate the mortality rate of the K-whz children treated as outpatients compared to those treated in the IPFs. Furthermore, addition of a low MUAC to those who already had a low WHZ and oedema (K-both) did not further augment the mortality rate over those with oedema and a low WHZ (K-whz). Thus, the presence or absence of a MUAC below 115 mm in the oedematous children appears to be without significance in terms of increasing their mortality risk; this is in marked contrast to WHZ where there was a profound increase in risk.

In comparison with those children with only a MUAC < 115 mm, each diagnostic category had a significantly higher relative CFR and RR (Figs. 2 & 3). In the case of the children with a WHZ < −3Z and oedema the death rate was between 6 to 12 times as high as those with

Table 2 Total numbers, deaths, case-fatality rates and relative risk of death of children with SAM by diagnostic criteria, treatment program and age group

SAM type	All patients							In patients (IPF)							Outpatients (OTP)							SFC				
Age group	Total	Dead	*CFR*	RR	95% CI	RR	95% CI	Total	Dead	*CFR*	RR	95% CI	RR	95% CI	Total	Dead	*CFR*	RR	95% CI	RR	95% CI	Total	Dead	*CFR*	RR	95% CI
6–60 m	#	#	%					#	#	%					#	#	%					#	#	%		
M-muac	7191	56	*0.78*	Ref.	—	—	—	759	21	*2.77*	Ref.	—	—	—	780	9	*1.15*	Ref.	—	—	—	5652	26	*0.46*	Ref.	—
M-whz	16,531	332	*2.01*	2.58	1.9–3.4	—	—	674	27	*4.01*	1.45	0.8–2.5	—	—	10,126	280	*2.77*	2.40	0.8–2.5	—	—	5731	25	*0.44*	0.95	0.5–1.6
M-both	40,309	2000	*4.96*	6.37	4.9–8.3	—	—	5985	559	*9.34*	3.38	2.2–5.2	—	—	29,119	1381	*4.74*	4.11	2.2–5.2	—	—	5205	60	*1.15*	2.51	1.6–4.0
Kwash	5882	337	*5.73*	7.36	5.6–9.7	Ref.	—	3735	262	*7.01*	2.54	1.6–3.9	Ref.	—	2147	75	*3.49*	3.03	1.6–3.9	Ref.	—	—	—	—	—	—
K-muac	1669	118	*7.07*	9.08	6.6–12	1.23	1.0–1.5	1138	100	*8.79*	3.18	2.0–5.0	1.25	1.0–1.6	531	18	*3.39*	2.94	2.0–5.0	0.97	0.6–1.6	—	—	—	—	—
K-whz	1088	169	*15.53*	19.95	15–27	2.71	2.3–3.2	465	77	*16.56*	5.98	3.7–9.6	2.36	1.9–3.0	623	92	*14.77*	12.80	3.7–9.6	4.23	3.2–5.6	—	—	—	—	—
K-both	4217	576	*13.66*	17.54	13–23	2.38	2.1–2.7	2179	367	*16.84*	6.09	4–9.4	2.40	2.1–2.8	2038	209	*10.26*	8.89	4–9.4	2.94	2.3–3.8	—	—	—	—	—
Total	76,887	3588	*4.67*					14,935	1413	*9.46*					45,364	2064	*4.55*					16,588	111	*0.67*		
6 - < 18 m	#	#	%					#	#	%					#	#	%					#	#	%		
M-muac	4650	32	*0.69*	Ref.	—	—	—	246	8	3.25	Ref.	—	—	—	298	5	*1.68*	Ref.	—	—	—	4106	19	*0.46*	Ref.	—
M-whz	5906	124	*2.10*	3.05	2.1–4.5	—	—	208	13	6.25	1.92	0.8–4.5	—	—	2901	94	*3.24*	1.93	0.8–4.7	—	—	2797	17	*0.61*	1.31	0.7–2.5
M-both	21,095	1073	*5.09*	7.39	5.2–10	—	—	2703	307	11.37	3.50	1.8–7.0	—	—	14,416	721	*5.00*	2.98	1.2–7.1	—	—	3976	45	*1.13*	2.45	1.4–4.2
Kwash	667	33	*4.95*	7.19	4.5–12	Ref.		290	17	5.86	1.80	0.8–4.1	Ref.		377	16	*4.24*	2.53	0.9–6.8	Ref.		—	—	—	—	—
K-muac	462	20	*4.33*	6.29	3.6–11	0.87	0.5–1.5	231	16	6.93	2.13	0.9–4.9	1.18	0.6–2.3	231	4	*1.73*	1.03	0.3–3.8	0.41	0.1–1.2	—	—	—	—	—
K-whz	194	26	*13.40*	19.47	12–32	2.71	1.7–4.4	63	10	15.87	4.88	2.0–12	2.71	1.3–5.6	131	16	*12.21*	7.28	2.7–19	1.63	0.8–3.2	—	—	—	—	—
K-both	1264	155	*12.26*	17.82	12–26	2.48	1.7–3.6	579	90	15.54	4.78	2.4–9.7	2.65	1.6–4.4	685	65	*9.49*	5.66	2.3–14	2.24	1.3–3.8	—	—	—	—	—
Total	34,238	1463	*4.27*					4320	461	*10.68*					19,039	921	*4.84*					10,879	81	*0.74*		
18 - < 36 m	#	#	%					#	#	%					#	#	%					#	#	%		
M-muac	1973	16	*0.81*	Ref.	—	—	—	242	8	*3.31*	Ref.	—	—	—	376	2	*0.53*	Ref.	—	—	—	1355	6	*0.44*	Ref.	—
M-whz	8044	171	*2.13*	2.62	1.6–4.4	—	—	242	7	*2.89*	0.88	0.3–2.4	—	—	6143	158	*2.57*	4.84	1.2–19	—	—	1659	6	*0.36*	0.82	0.3–2.5
M-both	16,506	774	*4.69*	5.78	3.5–9.5	—	—	2110	169	*8.01*	2.42	1.2–4.9	—	—	13,289	594	*4.47*	8.40	2.1–34	—	—	1107	11	*0.99*	2.24	0.8–6.0
Kwash	2510	138	*5.50*	6.78	4.1–11	Ref.		1393	99	*7.11*	2.15	1.1–4.4	Ref.		1117	39	*3.49*	6.56	1.6–27	Ref.		—	—	—	—	—
K-muac	655	43	*6.56*	8.10	4.6–14	1.19	0.8–1.7	444	35	*7.88*	2.38	1.1–5.1	1.11	0.8–1.6	211	8	*3.79*	7.13	1.5–33	1.09	0.5–2.3	—	—	—	—	—
K-whz	574	83	*14.46*	17.83	11–30	2.63	2.0–3.4	173	32	*18.50*	5.60	2.6–12	2.60	1.8–3.7	401	51	*12.72*	23.91	5.9–97	3.64	2.4–5.4	—	—	—	—	—
K-both	2139	275	*12.86*	15.85	9.6–26	2.34	1.9–2.8	976	160	*16.39*	4.96	2.5–9.9	2.31	1.8–2.9	1163	115	*9.89*	18.59	4.6–75	2.83	2.0–4.0	—	—	—	—	—
Total	32,401	1500	*4.63*					5580	510	*9.14*					22,700	967	*4.26*					4121	23	*0.56*		

Table 2 Total numbers, deaths, case-fatality rates and relative risk of death of children with SAM by diagnostic criteria, treatment program and age group *(Continued)*

SAM type	All patients							In patients (IPF)							Outpatients (OTP)							SFC				
Age group	Total	Dead	*CFR*	RR	95% CI	RR	95% CI	Total	Dead	*CFR*	RR	95% CI	RR	95% CI	Total	Dead	*CFR*	RR	95% CI	RR	95% CI	Total	Dead	*CFR*	RR	95% CI
36–60 m	#	#	%					#	#	%					#	#	%					#	#	%		
M-muac	568	8	*1.41*	Ref.	—	—	—	271	5	*1.85*	Ref.	—	—	—	106	2	*1.89*	Ref.	—	—	—	191	1	*0.52*	Ref.	—
M-whz	2581	37	*1.43*	1.02	0.5–2.2	—	—	224	7	*3.13*	1.69	0.5–5.3	—	—	1082	28	*2.59*	1.37	0.3–5.7	—	—	1275	2	*0.16*	0.30	0.0–3.3
M-both	2708	153	*5.65*	4.01	2.0–8.1	—	—	1172	83	*7.08*	3.84	1.6–9.4	—	—	1414	66	*4.67*	2.47	0.6–10	—	—	122	4	*3.28*	6.26	0.7–55
Kwash	2705	166	*6.14*	4.36	2.2–8.8	Ref.	—	2052	146	*7.12*	3.86	1.6–9.3	Ref.	—	653	20	*3.06*	1.62	0.4–6.8	Ref.	—	—	—	—	—	—
K-muac	552	55	*9.96*	7.07	3.4–15	1.62	1.2–2.2	463	49	*10.58*	5.74	2.3–14	1.49	1.2–2.0	89	6	*6.74*	3.57	0.7–17	2.20	0.9–5.3	—	—	—	—	—
K-whz	320	60	*18.75*	13.31	6.4–27	3.06	2.3–4.0	229	35	*15.28*	8.28	3.3–21	2.15	1.5–3.0	91	25	*27.47*	14.56	3.5–60	8.97	5.2–15	—	—	—	—	—
K-both	814	146	*17.94*	12.73	6.3–26	2.92	2.4–3.6	624	117	*18.75*	10.16	4.2–25	2.64	2.1–3.3	190	29	*15.26*	8.09	2.0–33	4.98	2.9–8.6	—	—	—	—	—
Total	10,248	625	*6.10*					5035	442	*8.78*					3625	176	*4.86*					1588	7	*0.44*		

IPF In-patient Facility (Hospital. Therapeutic Feeding Center); *OTP* Out-patient treatment program (Home treatment); *SFC* Supplementary Feeding Center; *M-muac* MUAC < 115 mm with WHZ ≥ −3Z and no oedema (marasmus by MUAC only); *M-whz* WHZ < −3Z with MUAC ≥115 mm and no oedema (marasmus by WHZ only); *M-Both* MUAC < 115 mm & WHZ < −3Z and no oedema (marasmus by both diagnostic criteria); *Kwash* nutritional oedema/Kwashiorkor without meeting either MUAC or WHZ criteria; *K-muac* oedema & MUAC < 115 mm with WHZ ≥ −3Z (marasmic kwashiorkor by MUAC only); *K-whz* oedema & WHZ < −3Z with MUAC ≥115 mm (marasmic kwashiorkor by WHZ only); *K-Both* oedema & MUAC < 115 mm & WHZ < −3Z (marasmic kwashiorkor by both diagnostic criteria); *CFR* Case Fatality Rate %; *RR* Relative Risk of death; *95% CI* 95% Confidence interval. Significance tests are given in Table 3

Table 3 Significance levels of comparisons between diagnostic groups using Marascuilo post-hoc analysis procedure

Children with marasmus				
Comparisons	All	IPF	OTP	SFC
0–60 m	p	p	p	p
muac v whz	0.000	ns	0.001	ns
muac v both	0.000	0.000	0.000	0.000
whz v both	0.000	0.000	0.000	0.000
6 - < 18 m				
muac v whz	0.000	ns	ns	ns
muac v both	0.000	0.000	0.000	0.003
whz v both	0.000	0.017	0.000	ns
18 - < 36 m				
muac v whz	0.000	ns	0.000	ns
muac v both	0.000	0.001	0.000	ns
whz v both	0.000	0.000	0.000	ns
36–60 m				
muac v whz	ns	ns	ns	ns
muac v both	0.000	0.000	ns	ns
whz v both	0.000	0.017	0.019	ns
Children with kwashiorKor/marasmic-kwashiorKor				
Comparisons	All	IPF	OTP	
0–60 m	*p*	*p*	*p*	
K-muac v Kwash	ns	ns	ns	
K-whz v Kwash	0.000	0.000	0.000	
K-both v Kwash	0.000	0.000	0.000	
K-muac v K-whz	0.000	0.001	0.000	
K-muac v K-both	0.000	0.000	0.000	
K-whz v K-both	ns	ns	0.041	
6 - < 18 m				
K-muac v Kwash	ns	ns	ns	
K-whz v Kwash	0.014	ns	ns	
K-both v Kwash	0.000	0.000	ns	
K-muac v K-whz	0.007	ns	0.006	
K-muac v K-both	0.000	0.002	0.000	
K-whz v K-both	ns	ns	ns	
18 - < 36 m				
K-muac v Kwash	ns	ns	ns	
K-whz v Kwash	0.000	0.003	0.000	
K-both v Kwash	0.000	0.000	0.000	
K-muac v K-whz	0.000	0.012	0.001	
K-muac v K-both	0.000	0.000	0.002	
K-whz v K-both	ns	ns	ns	
36–60 m				
K-muac v Kwash	0.047	ns	ns	
K-whz v Kwash	0.000	0.011	0.000	

Table 3 Significance levels of comparisons between diagnostic groups using Marascuilo post-hoc analysis procedure *(Continued)*

Children with marasmus				
Comparisons	All	IPF	OTP	SFC
K-both v Kwash	0.000	0.000	0.000	
K-muac v K-whz	0.007	ns	0.002	
K-muac v K-both	0.000	0.002	ns	
K-whz v K-both	ns	ns	ns	

Abbreviations are given in Table 2; *ns* not significant at $p < 0.05$

only a MUAC < 115 mm. These observations did not change by age group, although the numbers of deaths in the older age group and in the children admitted to SFC was insufficient to reach significance.

Meta-analysis showing regional differences

Figure 4 shows the forest-plot of the meta-analysis by programs from the different regions of Africa comparing WHZ-only with MUAC-only. The countries that constituted each of the regions are given in Additional file 4: Table S4 (OTP of oedematous children from West Africa is omitted from the plot for formatting reasons. The odds ratio in favour of K-whz over K-muac was very high – 17.8, CI = 7.5–41.9 – but is included in the statistics and sensitivity analyses given in Additional file 5: Table S5). Overall the odds ratio of death was 1.7 times higher for the children with only a WHZ < −3Z that those with only a MUAC < 115 mm. There were regional differences; for each of the modes of treatment (IPF, OTP, SFC) WHZ carried a higher risk of death than MUAC in the Central, West and Sahelian countries for both non-oedematous and oedematous children. In contrast, marasmic children in the East African group (Kenya, Tanzania, Uganda, Ethiopia) had a lower risk of death with WHZ than with MUAC, albeit not significantly.

The same data are analysed by oedema status and presented in Fig. 5. They show that for marasmic children the odds ratio is marginally significant at 1.37 (95% CI, 0.99–1.90) whereas for oedematous children the odds ratio for death with K-whz is twice that of K-muac (2.03, CI 1.50–2.75). The East African data in particular shows a discordance between the children without oedema and those with oedema.

Simpson's paradox

In Table 4 the case fatality rates for the patients with MUAC-alone, WHZ-alone and both combined are shown and compared with all the cases with a low MUAC (All-muac = M-muac + M-both) and all the WHZ cases (All-whz = M-whz + M-both). As shown in Table 2, for marasmic cases each comparison is highly

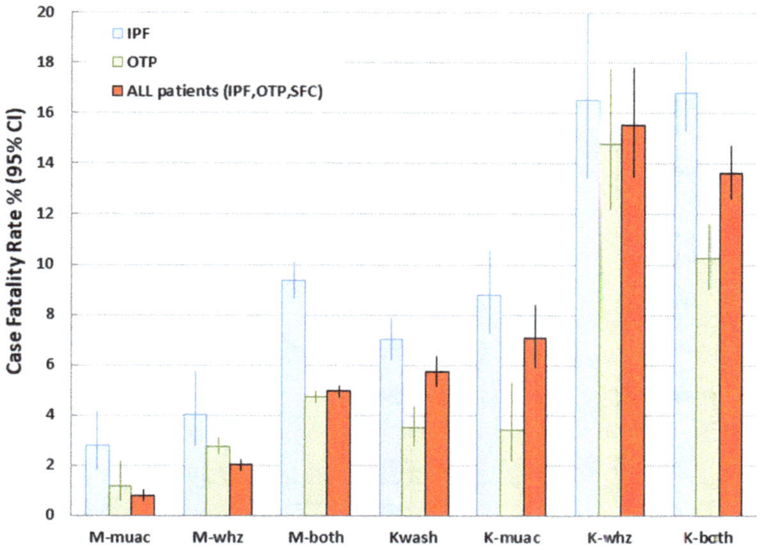

Fig. 2 Case-fatality rates of children with SAM aged 6–60 by diagnostic criteria and treatment program. *IPF* In-patient Facility; *OTP* Out-patient Treatment Program; *All patients* refers to the combined totals of children in the IPF, OTP and the SFC (Supplementary Feeding Center); *M-muac* MUAC < 115 mm with WHZ ≥ −3Z and no oedema; *M-whz* WHZ < −3Z with MUAC ≥115 mm and no oedema; *M-both* MUAC < 115 mm & WHZ < −3Z and no oedema; *Kwash* nutritional oedema/Kwashiorkor without meeting either MUAC or WHZ criteria; *K-muac* oedema & MUAC < 115 mm with WHZ ≥ −3Z; *K-whz* oedema & WHZ < −3Z with MUAC ≥115 mm; *K-both* oedema & MUAC < 115 mm & WHZ < −3Z; *CFR* Case fatality rate

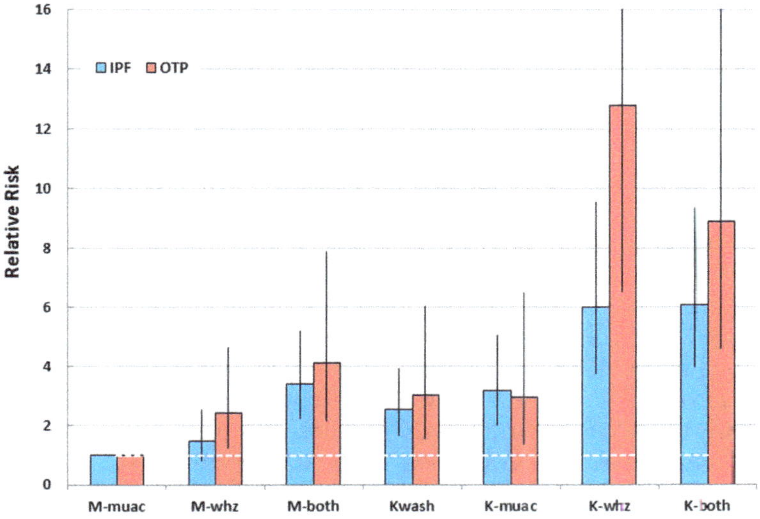

Fig. 3 Relative Risks of death (RR) of children with SAM aged 6–60 months by diagnostic criteria and treatment program. The relative risks of death are calculated against marasmic children by MUAC only (M-muac). The error bars are the 95% confidence intervals. *IPF* In-patient Facility; *OTP* Out-patient Treatment Program; *M-muac* MUAC < 115 mm with WHZ ≥ −3Z and no oedema; *M-whz* WHZ < −3Z with MUAC ≥115 mm and no oedema; *M-both* MUAC < 115 mm & WHZ < −3Z and no oedema; *Kwash* nutritional oedema/Kwashiorkor without meeting either MUAC or WHZ criteria; *K-muac* oedema & MUAC < 115 mm with WHZ ≥ −3Z; *K-whz* oedema & WHZ < −3Z with MUAC ≥115 mm; *K-both* oedema & MUAC < 115 mm & WHZ < −3Z; *RR* Relative Risk of death

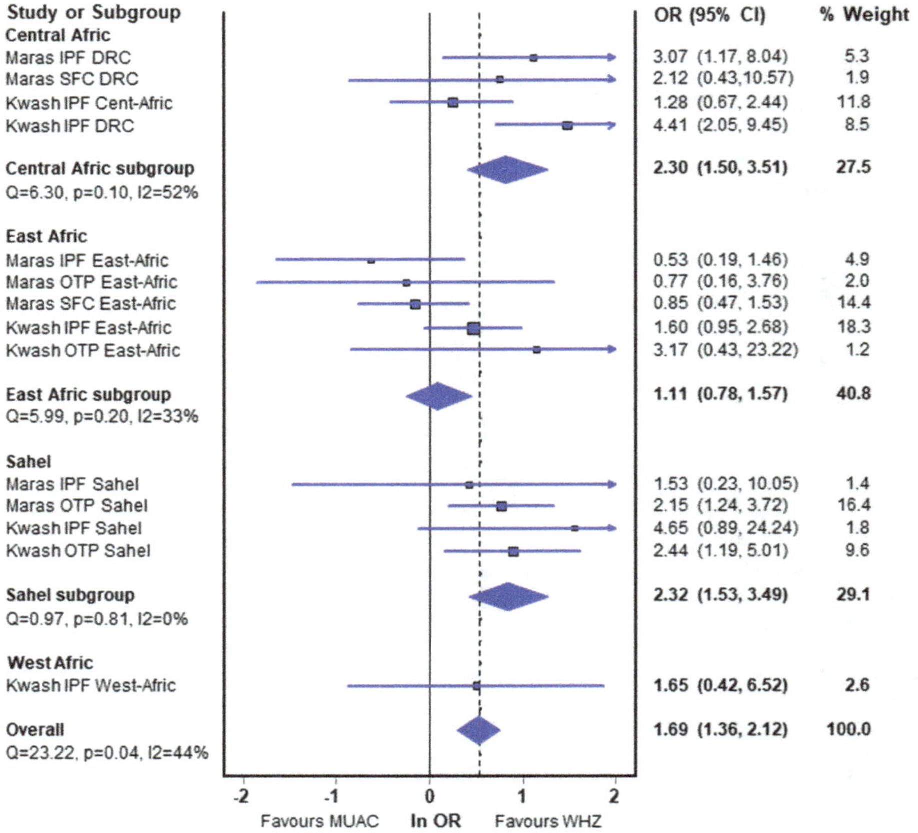

Fig. 4 Forest plot by region comparing Odds ratios of the risk of death of M-muac v M-whz. *Maras* Marasmus (M-muac vs M-whz); *Kwash* nutritional oedema (K-muac vs K-whz); *IPF* In-patient Facility; *OTP* Out-patient Treatment Program; *SFC* Supplementary Feeding Center; *DRC* Democratic Republic of Congo. The countries contributing data from each region are given in Additional file 2: Table S3. The statistical data are given in Additional file 4: Table S4 and the sensitivity analysis in Additional file 5: Table S5. Please note that the data for OTP West Africa has been omitted from this plot due to issues of presentation, but the data including this program is given in the additional files. In each of the forest plots "favours WHZ" indicates that the Odds ratio for death is higher in children with WHZ < −3Z than with a MUAC of < 115 mm; "favours MUAC" indicates that the Odds ratio for children with a MUAC < 115 mm is higher than those with WHZ < −3Z

significant with WHZ having a higher mortality than MUAC when the children fulfilling each criterion alone are considered. Table 4 shows that when the children with both defects are added to the WHZ and the MUAC categories not only is the difference now non-significant, but the CFR is *reversed* so that MUAC now appears to have a *higher* mortality than WHZ. For the oedematous children the ratio is not quite reversed, but the apparent mortality of MUAC has increased and that of WHZ decreased. When all the SAM children are considered, that is oedematous and non-oedematous SAM combined, again the relative mortality is significantly higher in children with a low WHZ when considered alone, but this is reversed when the children with both criteria are incorporated into the MUAC and the WHZ groups.

This is an example of extreme confounding, in this case due to mathematical coupling, leading to Simpson's paradox where there is a paradoxical reversal of the estimated mortality risk to give an erroneous result when groups of children are inappropriately combined.

Discussion

To judge whether using any of the 3 recognised WHO diagnostic criteria for SAM can be dropped, the critical factor is to focus on the potential fate of those children who would then become systematically ineligible for treatment and omitted from care. About 45% of SAM children in the community fulfil the WHZ but not the MUAC criterion [42]. Any advocates that propose elimination of children fulfilling WHZ criteria from treatment should demonstrate that both their risk of death and the other detrimental effects of being severely malnourished are trivial or at least substantially lower than those diagnosed using MUAC. Our data demonstrate that children with a WHZ less than -3Z but a MUAC of above 115 mm are at high risk of death, at least as high as or

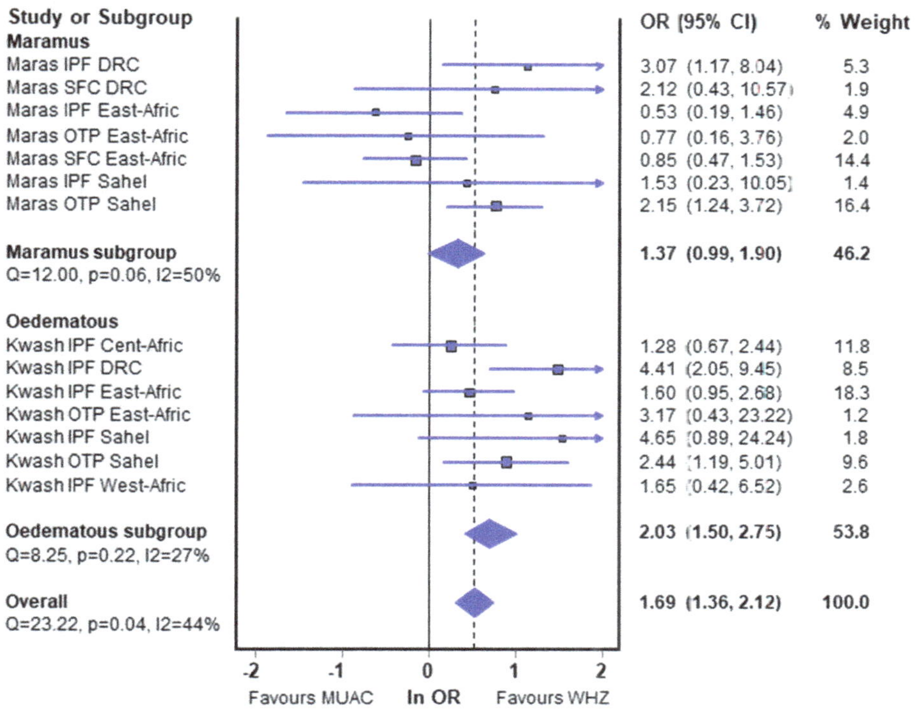

Fig. 5 Forest plot by oedema status (marasmus vs kwasiorkor) region comparing Odds ratios of the risk of death of children admitted with WHZ < −3Z only against MUAC < 115 mm only. *Maras* Marasmus (M-muac vs M-whz); *Kwash* nutritional oedema (K-muac vs K-whz); *IPF* In-patient Facility; *OTP* Out-patient Treatment Program; *SFC* Supplementary Feeding Center; *DRC* Democratic Republic of Congo

higher than those with a low MUAC across each of the age groups. On this evidence there is no place to cease the use of WHZ as an independent criterion for the admission and treatment of SAM children; agencies and governments that have adopted a MUAC-only policy should reflect upon the provisions of their guidelines, and where appropriate reverse the MUAC-only policy and maintain using the current WHO guidance.

It would appear that the contentions put forward by Briend et al. and others [43, 46, 49–51] are incorrect (see also the companion paper [60] where the literature is reviewed). In particular the contention that children with a WHZ below -3Z are relatively healthy with a low risk of death. This is justified by reference to a review on leg length and beauty which does not mention wasting let alone marasmus [64]. This contention is without evidence and contrary to common sense and clinical experience in all age groups [65]. In fact there are abundant data to confirm that low WHZ itself caries a substantial risk of death [66–78]. Although none of these papers also measured MUAC to determine whether the deaths occurred in patients that had a concomitant low MUAC and would therefore be identified by both criteria. Given the low rate of concordance it is unlikely that the majority of deaths occurred in children with both deficits. Of interest is the paper by Katz et al. [72] who show a much higher mortality risk for WHZ (< 80% NCHS) in older than younger children, when they are less likely to have a low MUAC. Briend is a co-author on O'Neill et al's paper [76] where BMI-for-age (closely related to WHZ) is a better predictor of mortality than MUAC and WHZ itself has a dramatic impact on mortality.

Briend et al. also assert that the discrepancy is simply because children with a low WHZ have longer legs, whereas the only papers that have addressed this issue show this is, at best, a minor contributor [32, 42, 79] and the original authors are clear that long legs do not explain the discrepancy between WHZ and MUAC. Long legs do not account for the fact that in most surveys different children are identified by WHZ and MUAC. The discrepancy is more likely due to differences in body build, rather than linear growth; a concern of auxologists in early studies which has not been considered in deriving modern standards [9, 80]. What is not clear is whether endomorphic children, with narrow torsos, who are more likely to have a lower WHZ, have a different risk of death than exomorphic children. We speculate that endomorphic children have a higher risk of death than exomorphic children, in the

Table 4 Effect of combining the diagnostic groups together to show Simpson's paradox

Effect of combining diagnostic groups					
Subgroups	Total #	dead #	CFR %	comparisons	*p*
All-muac v All-whz without oedeam					
M-muac	7191	56	0.78	muac v whz	0.000
M-whz	16,530	332	2.01	muac v both	0.000
M-both	40,307	2000	4.96	whz v both	0.000
				Cramer's V	0.044
M-All-muac	47,498	2056	4.33	$\chi^2 = 3.01$	0.083
M-All-whz	56,837	2332	4.10	Cramer's V	0.005
All-muac v All-whz with oedema					
K-muac	1669	118	7.07	muac v whz	0.000
K-whz	1088	169	15.53	muac v both	0.000
K-both	4217	576	13.66	whz v both	0.411
				Cramer's V	0.115
K-All-muac	5886	694	11.79	$\chi^2 = 9.75$	0.002
K-All-whz	5305	745	14.04	Cramer's V	0.028
All-muac v All-whz with and without oedema					
M + K-muac	8860	174	1.96	muac v whz	0.000
M + K-whz	17,618	501	2.84	muac v both	0.000
M + K-both	44,524	2576	5.79	whz v both	0.000
				Cramer's V	0.025
M + K - All-muac	53,384	2750	5.15	$\chi^2 = 2.16$	0.141
M + K - All-whz	62,142	3077	4.95	Cramer's V	0.004

The effect of grouping M-both and K-both with the single deficits to produce erroneous results due to mathematical coupling. *All-muac* is defined as M-muac + M-both or K-muac + K-both; *All-whz* is defined as M-whz + M-both or K-whz + K-both; *Cramer's V* (a measure of the degree to which the two categories are associated, 0 = no association, 1 = identity) calculated for MUAC v WHZ only

face of privation, as their body fat and muscle mass is relatively low; however, there are no data to support or refute such an hypothesis.

Briend et al. also dispute that the deficits are additive or that the two diagnostic criteria are complementary. Our data also show that this assertion to be false. Those with both deficits had over twice the mortality of those with a MUAC< 115 mm alone. Indeed, some of the data suggests that the deficits might by synergistic. Even WHZ and stunting (height-for-age) combined show an additive effect [74]. Although stunting has not been taken into account in our analysis it is another confounder for all prognostic assessments of SAM. In our companion paper [60] we present a literature review of studies comparing WHZ and MUAC to predict death of malnourished children; the conclusions reached are in broad agreement with the present study.

Confounding and Simpson's paradox

Simpson's paradox is an example of extreme confounding where the actual results of a comparison can be reversed resulting in the less important variable becoming the dominant variable. This can occur with all analyses of categorical data, including simple Chi-squared analyses, logistic regression and ROC curve analyses. When categorical and continuous/ordinal data are combined the same phenomena can also occur and is then termed Lord's paradox and when both sets of data are continuous "suppression effects". They all have the same basis and are due to inadequate categorisation of subjects, confounding, mathematical coupling, inappropriate adjustment and unmeasured effects [81]. Even if the results are not actually reversed, mathematical coupling and the other confounders give erroneous results. The classical examples compare surgical operations for renal stones, psychiatric hospital admissions and death from diabetes [82] where those with more severe disease are not analysed separately from those with milder forms of a condition. Combining patients inappropriately led to erroneous statics and conclusions in each case. In the case of SAM, the same phenomenon occurs when children with both deficits, who have a higher mortality risk, are combined with those with single deficits who have a lower mortality risk, particularly when WHZ children are at higher risk of death than those with a low MUAC. Thus, inappropriate categorisation of patients, the presence of confounding or data from patients that are included in both arms of a comparison, even if the results are not completely reversed the magnitude of the difference in mortality can be grossly in error. Stochastic studies that relate subsequent events to antecedent parameters (such as subsequent death to antecedent anthropometry or adult blood pressure to birth weight etc. [83]) are particularly liable to error by confounding, sometimes to the extent of paradoxical reversal.

Consider Table 5. Here we present comparison of two criteria X and Y, with different numbers of subjects and deaths (the table can be reproduced in a spreadsheet to examine the paradox). In scenario A, there are no deaths at all in children with X alone, but when combined with children with both X and Y, the two deficits appear to have exactly the same mortality risk. In scenario B there is a lower CFR with X than with Y, but when those with both deficits are added the apparent CFR is reversed. In scenario C the two deficits have the same morality risk, but when combined with those with both deficits X appears to have a higher mortality. The percentage of total deaths identified using criterion X is much lower than with Y in each scenario even though the CFR with X appears to be higher when those with both groups are incorporated. In this case the error is due to mathematical coupling.

Table 5 The effect of group combination on the proportion of deaths identified by X or Y criteria

	Total #	Dead #	CFR %	CFR X/Y	X deaths %	Y deaths %
			Scenario A			
X	500	0	0.0			
Y	1500	30	2.0	0.0		
Both X & Y	500	30	6.0			
Total	2500	60	2.4			
All-X	*1000*	*30*	3.0		50%	
All- Y	*2000*	*60*	3.0	1.0		100%
			Scenario B			
X	500	6	1.2			
Y	1500	30	2.0	0.6		
Both X & Y	500	30	6.0			
Total	2500	66	2.6			
All- X	*1000*	*36*	3.6		55%	
All- Y	*2000*	*60*	3.0	1.2		91%
			Scenario C			
X	500	10	2.0			
Y	1500	30	2.0	1.0		
Both X & Y	500	30	6.0			
Total	2500	70	2.8			
All- X	*1000*	*40*	4.0		57%	
All- Y	*2000*	*60*	3.0	1.3		86%

In Scenario A, X does not have any mortality by itself, but when the subjects with both criteria are included X and Y appear to have the same mortality rate. Using only criterion X would select those children with zero mortality and those with both X and Y criteria and miss all the deaths related to criterion Y
In Scenario B, there is a lower mortality with criterion X, however when the subjects fulfilling both criteria are included the relative case fatality rates are reversed so it appears now that X is a superior diagnostic parameter than Y. Yet its use only identifies 55% of the deaths
In Scenario C, both X and Y have the same mortality rates but when the subjects with both criteria are included Y appears to be a superior diagnostic criterion. Yet this only leads to identification of 57% of deaths
The columns % deaths shows the percentage of all deaths that would occur in children with criterion X or criterion Y as the single diagnostic tool. Criterion Y identifies more deaths than criterion X, but when the children with both criteria are included criterion X appears to have a higher case fatality rate

Mathematical coupling occurs where *"one variable directly or indirectly contains the whole or part of another, and the two variables are analysed using standard statistical techniques"* [84, 85]. This nearly always results in erroneous results and appears to be the case in all the papers where children with M-both or K-both have been incorporated into the data analysed (see companion paper II [60]) and is the case with our patient's data (Table 4). It is for this reason that we have not used the children with both deficits in the meta-analysis and separated them in Table 2. Other types of confounding can also cause errors and even generate Simpson's paradox. Some are know; for example, the meta-analysis showed that MUAC had a higher risk of death for marasmic children in three different programs in East Africa and the combined risk is marginally in favour of WHZ, but when the children with oedema are added to the them Fig. 5 shows that the risk is changed so that overall WHZ has a significantly higher mortality. Some confounders have not been recorded in our data such as HIV, diarrhoea and family circumstances; and some are unknown such as birth weight. The use of such data to guide policy must be circumspect and confirmed. These problems are usually described in regression or correlation analyses, but the phenomenon also applies to logistic regression and ROC curve analysis.

ROC curves

Comparison of WHZ and MUAC related all-cause mortality using ROC curve comparisons generally show that the area under the curve is greater with MUAC than WHZ and is the only reason why MUAC is considered to be a "superior" prognostic of death than WHZ [51, 68, 86–88]. The question arises as to why these ROC curves have provided the opposite results to the findings in the present analysis. We have discussed many problems of ROC curve interpretation in relation to MUAC and WHZ assessment of future all-cause mortality elsewhere [52]. In particular, if they identify mostly or completely different children at high risk of death we argue that they are complementary and are not competing to identify the same child deaths. Thus, even if one diagnostic has a higher mortality risk than the other, if different deaths are identified, they are both useful prognostic indicators. If the objective of treatment is to try to prevent all the deaths and not only deaths which are related to one or the other diagnostic criterion both diagnostic criteria must be used. This is despite the fact that none of the anthropometric criteria are very good prognostic indicators and the differences between them are marginal. Each relates poorly to clinical or physiological abnormalities [89–92].

There has been a debate in the statistical literature about the problems of bias in ROC curves [93] which are particularly relevant to prognostic models of stochastic data (i.e. a future event) [94–96]. There have been attempts to combine time-to-event analysis with ROC curve analysis [97] and also comparison of crude data against smoothed data analysis with small sample sizes of individuals [98], but frequently there are anomalous results [99]. It is noteworthy that most of the papers presenting ROC curves of WHZ and MUAC have not given the confidence intervals of the curves [100].

The ROC curves that have been published in support of MUAC being "superior" to WHZ are all subject to Simpson's paradox because the children with both defects have not been analysed separately. They are also confounded due to the presence of oedema, HIV, convulsions, measles and other biases that affect children with a low MUAC and WHZ differently. As Tu et al. [81] state: *"Incorrect use of statistical models might produce consistent, replicable, yet erroneous results"*. We contend that this stricture applies to each of the reports using ROC curve analysis and the conclusions based upon these data are consistently erroneous. When we separate those children with both defects from those with either one or the other we reach quite the opposite conclusion; WHZ < –3Z has a higher mortality risk than MUAC < 115 mm.

When the WHZ ROC curve has a greater area under the curve than the MUAC curve, the data are not presented as the authors consider there has been a mistake [101]. When sensitivity is compared there are some situations where WHZ out performs MUAC [39]; this is uncommon with combined data but is usually ignored. Although papers, with completely inadequate data are erroneous and have been heavily criticised [102], they are still being quoted to justify a MUAC-only policy [103].

Marasmic-kwashiorkor

The finding of an exceptionally high mortality among children with oedema and a WHZ < –3Z, but no augmentation of mortality in those with oedema and a MUAC < 115 mm, is an unexpected new finding which to our knowledge has not been previously reported. The only explanation we can think of is that the weight of the oedema fluid will increase the WHZ so that the oedema-free WHZ may be much less than -3Z. However, the fact that the high mortality occurred in the OTP, with mild to moderate oedema, as well as the IPF with more severe oedema is against this as a complete explanation. The severity of the oedema does not appear to substantially affect the increased mortality risk when combined with a WHZ < –3Z. It appears that there is a qualitative difference between oedematous SAM related to a low WHZ and a low MUAC. The effect is seen in both younger and older children, so that age is not a satisfactory explanatory factor. Nevertheless, this observation may explain a controversy surrounding the relative increase in risk of children with marasmic-kwashiorkor over those with either marasmus or kwashiorkor alone. The WHO guidelines state that children who have been selected by screening children with MUAC and have mild or moderate oedema can be safely treated as outpatients [104], whereas clinicians treating children admitted using WHZ criteria maintain that children who also have oedema are at very high risk of death. Our data may reconcile this difference as the difference appears to depend upon whether a child has been diagnosed using the WHZ or the MUAC criterion. It should be noted that the high mortality in our data for oedema plus WHZ < –3Z was for both children with a MUAC of more and less than 115 mm. As the two anthropometric parameters appear to identify different risks of death, we suggest that all oedematous children should have their WHZ assessed and if they have marasmic-kwashiorkor with a WHZ of less than -3Z they should be treated as in-patients, whereas if their only anthropometric deficit is a low MUAC they can continue to be treated as out-patients.

Limitations of the study

Although there were a very large number of children's data amassed for this analysis, when those with "both" criteria were omitted from the analyses there were few deaths in some of the categories of interest, making it necessary to combine data from different sites. This could have resulted in a "clustering" effect. However, the large number of sites contributing data should have ameliorated such effects.

The percent of children with both WHZ and MUAC criteria without oedema in the IPF, OTP and SFC is 81, 73 and 31% respectively; for those with oedema the overlap was 58 and 64%. Compared to the overlap of SAM children identified in nutritional surveys (16.5%) in the community there is an excess of children fulfilling both criteria. There is a clear ascertainment bias as well as potential co-morbidity and stochastic biases [52]. The increase is numbers of children with both criteria may have contributed to the appearance of Simpson's paradox. The increase in the degree of overlap going from the least to the most intensive management reflects the severity of the cases being admitted as well as the diagnostic procedures and policy of the institutions/agencies involved. As a child deteriorates s/he is more likely to be complicated, to fulfil more than one diagnostic category and to be admitted for more intensive treatment. The ascertainment bias indicates that the data do not reflect the children with SAM in the community and disproportionally describes the experience of more severely affected children than are generally found during a community survey. Nevertheless, by dividing the children into the 7 different diagnostic categories, and omitting those satisfying both criteria from comparison of MUAC and WHZ CFRs, we consider that this bias has been ameliorated; thus, the M-muac and M-whz children included are more likely to represent the M-muac and M-whz children found in the community than the M-both children. Ascertainment bias is likely to be a more important consideration in studies that fail to separate the categories of patients and also those that include oedematous children in the analysis.

The fact that similar results were obtained in each mode of treatment supports the conclusion that children with a low WHZ have a higher mortality risk than those with a low MUAC, in all age groups and modes of treatment irrespective of the criterion used to admit the child for treatment initially. The fact that similar results were obtained with the three modes of treatment, each with a different degree of overlap, indicates that this is not a primary cause for the paradoxical results found.

We did not have data for other potential confounding influences on our analyses; in particular variables such as infection rates (TB, HIV, malaria etc.), socio-economic status, birth weight etc. all of which could confound studies of this nature. Furthermore, the causes of death were not clear, but were presumed to be related to their severe acute malnutrition.

There were a considerable numbers of defaulters from all the programs (Table 1). We included them in our study because they were at risk of death up to the time they defaulted and defaulting generally occurs after most of the deaths due to SAM have taken place [56]. However, this applies mainly to the IPF patients were it is know for certain whether a child has died or not prior to default. The patients in OTP and SFC are at home and attend the program sites weekly or less often; they are declared defaulters if they do not attend for two consecutive visits. As home visits are rarely performed, a proportion of these "defaulters" will have died; thus, the OTP and SFC's mortality rates should be regarded as minimum mortality rates and not actual mortality rates. For this reason defaulting is a potential major bias particularly for the OTP and SFC data. Table 6 shows the percent of defaulting by category and treatment mode. There was no difference in the rate of defaulting for children with M or K muac and whz in the IPF. However, in the OTP and SFC the difference was significant; children with M-muac had a higher percent of defaults than those with M-whz. If the same proportion of defaulting children died with each criterion, then there would be more deaths added to the M-muac group which would increase their CFR. With the oedematous children in the OTP the defaulting rate difference was the opposite so that this would increase the oedematous children's K-whz CFR more than the K-muac rate. For these reasons the OTP and SFC data are less reliable than the IPF data. This criticism applies to all studies of patients attending OTP programs unless there is universal home-visiting follow-up to ascertain the reason for the patient not attending the OTP/SFC site. This is very rarely done. One study from Niger (Médecins Sans Frontières personal communication) indicated that about 10% of "defaults" could be reclassified as deaths, but this figure is likely to be context specific, so we have not assumed any particular "correction" factor for our analyses.

Oedema is rarely seen during a nutritional survey because the time course of kwashiorkor is brief relative to marasmus; thus, even if the prevalence is low during a survey, the incidence can be considerable; this is evident from the high proportion of oedematous cases in some of the IPF studies. The ratios of oedematous SAM to non-oedematous SAM in treatment facilities always greatly exceed those in surveys.

In order to choose an appropriate admission policy that avoids death due to SAM, children should be categorised in the analysis into those with each criterion alone or both separately and those who have oedema or death from diseases not related to their nutritional status should be analysed separately.

Conclusions

Some within the nutritional community has been deceived by replicated ROC analyses because of mathematical coupling and confounding which may even lead to Simpson's paradox. Children with a low weight-for-height are at substantial risk of death at least as great as those with a low MUAC. But, because the two parameters identify different children they cannot be fairly compared as diagnostic markers for the *same* risks so that the comparison of areas under ROC curves, even if this were statistically a legitimate comparison, is largely meaningless. In studies of cancer, for example, one would not compare the ROC curves of all-cause

Table 6 Percent of patients who defaulted by diagnostic category and treatment

	IPF		OTP		SFC	
Category	%	χ2 P Cramer's V	%	χ2 P Cramer's V	%	χ2 P Cramer's V
M-muac	10.5	0.015	7.4	10.6	22.3	29.4
M-whz	10.8	*0.901*	4.7	*0.001*	17.2	*0.000*
		0.003		0.031		0.048
K-muac	12.6	1.735	4.5	6.953		
K-whz	15.7	*0.188*	8.7	*0.008*		
		0.032		0.076		
M-both	17.1		12.3		18.5	
K-both	14.1		13.8			

Abbreviations are given in Table 2

mortality in patients with bladder and renal cancer and decide, because one curve was "superior" to drop attempts to diagnose the other condition.

MUAC-only programs will fail to identify up to 45% of SAM children at high risk of death without the possibility of their being diagnosed or treated, and this omission will fail to be recognised by "coverage surveys" using MUAC screening alone. In our opinion MUAC-only programs are unethical wherever it is possible to also measure WHZ because they contravene the dictates of Hippocrates. In emergency situations where health services are overwhelmed MUAC- only programs could be justified at the outset of the emergency; however, in emergencies older children have a proportionately higher increase in prevalence of SAM (unpublished) than younger children and emergency interventions should not neglect this group of children. The research priority should be to develop innovative ways of identifying those children with a low WHZ in community screening programs. Stereo-photography has been used for many years [105] but with modern technology this has become practical [106–109]. Such data may also solve the problems of body build in determination of the difference between those with a low WHZ and a low MUAC and explore the relative risks of endomorphic and exomorphic children. In the meantime WHZ should continue to be used in all health facilities to identify and treat all those children with SAM by WHZ only.

Our data also suggest that those children with oedema and a low WHZ, but not those with a low MUAC, are at very high risk of death and should be referred to an IPF for initial treatment; they should form a separate diagnostic category and considered to be a very high risk group.

Both a WHZ < −3Z and MUAC < 115 mm must be retained as diagnostic criteria for SAM.

Additional files

Additional file 1: Table S1. Regional grouping of data from countries for meta-analysis.

Additional file 2: Table S2. Admission diagnostic criteria by country and admission facility.

Additional file 3: Table S3. Analysis of IPF and OTP patients combined.

Additional file 4: Table S4. Statistical data on the meta-analysis comparing WHZ-only vs MUAC-only by Region, oedema and treatment facility/program.

Additional file 5: Table S5. Sensitivity statistics for meta-analysis of WHZ-only vs MUAC-only, by oedema, Region and treatment facility/program.

Abbreviations

CFR: Case fatality rate; IPFs: In-patient treatment facilities; MAM: Moderate acute malnutrition; MUAC: Mid-upper-arm-circumference; NGOs: Non-governmental organisations; OR: Odds ratios; OTPs: Out-patient treatment programs; ROC curve: Receiver operating characteristic curve; RR: Relative risks; SAM: Severe acute malnutrition; SFCs: Supplementary feeding centres; WHZ: Weight-for-height Z-score

Acknowledgements

We would like to acknowledge Action Contre le Faim, Médecins Sans Frontières, Save the Children, Concern International, UNICEF and the National Governments of the countries from which we obtained data. We would also like to thank the following reviewers of the initial submission, Alan Jackson, Dominique Roberfroid and Geraldine Lo Siou for their very careful and useful comments; they have led to real improvement of our paper.

Funding

Nutriset provided a PhD fellowship to Université Libre de Bruxelles in support of EG. Nutriset had no role in any aspect of this research including data collection, design, analysis, interpretation or writing the article. MHG received no support.

Authors' contributions

EG & MHG were involved in all stages from the conception and design, data acquisition, analysis and interpretation. Both authors approved the final version of the article.

Competing interests

The authors declare that they have no competing interests.

Author details

[1]Research Center Health Policy and Systems - International Health, School of Public Health, Université Libre de Bruxelles, Bruxelles, Belgium. [2]Department of Medicine and Therapeutics, University of Aberdeen, Aberdeen, Scotland.

References

1. Black RE, Victora CG, Walker SP, Bhutta ZA, Christian P, De Onis M, et al. Maternal and child undernutrition and overweight in low-income and middle-income countries. Lancet. 2013;382:427–51. http://www.sciencedirect.com/science/article/pii/S014067361360937X
2. Grellety E, Golden MH. The effect of random error on diagnostic accuracy illustrated with the anthropometric diagnosis of malnutrition. PLoS One. 2016;11:e0168585. http://journals.plos.org/plosone/article?id=10.1371/journal.pone.0168585.
3. Isanaka S, O'Neal Boundy E, Grais RF, Myatt M, Briend B. Improving estimates of numbers of children with severe acute malnutrition using cohort and survey data. Am J Epidemiol. 2016;184(12):861–9. https://doi.org/10.1093/aje/kww129.
4. Gomez F, Galvan RR, Cravioto J, Frenk S. Malnutrition in infancy and childhood, with special reference to kwashiorkor. Adv Pediatr. 1955;7:131–69.
5. Anonymous. Classification of infantile malnutrition. Lancet. 1970;2:302–3.
6. Gopalan C, Rao KSJ. Classifications of undernutrition? Their limitations and fallacies. J Trop Pediatr. 1984;30:7–10.
7. Dugdale AE. An age-independent anthropometric index of nutritional status. Am J Clin Nutr. 1971;24:174–6. http://ajcn.nutrition.org/content/24/2/174.full.pdf+html
8. Waterlow JC. Classification and definition of protein-calorie malnutrition. Br Med J. 1972;3:566–9. https://www.bmj.com/content/bmj/3/5826/566.full.pdf.
9. Pryor HB, Stolz HR. Determining appropriate weight for body build. J Pediatr. 1933;3:608–22. http://www.sciencedirect.com/science/article/pii/S0022347633801284
10. Stuart HC, Stevenson SS, Nelson WE. Textbook of pediatrics. In: Textbook of pediatrics. Philadelphia: Saunders; 1959. p. 50–1.
11. Hamill PV, Drizd TA, Johnson CL, Reed RB, Roche AF. NCHS growth curves for children birth-18 years. United States, Vital and health statistics. Series 11, Data from the National Health Survey edn. 1977. http://www.dtic.mil/dtic/tr/fulltext/u2/a433981.pdf

12. Kuczmarski RJ, Ogden CL, Grummer-Strawn LM, Flegal KM, Guo SS, Wei R et al. CDC growth charts: United States. Advance data [314], 1–27. 2000. https://stacks.cdc.gov/view/cdc/11267
13. WHO. The WHO Child Growth Standards. 2006. http://www.who.int/childgrowth/standards/en/
14. De Onis M, Garza C, Onyango AW, Borghi E. Comparison of the WHO child growth standards and the CDC 2000 growth charts. J Nutr. 2007;137:144–8. http://jn.nutrition.org/content/137/1/144.full
15. WHO, Unicef. WHO child growth standards and the identification of severe acute malnutrition in infants and children: a joint statement by the World Health Organization and the United Nations Children's fund. 2009. http://www.who.int/nutrition/publications/severemalnutrition/9789241598163_eng.pdf
16. Myatt M, Khara T, Collins S. A review of methods to detect cases of severely malnourished children in the community for their admission into community-based therapeutic care programs. Food Nutr Bull. 2006;27:S7–23. http://archive.unu.edu/unupress/food/FNB_v27n3_suppl.pdf#page=7
17. Ale FG, Phelan KP, Issa H, Defourny I, Le Duc G, Harczi G, et al. Mothers screening for malnutrition by mid-upper arm circumference is non-inferior to community health workers: results from a large-scale pragmatic trial in rural Niger. Arch Public Health. 2016;74:38. https://archpublichealth.biomedcentral.com/track/pdf/10.1186/s13690-016-0149-5?site=archpublichealth.biomedcentral.com
18. Briend A, Lacsala R, Prudhon C, Mounier B, Grellety Y, Golden MH. Ready-to-use therapeutic food for treatment of marasmus. Lancet. 1999; 353:1767–8. http://www.thelancet.com/journals/lancet/article/PIIS0140-6736(99)01078-8/abstract
19. Collins S, Yates R. The need to update the classification of acute malnutrition. Lancet. 2003;362:249. http://www.thelancet.com/pdfs/journals/lancet/PIIS014067360313927X.pdf
20. Collins S, Dent N, Binns P, Bahwere P, Sadler K, Hallam A. Management of severe acute malnutrition in children. Lancet. 2006;368:1992–2000. http://www.sciencedirect.com/science/article/pii/S0140673606694439
21. Epicentre. Open review of coverage methodologies. 2015. http://www.coverage-monitoring.org/wp-content/uploads/2015/03/Open-Review-of-Coverage-Methodologies-Questions-Comments-and-Way-Forwards.pdf
22. WHO. Updates on the management of severe acute malnutrition in infants and children. 2013. http://www.who.int/nutrition/publications/guidelines/updates_management_SAM_infantandchildren/en/
23. Goossens S, Bekele Y, Yun O, Harczi G, Ouannes M, Shepherd S. Mid-upper arm circumference based nutrition programming: evidence for a new approach in regions with high burden of acute malnutrition. PLoS One. 2012;7:e49320. http://journals.plos.org/plosone/article?id=10.1371/journal.pone.0049320
24. John C, Ocheke IE, Diala U, Adah RO, Envuladu EA. Does mid upper arm circumference identify all acute malnourished 6-59 month old children, in field and clinical settings in Nigeria? South Afr J Clin Nutr. 2016:1–5. http://www.tandfonline.com/doi/abs/10.1080/16070658.2016.1255486
25. Manyike PC, Chinawa JM, Ubesie A, Obu HA, Odetunde OI, Chinawa AT. Prevalence of malnutrition among pre-school children in. South-east Niger Ital J Pediatr. 2014;40:75. https://www.ijponline.biomedcentral.com/articles/10.1186/s13052-014-0075-5
26. Gayle HD, Binkin NJ, Staehling NW, Trowbridge FL. Arm circumference v. Weight-for-height in nutritional assessment: are the findings comparable? J Trop Pediatr. 1988;34:213–7. https://www.academic.oup.com/tropej/article-abstract/34/5/213/1632459/Arm-Circumference-v-Weight-for-Height-in.
27. Ross DA, Taylor N, Hayes R, McLean M. Measuring malnutrition in famines: are weight-for-height and arm circumference interchangeable? Int J Epidemiol. 1990;19:636–45. https://www.academic.oup.com/ije/article-abstract/19/3/636/760605/Measuring-Malnutrition-in-Famines-Are-Weight-for
28. Bern C, Nathanail L. Is mid-upper-arm circumference a useful tool for screening in emergency settings? Lancet. 1995;345:631–3. http://www.sciencedirect.com/science/article/pii/S0140673695905278
29. Rees DG, Henry CJK, Diskett P, Shears P. Measures of nutritional status: survey of young children in north-East Brazil. Lancet. 1987;329:87–9. http://www.sciencedirect.com/science/article/pii/S0140673687919209
30. Hop LT, Gross R, Sastroamidjojo S, Giay T, Schultink W. Mid-upper-arm circumference development and its validity in assessment of undernutrition. Asia Pac J Clin Nutr. 1998;7:65–9. http://indianpediatrics.net/feb2016/166.pdf.
31. Tripathy JP, Sharma A, Prinja S. Is mid-upper arm circumference alone sufficient to identify severe acute malnutrition correctly. Indian Pediatr. 2016;53:166–7. http://indianpediatrics.net/feb2016/166.pdf
32. Roberfroid D, Huybregts L, Lachat C, Vrijens F, Kolsteren P, Guesdon B. Inconsistent diagnosis of acute malnutrition by weight-for-height and mid-upper arm circumference: contributors in 16 cross-sectional surveys from South Sudan, the Philippines, Chad, and Bangladesh. Nutr J. 2015;14:1. https://nutritionj.biomedcentral.com/articles/10.1186/s12937-015-0074-4
33. Dasgupta R, Sinha D, Jain SK, Prasad V. Screening for SAM in the community: is MUAC a simple tool? Indian Pediatr. 2013;50:154–5. http://link.springer.com/article/10.1007/s13312-013-0032-1
34. Fernandez MA, Delchevalerie P, Van HM. Accuracy of MUAC in the detection of severe wasting with the new WHO growth standards. Pediatrics. 2010;126:e195–201. http://citeseerx.ist.psu.edu/viewdoc/download?doi=10.1.1.919.6180&rep=rep1&type=pdf
35. Carter EP. Comparison of weight: height ratio and arm circumference in assessment of acute malnutrition. Arch Dis Child. 1987;62:833–5. https://adc.bmj.com/content/62/8/833.short.
36. Laillou A, Prak S, de Groot R, Whitney S, Conkle J, Horton L, et al. Optimal screening of children with acute malnutrition requires a change in current WHO guidelines as MUAC and WHZ identify different patient groups. PLoS ONE. 2014;9:e101159. https://bmcnutr.biomedcentral.com/articles/10.1186/s40795-016-0049-7
37. Grellety E, Krause LK, Shams EM, Porten K, Isanaka S. Comparison of weight-for-height and mid-upper arm circumference (MUAC) in a therapeutic feeding programme in South Sudan: is MUAC alone a sufficient criterion for admission of children at high risk of mortality? Public Health Nutr. 2015;18: 2575–81. http://www.epicentre.msf.org/sites/preprod.epicentre.actency.fr/files/661_Comparison%20of%20weight-for-height.pdf
38. Talapalliwar MR, Garg BS. Diagnostic accuracy of mid-upper arm circumference (MUAC) for detection of severe and moderate acute malnutrition among tribal children in Central India. Int J Med Sci Public Health. 2016;5:1317–21. http://www.ejmanager.com/mnstemps/67/67-1441365239.pdf
39. Dukhi N, Sartorius B, Taylor M. Mid-upper arm circumference (MUAC) performance versus weight for height in south African children (0-59 months) with acute malnutrition. S Afr J Clin Nutr. 2017:1–6. http://www.tandfonline.com/doi/abs/10.1080/16070658.2016.1255483
40. Fiorentino M, Sophonneary P, Laillou A, Whitney S, de Groot R, Perignon M, et al. Current MUAC Cut-Offs to Screen for Acute Malnutrition Need to Be Adapted to Gender and Age: The Example of Cambodia. PLoS ONE. 2016; 11:e0146442. http://journals.plos.org/plosone/article/file?id=10.1371/journal.pone.0146442&type=printable
41. Tadesse AW, Tadesse E, Berhane Y, Ekstrom EC. Comparison of mid-upper arm circumference and weight-for-height to diagnose severe acute malnutrition: a study in southern Ethiopia. Nutrients. 2017;9:267. http://www.mdpi.com/2072-6643/9/3/267/htm
42. Grellety E, Golden MH. Weight-for-height and mid-upper-arm circumference should be used independently to diagnose acute malnutrition: policy implications. BMC Nutr. 2016;2:10. https://bmcnutr.biomedcentral.com/articles/10.1186/s40795-016-0049-7
43. Briend A, Alvarez JL, Avril N, Bahwere P, Bailey J, Berkley JA, et al. Low mid-upper arm circumference identifies children with a high risk of death who should be the priority target for treatment. BMC Nutr. 2016;2:63. https://bmcnutr.biomedcentral.com/articles/10.1186/s40795-016-0101-7
44. Hammond W, Badawi AE, Deconinck H. Detecting severe acute malnutrition in children under five at scale. The Challenges of Anthropometry to Reach the Missed Millions Ann Nutr Disord & Ther. 2016;3:1030. http://austinpublishinggroup.com/nutritional-disorders/fulltext/andt-v3-id1030.php#Top
45. Garenne M, Maire B, Fontaine O, Briend A. Adequacy of child anthropometric indicators for measuring nutritional stress at population level: a study from Niakhar, Senegal. Public Health Nutr. 2013;16:1533–9. https://www.cambridge.org/core/services/aop-cambridge-core/content/view/S136898001200448X
46. Briend, A. Use of MUAC for severe acute malnutrition. CMAM forum 2012. http://citeseerx.ist.psu.edu/viewdoc/download?doi=10.1.1.662.303&rep=rep1&type=pdf
47. Taren D, de Pee S. The Spectrum of Malnutrition. In Nutrition and Health in a Developing World. Springer. 2017:91–117.
48. Deconinck H. Understanding pathways of integrating severe acute malnutrition interventions into national health systems in low-income

countries. Doctoral dissertation. Université catholique de Louvain; 2017. https://dial.uclouvain.be/pr/boreal/object/boreal%3A183112/datastream/PDF_02/view
49. EN-Net. WFH versus MUAC. 2015. Emergency Nutrition Network. http://www.en-net.org/question/1915.aspx
50. EN-Net. Only MUAC for admission and discharge? 2015. Emergency Nutrition Network. http://www.en-net.org/question/1922.aspx
51. Briend A, Maire B, Fontaine O, Garenne M. Mid-upper arm circumference and weight-for-height to identify high-risk malnourished under-five children. Matern Child Nutr. 2012;8:130–3. http://onlinelibrary.wiley.com/doi/10.1111/j.1740-8709.2011.00340.x/full
52. Grellety E, Golden MH. Response to Briend et al "low mid-upper-arm-circumference identifies children with a high risk of death and should be the priority target for treatment". BMC Nutr. 2016;2-63:1–12. https://bmcnutr.biomedcentral.com/articles/10.1186/s40795-016-0101-7
53. WHO. Management of severe malnutrition: a manual for physicians and other senior health workers. World Health Organization; 1999. http://apps.who.int/iris/handle/10665/41999
54. Golden MH, Grellety Y. Integrated Management of Acute Malnutrition (IMAM) Generic Protocol ENGLISH version 6.6.2. 2011. https://doi.org/10.13140/RG.2.1.3511.1448
55. Concern Worldwide, FANTA, UNICEF and Valid International. Training Guide for Community-Based Management of Acute Malnutrition (CMAM). Washington, DC: FANTA FHI360; 2008. https://www.fantaproject.org/focus-areas/nutrition-emergencies-mam/cmam-training
56. Grellety Y. The management of severe malnutrition in Africa.Ph.D. University of Aberdeen; 2000. https://www.ennonline.net/managementsamafrica.
57. Erhardt J, Golden MH, Seaman J, Bilukha O. Software for emergency nutrition assessment (ENA for SMART). SMART 2011. http://smartmethodology.org/survey-planning-tools/smart-emergency-nutrition-assessment/
58. Marascuilo LA. Large-sample multiple comparisons. Psychol Bull. 1966;65:280.
59. Wagh ST, Razvi NA. Marascuilo method of multiple comparisons (an analytical study of caesarean section delivery). Int J Contemp Med Res. 2016;3:1137–40. https://www.ijcmr.com/uploads/7/7/4/6/77464738/_marascuilo_method_of_multiple_comparisons__an_analytical_study_of_caesarean_section_delivery___.pdf
60. Grellety E, Golden MH. Severely malnourished children with a low weight-for-height have a higher mortality than those with a low mid-upper-arm-circumference: II. Systematic literature review and meta-analysis. Nutr J. 2018. https://doi.org/10.1186/s12937-018-0383-5
61. Barendregt JJ, Doi SA. Meta XL. 5.32 [computer program]. EpiGear International Pty Ltd: Queensland, Australia; 2016. https://www.epigear.com/index_files/metaxl.html
62. Peto R. Why do we need systematic overviews of randomized trials? Stat Med. 1987;6:233–40. https://doi.org/10.1002/sim.4780060306.
63. The Sphere Project. Humanitarian Charter and Minimum Standards in Disaster Response, 2 edn. Geneva, Switzerland; 2011. http://www.sphereproject.org/resources/download-publications/?search=1&keywords=&language=English&type=0&category=22
64. Bogin B, Varela-Silva MI. Leg length, body proportion, and health: a review with a note on beauty. Int J Environ Res Public Health. 2010;7:1047–75. http://www.mdpi.com/1660-4601/7/3/1047/htm
65. Signorini A, De Filippo E, Panico S, De Caprio C, Pasanisi F, Contaldo F. Long-term mortality in anorexia nervosa: a report after an 8-year follow-up and a review of the most recent literature. Eur J Clin Nutr. 2007;61:119–22. http://www.nature.com/ejcn/journal/v61/n1/abs/1602491a.html
66. Van Den Broeck J, Eeckels R, Vuylsteke J. Influence of nutritional status on child mortality in rural Zaire. Lancet. 1993;341:1491–5. http://www.sciencedirect.com/science/article/pii/014067369390632Q
67. Lindskog U, Lindskog P, Carstensen J, Larsson Y, Gebre-Medhin M. Childhood mortality in relation to nutritional status and water supply--a prospective study from rural Malawi. Acta Paediatr Scand. 1988;77:260–8. http://www.ircwash.org/sites/default/files/203.1-88CH-18814.pdf.
68. Pelletier DL. The relationship between child anthropometry and mortality in developing countries: implications for policy, programs and future research. J Nutr. 1994;124:2047S–81S. https://sites.google.com/site/mfkdocsexternal/Home/articles/Childanthropometryandmortality_Pelletier_1994.pdf
69. Olofin I, McDonald CM, Ezzati M, Flaxman S, Black RE, Fawzi WW, et al. Associations of suboptimal growth with all-cause and cause-specific mortality in children under five years: a pooled analysis of ten prospective studies. PLoS One. 2013;8:e64636. http://journals.plos.org/plosone/article?id=10.1371/journal.pone.0064636
70. Acevedo P, Esteban MTG, Lopez-Ejeda N, Gomez A, Marrodan MD. Influence of malnutrition upon all-cause mortality among children in Swaziland. Endocrinologia, Diabetes y Nutricion 2017. https://doi.org/10.1016/j.endinu.2017.01.008
71. Fawzi WW, Herrera MG, Spiegelman DL, el Amin A, Nestel P, Mohamed KA. A prospective study of malnutrition in relation to child mortality in the Sudan. Am J Clin Nutr. 1997;65:1062–9. http://ajcn.nutrition.org/content/65/4/1062.short
72. Katz J, West KP, Tarwotjo I, Sommer A. The importance of age in evaluating anthropometric indices for predicting mortality. Am J Epidemiol. 1989;130:1219–26. https://doi.org/10.1093/oxfordjournals.aje.a115450
73. Lawrence M, Yimer T, O'Dea JK. Nutritional status and early warning of mortality in southern Ethiopia, 1988–1991. Eur J Clin Nutr. 1994;48:38–45. PM:8200328
74. McDonald CM, Olofin I, Flaxman S, Fawzi WW, Spiegelman D, Caulfield LE, et al. The effect of multiple anthropometric deficits on child mortality: meta-analysis of individual data in 10 prospective studies from developing countries. Am J Clin Nutr. 2013;97:896–901. http://ajcn.nutrition.org/content/97/4/896.full
75. Nieburg P, Person-Karell B, Toole MJ. Malnutrition-mortality relationships among refugees. J Refug Stud. 1992;5:247–56. https://academic.oup.com/jrs/article-abstract/5/3-4/247/1522998/Malnutrition-Mortality-Relationships-among
76. O'Neill SM, Fitzgerald A, Briend A, Van Den Broeck J. Child mortality as predicted by nutritional status and recent weight velocity in children under two in rural Africa. J Nutr. 2012;142:520–5. PM:22259194
77. Yambi O, Latham MC, Habicht JP, Haas JD. Nutrition status and the risk of mortality in children 6-36 months old in Tanzania. Food Nutr Bull. 1991;13:6.
78. Roberfroid D, Hammami NM, Lachat C, Prinzo ZW, Sibson V, Guesdon B, et al. Utilization of mid-upper arm circumference versus weight-for-height in nutritional rehabilitation programmes: a systematic review of evidence. Geneva: World Health Organization; 2013. www.who.int/entity/nutrition/publications/guidelines/updates_management_SAM_infantandchildren_review1.pdf?ua=1
79. Post CL, Victora CG. The low prevalence of weight-for-height deficits in Brazilian children is related to body proportions. J Nutr. 2001;131:1290–6. http://jn.nutrition.org/content/131/4/1290.full
80. Manuel HT. Physical Measurements of Mexican Children in American Schools 1934, 5: 237–252. http://www.jstor.org/stable/1125742
81. Tu YK, Gunnell D, Gilthorpe MS. Simpson's paradox, Lord's paradox, and suppression effects are the same phenomenon - the reversal paradox. Emerg Themes Epidemiol. 2008;5:2. https://ete-online.biomedcentral.com/articles/10.1186/1742-7622-5-2
82. Julious SA, Mullee MA. Confounding and Simpson's paradox. Br Med J. 1994;309:1480–1. https://www.bmj.com/content/309/6967/1480.full.pdf+html
83. Tu YK, Tilling K, Sterne JA, Gilthorpe MS. A critical evaluation of statistical approaches to examining the role of growth trajectories in the developmental origins of health and disease. Int J Epidemiol 2013, dyt157. http://citeseerx.ist.psu.edu/viewdoc/download?doi=10.1.1.923.9437&rep=rep1&type=pdf
84. Archie JP Jr. Mathematic coupling of data: a common source of error. Ann Surg. 1981;193:296. http://journals.lww.com/annalsofsurgery/abstract/1981/03000/mathematic_coupling_of_data__a_common_source_of.8.aspx
85. Tu YK, Maddick IH, Griffiths GS, Gilthorpe MS. Mathematical coupling can undermine the statistical assessment of clinical research: illustration from the treatment of guided tissue regeneration. J Dent. 32:133–42. https://doi.org/10.1016/j.jdent.2003.10.001
86. Berkley J, Mwangi I, Griffiths K, Ahmed I, Mithwani S, English M, et al. Assessment of severe malnutrition among hospitalized children in rural Kenya: comparison of weight for height and mid upper arm circumference. Jama. 2005;294:591–7. http://jamanetwork.com/journals/jama/fullarticle/201328
87. Chiabi A, Mbanga C, Mah E, Nguefack DF, Nguefack S, Fru F, et al. Weight-for-Height Z Score and Mid-Upper Arm Circumference as Predictors of Mortality in Children with Severe Acute Malnutrition. J Trop Pediatr. 2017;63:260–6.
88. Sachdeva S, Dewan P, Shah D, Malhotra RK, Gupta P. Mid-upper arm circumference v. weight-for-height Z-score for predicting mortality in hospitalized children under 5 years of age. Public Health Nutr. 2016:1–8. https://www.cambridge.org/core/services/aop-cambridge-core/content/view/S1368980016000719
89. Brasseur D, Hennart P, Dramaix M, Bahwere P, Donnen P, Tonglet R, et al.

Biological risk factors for fatal protein energy malnutrition in hospitalized children in Zaire. J Pediatr Gastroenterol Nutr. 1994;18:220–4. http://journals.lww.com/jpgn/Abstract/1994/02000/Biological_Risk_Factors_for_Fatal_Protein_Energy.16.aspx

90. Van Den Broeck J, Meulemans W, Eeckels R. Nutritional assessment: the problem of clinical-anthropometrical mismatch. Eur J Clin Nutr. 1994;48:60–5. PM:8200330
91. Dramaix M, Hennart P, Brasseur D, Bahwere P, Mudjene O, Tonglet R, et al. Serum albumin concentration, arm circumference, and oedema and subsequent risk of dying in children in Central Africa. Br Med J. 1993;307:710–3. https://www.bmj.com/content/307/6906/710.abstract.
92. Dramaix M, Brasseur D, Donnen P, Bawhere P, Porignon D, Tonglet R, et al. Prognostic indices for mortality of hospitalized children in central Africa. Am J Epidemiol. 1996;143:1235–43. PM:8651222
93. Whiting P, Rutjes AW, Reitsma JB, Glas AS, Bossuyt PM, Kleijnen J. Sources of variation and bias in studies of diagnostic accuracy: a systematic review. Ann Intern Med. 2004;140:189–202. http://citeseerx.ist.psu.edu/viewdoc/download?doi=10.1.1.833.9748&rep=rep1&type=pdf#page=46
94. Coggon DIW, Martyn CN. Time and chance: the stochastic nature of disease causation. Lancet. 2005;365:1434. http://www.thelancet.com/pdfs/journals/lancet/PIIS0140673605663805.pdf
95. Cook NR. Use and misuse of the receiver operating characteristic curve in risk prediction. Circulation. 2007;115:928–35. http://citeseerx.ist.psu.edu/viewdoc/download?doi=10.1.1.324.758&rep=rep1&type=pdf
96. Cook NR. Statistical evaluation of prognostic versus diagnostic models: beyond the ROC curve. Clin Chem. 2008;54:17–23. http://citeseerx.ist.psu.edu/viewdoc/download?doi=10.1.1.325.269&rep=rep1&type=pdf
97. Lorent M, Giral M, Foucher Y. Net time-dependent ROC curves: a solution for evaluating the accuracy of a marker to predict disease-related mortality. Stat Med. 2014;33:2379–89. http://onlinelibrary.wiley.com/doi/10.1002/sim.6079/full
98. Pepe MS, Janes H, Longton G, Leisenring W, Newcomb P. Limitations of the odds ratio in gauging the performance of a diagnostic, prognostic, or screening marker. Am J Epidemiol. 2004;159:882–90. http://citeseerx.ist.psu.edu/viewdoc/download?doi=10.1.1.547.5511&rep=rep1&type=pdf
99. Van Calster B, Steyerberg EW, D'Agostino RB, Pencina MJ. Sensitivity and specificity can change in opposite directions when new predictive markers are added to risk models. Med Decis Mak. 2014;34:513–22. http://journals.sagepub.com/doi/abs/10.1177/0272989X13513654
100. Westover MB, Westover KD, Bianchi MT. Significance testing as perverse probabilistic reasoning. BMC Med. 2011;9:20. https://bmcmedicine.biomedcentral.com/articles/10.1186/1741-7015-9-20
101. Lapidus N, Luquero FJ, Gaboulaud VR, Shepherd S, Grais RF. Prognostic accuracy of WHO growth standards to predict mortality in a large-scale nutritional program in Niger. PLoS Med. 2009;6:e1000039. http://journals.plos.org/plosmedicine/article?id=10.1371/journal.pmed.1000039
102. Golden MH. Comment on WHZ and MUAC for diagnosis of severe malnutrition by Chiabi a et al. J Trop Pediatr 2017;0:1–2. doi: https://doi.org/10.1093/tropej/fmx008.
103. Heikens GT, Manary MJ, Trehan I. African children with severe pneumonia remain at high risk for death even after discharge. Paediatr Perinat Epidemiol. 2017; http://onlinelibrary.wiley.com/doi/10.1111/ppe.12350/full
104. WHO. Guideline: Updates on the management of severe acute malnutrition in infants and children. Geneva: World Health Organization; 2013. http://www.who.int/nutrition/publications/guidelines/updates_management_SAM_infantandchildren/en/
105. Piebson WR. Monophotogrammetric determination of body volume. Ergonomics. 1961;4:213–8. http://www.tandfonline.com/doi/abs/10.1080/00140136108930521
106. Wells JCK, Ruto A, Treleaven P. Whole-body three-dimensional photonic scanning: a new technique for obesity research and clinical practice. Int J Obes. 2008;32:232–8. http://www.nature.com/ijo/journal/v32/n2/abs/0803727a.html
107. Yu W. Development of a three-dimensional anthropometry system for human body composition assessment. The University of Texas at Austin; 2008. https://repositories.lib.utexas.edu/bitstream/handle/2152/17838/yuw.pdf%3Bjsessionid%3D61F89DE75AA927339A6A0909C615A7FE?sequence%3D2
108. Mikat RP. Chest, waist, and hip circumference estimations from stereo photographic digital topography. J Sports Med Phys Fitness. 2000;40:58.
109. Conkle J, Ramakrishnan U, Flores-Ayala R, Suchdev PS, Martorell R. Improving the quality of child anthropometry: manual anthropometry in the body imaging for nutritional assessment study (BINA). PLoS One. 2017;12(12):e0189332. http://journals.plos.org/plosone/article?id=10.1371/journal.pone.0189332

8

Fortified food supplementation in children with reduced dietary energy and micronutrients intake in Southern Mexico

Gabriela Añorve-Valdez[1,2], Amado David Quezada-Sánchez[5], Fabiola Mejía-Rodríguez[1,4*], Armando García-Guerra[1] and Lynnette Marie Neufeld[3]

Abstract

Background: Nutritional supplements are an important source of complementary food for young children, since they may either complement or substitute nutrients obtained from other food sources. Assessing how the introduction of different types of supplements modifies the consumption of other food sources may help in designing supplementation programs that aim to improve the nutrition of vulnerable populations.
The objetive is to quantify dietary energy and nutrient intake among children aged 6–12 months who received one of three nutritional supplements.

Methods: A cluster-randomized trial was conducted from 2005 to 2007. Urban communities were randomly allocated to one of three intervention groups receiving one of the following: a milk-based fortified food, micronutrient powders, or syrup. Each supplement was fortified with equal amounts of micronutrients. Dietary intake was estimated using a food frequency questionnaire (FFQ) to reflect the average consumption over the month prior to the interview. Children between 6 and 12 months of age were recruited. Median regression was performed with adjusted standard errors for clustered data, and the linear predictors for the median included the study group, study stage and their interaction. Adjusted medians by study group and study stage were obtained as post-estimations.

Results: No statistically significant differences between study groups were observed at baseline. After four months of supplementation, the children in the fortified food group had a smaller increase in median dietary energy (183.7 kcal, CI95%: 59.9, 307.5) and dietary protein (6.6 g, CI95%: 2.6, 10.6) intake from their home diet than those in the syrup group ($p < 0.05$). These differences remained significant after adjusting for group differences at baseline. Regarding covariate-adjusted median changes from baseline to follow-up at 10 months, the children in the fortified food group had a smaller median increase in dietary energy intake than those in the syrup group (698 vs 915 kcal), with a difference of 217.9 kcal (CI95%: 20.4, 415.4).

Conclusion: Children in the fortified food group consumed less dietary energy, protein, and micronutrients than those in the micronutrient powder and syrup groups. It is possible that absolute nutrient intake may be overestimated by the FFQ, but this possibility does not compromise the ability to compare study groups. Given the observed differences in dietary energy consumption among the three supplemented groups, it can be concluded that supplementation with micronutrient powders is an adequate option for urban children who have met their minimum energy and protein requirements.

Keywords: Children, Developing country, Dietary intake, Fortified food, Micronutrient powder, Supplementation

* Correspondence: fmejia@insp.mx
[1]Instituto Nacional de Salud Publica (INSP), Cuernavaca, Morelos, Mexico
[4]Center for Nutrition and Health Research, INSP, Avenida Universidad 655, Colonia Santa María Ahuacatitlán, Cuernavaca, Morelos, Mexico
Full list of author information is available at the end of the article

Background

Micronutrient deficiencies in early childhood (6 to 24 months) influence several functional outcomes, including linear growth, health, and immune function [1–9]. According to the 2006 National Health and Nutrition Survey (ENSANUT, by its Spanish acronym), 27.5% and 3.2% of children in Mexico under the age of five were zinc and folate deficient, respectively [10]. The prevalence of anemia in the 2012 ENSANUT survey was 38% in children aged 12–23 months [11]. Additionally, ENSANUT reported a prevalence of 9.7% for overweight-obesity in children under five years [11], raising serious concern about the changing dietary patterns of children.

The *PROSPERA Programa de Inclusión Social* (*PROSPERA*; formerly known as the *Oportunidades* Human Development Program [PDHO] and previously named *Progresa*) has been distributing complementary fortified food (FF) as part of the program's benefits for children aged 6 to 59 months since 1997. The FF supplement provides 100% of the daily micronutrients and 20% of the daily energy requirements of these children [12, 13] and is intended for daily consumption as a mush, colloquially referred to as papilla.

In an early evaluation, the original program had significant effects on child growth in rural and urban areas and on anemia in rural areas [12, 14]. In-depth ethnographic studies showed a high acceptance of the FF, but patterns of intra-household sharing resulted in young children consuming far less than the recommended amount [15, 16]. It is important to assess dietary intake to understand the patterns of supplement utilization and the extent to which their utilization results in modifications of dietary intake of home foods.

Dietary intake was assessed as part of a cluster-randomized trial comparing the impact of 3 different types of nutritional supplements for children on several nutritional outcomes. The objective of the analyses presented here was to quantify the dietary energy and nutrient intake of children aged 6–12 months who received one of three nutritional supplements.

Methods

The dietary intake and supplement consumption data reported here were collected as part of a cluster-randomized efficacy trial specifically designed to identify the best supplement for use in *PROSPERA* based on the comparative impact of selected nutritional outcomes, acceptance, consumption, and cost. The details of this intervention have been reported elsewhere, and the main results of the study have been published and presented at international conferences [12, 15, 17, 18].

Design and participants

We conducted a cluster-randomized trial from 2005 to 2007 in 54 urban communities in the Mexican states of Tabasco, Veracruz, Oaxaca and Puebla. Randomization was performed at the community level, and all *PROSPERA* beneficiaries who were children within the baseline age range in those communities were eligible to participate. Allocation was performed using a block design to ensure comparability between supplementation groups. The communities were split into 18 blocks of three communities each prior to randomization. The blocks were defined using community characteristics, such as 1) the degree of marginalization (low or medium) 2) the population size and 3) geographic proximity (to avoid large differences in altitude, climate, etc.). Within each block study group, communities were randomly assigned to receive one of the supplements: FF supplied by *PROSPERA*, a micronutrient syrup (syrup) or a micronutrient powder (MNP). The syrup and MNP were purposefully designed with a micronutrient content identical to that of FF. For this analysis, we restricted analyses to the sample of children whose dietary intake data were available at baseline and after four and ten months of supplementation (Fig. 1).

Study settings and intervention

Physicians and nurses at local healthcare centers and clinics identified PROSPERA beneficiaries for potential inclusion in our study and organized informational meetings regarding our objectives. Prior to initiation, all families in the selected communities had been regularly receiving the PROSPERA FF supplement and health education messages [13]. The nutritional supplements used in this study (FF, MNP and syrup) were delivered directly to the homes of our sample groups six days per week. We did not include a placebo or a no-intervention group because the program, by its rules of operation, includes the distribution of a supplement; therefore, elimination of the supplement was not among the programmatic alternatives to be explored.

The FF, MNP and syrup supplements contained equal amounts of selected micronutrients: elemental iron and zinc, as well as vitamins A, B2, B12, C, E and folic acid (Table 1). FF was formulated with dry whole-milk powder, sugar and maltodextrin; therefore, the children randomized to the FF group were also given 194 kcal of energy, 5.8 g of proteins, 27.9 g of carbohydrates and 6.6 g of lipids per serving.

The FF supplement was produced for PROSPERA by Liconsa Corporation, which is located in the Mexican state of Queretaro and was distributed in 264 g bags. Instructions for FF preparation consisted of mixing a daily 44 g dose of dry product with a small amount of water immediately prior to consumption. The MNP supplement was specifically produced for our study and purchased from Ped-Med Ltd. (Toronto, Canada). A

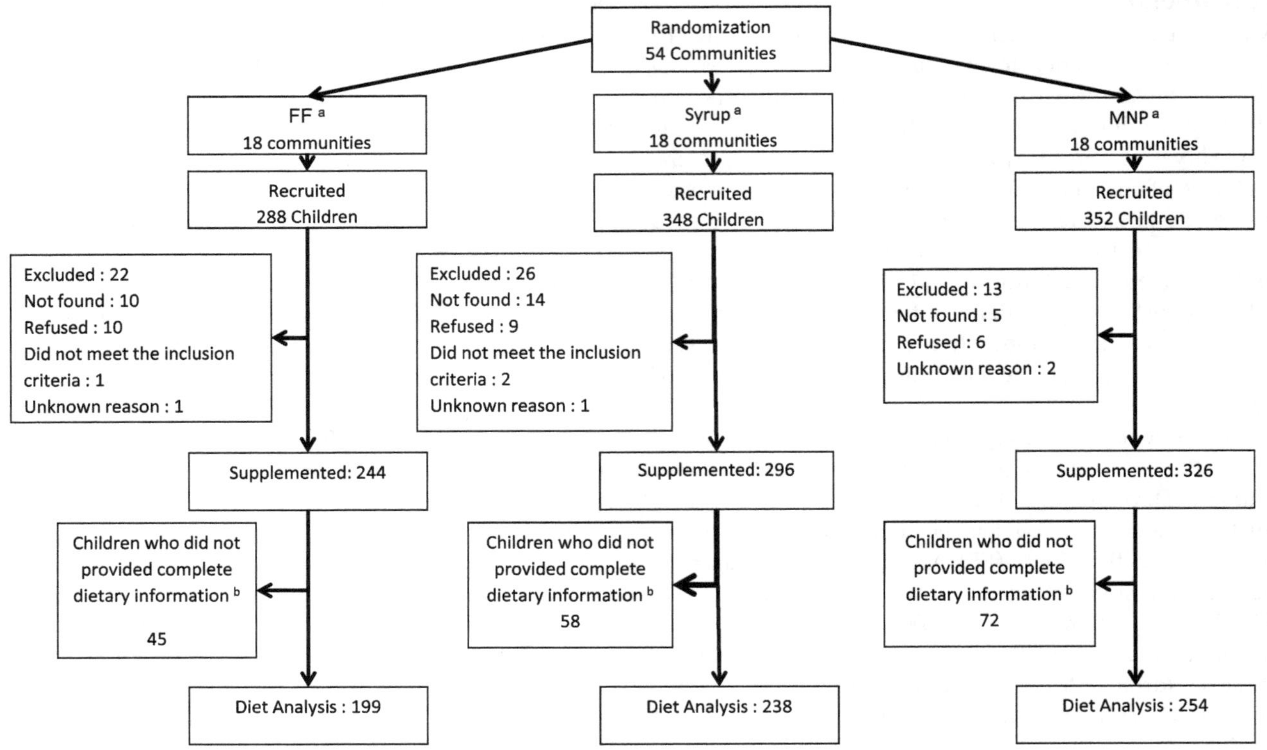

a. Fortified food (FF), Micronutrient powder (MNP), and Syrup (Syrup).
b. Baseline, 4 months of supplementation and 10 months of supplementation.

Fig. 1 Flowchart of children participating in the study

Table 1 Nutritional content per serving for the three nutritional supplements

Nutrient	FF[a] (44 g)	MNP[b] (1.0 g)	Syrup (5 mL)
Energy, kcal	194.0	–	–
Protein, g	5.8	–	–
Lipids, g	6.6	–	–
Carbohydrates, g	27.9	–	–
Sodium, mg	24.5	–	–
Iron, mg [δ]	10.0	10.0	10.0
Zinc, mg	10.0	10.0	10.0
Vitamin A, μg	400.0	400.0	400.0
Vitamin E, mg	6.0	6.0	6.0
Vitamin C, mg	50.0	50.0	50.0
Vitamin B2, mg	0.8	0.8	0.8
Vitamin B12, μg	0.7	0.7	0.7
Folic acid, μg	50.0	50.0	50.0

[a]Fortified Food (FF)
[b]Micronutrient Powder (MNP)
[δ]Gluconate ferrous in FF and Syrup; and fumarate ferrous in MNP

recommended daily dose of 1 g was provided in individual packs, and this was to be mixed with a small portion of the child's food immediately prior to consumption. The syrup supplement was also specifically developed for our project and was donated by Zerboni Laboratories in Mexico City, using a premix donated by DMS Nutritional Products (Mexico City). The syrup was distributed in 60 mL bottles, and a daily dose was 5 mL.

For the first 9 months of the study, the field staff visited each participant daily to distribute the supplement and observe its preparation and consumption. Subsequent visits were scheduled on a weekly basis. During each visit, the mother/caregiver registered the week's consumption on a self-administered form, which was designed to facilitate the recollection of routine consumption. At each weekly visit, the field staff reviewed and collected the form, gathered any remaining supplements from the previous week, and prepared the child's doses and form for the following week.

Data collection

Demographic characteristics

Demographic variables were obtained at baseline by means of home interviews with the child's mother/caregiver. The questionnaire, which was developed for previous studies in

Mexico [12], was used to collect information on maternal schooling, occupation, marital status, the family's socioeconomic status (SES), including housing characteristics, access to water and electricity services, and household possession of durable goods.

Dietary assessment

To estimate food consumption, we adapted a previously validated seven-day food frequency questionnaire (FFQ) [19]. The questionnaire was adapted by adding breast milk to the milk group and FF to the cereals group. Although 24-h recall questionnaires applied on nonconsecutive days have been proven to generate a more accurate estimation of individual dietary intake, we used the FFQ as our main objective was to assess patterns of dietary intake and supplement consumption across the groups. Our ability to use more robust dietary assessment methods was also limited by logistical and budgetary restrictions.

The FFQ registered the reported consumption of foods from a list for each child, including the amount consumed and the portion sizes. The questionnaire was administered by trained personnel, with standardized food units and measures, during in-person interviews with the child's mother/caregiver. The sessions were held at baseline and at follow-up after four and ten months. The FFQ included the 107 most frequently consumed foods according to sample age group in the study population and classified them into 15 groups, with an option to register additional foods not included in the list. The respondent was asked about the number of days and the number of times per day the child consumed each food item and about the amount consumed per serving. These amounts were recorded in different measurement units: ounce, teaspoon, tablespoon, serving tablespoon, drop, gram or milliliter, piece, cup, slice, and taste. During the initial FFQ interview, the mother/caregiver identified the appropriately sized spoons and measuring cups for portion-size estimation.

The number of grams of each food item consumed and its nutritional content were estimated based on the food composition tables of the *Instituto Nacional de Salud Pública* (INSP, according to its Spanish acronym), Mexico [20]. Outliers for plausible intake were excluded according to age and sex to minimize errors in estimating the grams of food consumed [21–23]. We analyzed energy and protein consumed because of their direct relationships with child growth and development. We analyzed iron, zinc and folic acid intake since serum deficiencies of these nutrients have been identified as serious public health concerns in Mexican children [24, 25].

Regarding breast milk, the mothers were asked to report only their breastfeeding status (Yes or No) because we did not attempt to quantify breast milk intake.

Supplement consumption

Compliance with supplement consumption recommendations was estimated by quarters (25%, 50%, 75%, and 100%) based on the reports provided by the field staff during home visits. For the FF and MNP supplements, the amounts of powder remaining in the individual portions of prepared food were evaluated (0% = all or almost all, 25% = more than half, 50% = approximately half, 75% = less than half, and 100% = nothing or almost nothing). For syrup, the approximate quantity of quarters consumed for portions of 5 mL of syrup was registered. During the first nine months, field staff performed daily visits and registered consumption compliance. Thereafter, field staff performed weekly visits, and forms were completed to cover the whole week. The information was collected weekly. We calculated supplement consumption and compliance during the week before the date of the dietary interviews.

Statistical analysis

Descriptive statistics were obtained to assess the balance between the study groups in terms of the general characteristics and nutritional status of participants. Means and standard deviations were calculated for quantitative variables, and percentages were calculated for categorical variables. All standard errors were adjusted for data dependencies at the community level using the Taylor Series linearization method [26]. Means were compared through analysis of pairwise differences between study groups using a t-test.

Dietary intake was assessed using median regression with adjusted standard errors for data dependencies at the community level [27]. The model included variables such as study stage, study group, and the interaction between these two parameters. Adjusted medians for each stage (baseline, four-month follow-up, and ten-month follow-up) and study group were obtained from the model equations.

Additional analyses were performed to adjust for variables with unbalanced means between study groups. All interactions of these variables with study stage and study group were included in the model. Adjusted medians were obtained by holding unbalanced covariates at their mean values. All statistical analyses were performed using Stata v.12.0 (Stata Corp. 2011, Stata Statistical Software: Release 12. College Station, TX: StataCorp LP).

Results

Of the 988 eligible children who completed the supplementation trial, 244 were in the FF group, 326 were in the MNP group, and 296 were in the syrup group. Those who did not provide full dietary data for the three time points (baseline, four months and ten months) were excluded from the analysis, leaving 199 in the FF group, 254 in the MNP group and 238 in the syrup group

(Fig. 1). There were no statistically significant differences among those who were included and not included in the analysis for selected characteristics (anthropometric measures, demographic characteristics and SES) (Table 2). No differences in age, sex or anthropometric indicators were observed among the study groups included in this analysis. However, the children in the syrup group began supplementation approximately one month after those in the FF and MNP groups (Table 2), and there was a significant difference in average SES between the FF and syrup groups ($p < 0.05$).

Dietary intake

At baseline, there were no significant differences between the study groups.

After four months of supplementation, the children in the FF group had smaller increases in median dietary energy (183.7 kcal, CI95%: 59.9, 307.5) and dietary protein (6.6 g, CI95%: 2.6, 10.6) intake from their home diet than those in the syrup group ($p < 0.05$) (Table 3). This energy difference remained significant after adjusting for group differences at baseline (Fig. 2). With regard to covariate-adjusted median changes from baseline to follow-up at 10 months, the children in the FF group had a smaller median increase in dietary energy intake than those in the syrup group (698 vs 915 kcal), with a difference of 217.9 kcal (CI95%: 20.4, 415.4).

Supplement compliance

The mean supplement compliance during the week before a dietary interview was 83.6% (CI95%: 76.9, 90.4) for the FF group, 84.4% (CI95%: 74.7, 94.1) for the syrup group, and 97.9% (CI95%: 96.5, 99.2) for the MNP group after 4 months of follow-up, and it was 83.7% (CI95%: 79.5, 88.0) for the FF group, 94.3% (CI95%: 91.5, 97.2) for the syrup group, and 93.0% (CI95%: 89.9, 96.1) for the MNP group after 10 months of follow-up.

Dietary intake with nutrient intake from supplements added to consumption

There were no significant differences between the groups at baseline. At four months of follow-up, the median increase in zinc consumption by the FF group was 2.0 mg (CI95%: 1.0, 2.9) lower than the median increase for the MNP group ($p < 0.05$) (Table 4). After adjusting for SES and supplement initiation age (Fig. 2), the median increase in iron intake after four months of follow-up was 1.1 mg (CI95%: 0.3, 1.9) lower in the FF group than in the MNP group. The median increase in zinc intake was also smaller for the FF group than for the MNP group, with a difference of 2.0 mg (CI95%: 0.9, 3.1). The same tendency for changes in median iron and zinc intake were observed after 10 months of follow-up.

Table 2 Baseline characteristics of children included and excluded in this analyses

Characteristics	Included				Excluded $n = 297$
	FF $n = 199$	Syrup $n = 238$	MNP $n = 254$	Total $n = 691$	
Infants					
Age, months	7.9 ± 2.5	8.2 ± 2.7	8.0 ± 2.5	8.0 ± 2.6	8.1 ± 2.5
Sex, % male	46.23	50.84	49.61	49.1	46.8
Weight, kg	7.9 ± 1.1	7.9 ± 1.2	7.9 ± 1.2	7.9 ± 1.2	7.9 ± 1.3
Length, cm	66.9 ± 4.1	67.3 ± 4.3	67.0 ± 4.1	67.1 ± 4.2	67.2 ± 4.6
Length/age, Z	− 1.0 ± 1.0	− 1.1 ± 1.1	− 1.1 ± 1.0	− 1.0 ± 1.1	−1.1 ± 1.1
Length/age, %	15.74	18.07	18.65	17.6	18.5
Starting age of supplementation, months	8.3 ± 2.6	$9.1^{a,c}$ ± 2.8	8.4 ± 2.5	8.6 ± 2.6	–
Mother					
Socioeconomic level	0.2 ± 1.0	-0.2^{b} ± 1.0	0.0 ± 1.0	0.0 ± 1.0	− 0.1 ± 1.0
Educational level of the mother, %					
None	12.6	10.5	12.2	11.7	7.7
Basic	41.2	45.8	52.4	46.9	50.5
High school	37.7	36.6	26.8	33.3	32.0
Secondary school or more	8.5	7.1	8.7	8.1	9.7

Fortified food (FF), Micronutrient powder (MNP), and Syrup (Syrup)
Mean ± standard deviation or percentages, are presented
$^{a}p < 0.05$ FF vs MNP
$^{b}p < 0.05$ FF vs Syrup
$^{c}p < 0.05$ Syrup vs MNP
No statistically significant differences were found between children who were the included and not included in the study

Table 3 Median intake of energy, protein, iron, zinc and folic acid, from diet at baseline, and changes from baseline to follow-up stages by supplementation group

Stage study	FF	Syrup	MNP	Syrup vs FF	MNP vs FF	MNP vs Syrup
	Diet					
Energy (kcal)						
Baseline	372.7 (258.8, 486.7)	463.1 (363.4, 562.8)	438.9 (333.1, 544.6)	90.4 (−61.0, 241.8)	66.1 (−89.3, 221.6)	− 24.2 (− 169.5, 121.1)
4 m - Baseline	262.4 (179.2, 345.7)	446.1 (354.5, 537.8)	352.2 (253.7, 450.7)	**183.7 (59.9, 307.5)**	89.8 (− 39.2, 218.8)	− 93.9 (− 228.5, 40.6)
10 m - Baseline	784.5 (683.1, 885.9)	955.4 (800.7, 1110.2)	831.9 (703.1, 960.6)	171.0 (− 14.1, 356.0)	47.4 (− 116.5, 211.3)	− 123.6 (− 324.9, 77.7)
Protein (g)						
Baseline	10.1 (7.0, 13.2)	11.8 (8.7, 14.9)	12.8 (9.8, 15.8)	1.7 (−2.7, 6.1)	2.7 (−1.7, 7.1)	1.0 (− 3.4, 5.4)
4 m - Baseline	9.7 (6.4, 13.1)	16.3 (14.1, 18.6)	13.9 (11.3, 16.6)	**6.6 (2.6, 10.6)**	4.2 (− 0.1, 8.5)	−2.4 (− 5.9, 1.1)
10 m - Baseline	28.8 (25.5, 32.1)	32.5 (26.8, 38.2)	28.9 (24.9, 32.9)	3.7 (−2.9, 10.3)	0.1 (−5.1, 5.3)	−3.6 (− 10.6, 3.4)
Iron (mg)						
Baseline	1.9 (1.0, 2.7)	2.0 (1.5, 2.5)	2.2 (1.6, 2.9)	0.2 (−0.8, 1.1)	0.4 (− 0.7, 1.5)	0.2 (− 0.6, 1.1)
4 m - Baseline	1.1 (0.6, 1.6)	1.9 (1.3, 2.6)	1.3 (0.6, 2.1)	0.8 (−0.0, 1.6)	0.2 (−0.7, 1.1)	− 0.6 (− 1.6, 0.4)
10 m - Baseline	4.0 (3.5, 4.6)	4.6 (3.5, 5.8)	4.0 (2.8, 5.2)	0.6 (−0.7, 1.9)	0.0 (− 1.3, 1.3)	−0.6 (−2.3, 1.0)
Zinc (mg)						
Baseline	2.2 (1.5, 2.9)	2.5 (1.8, 3.2)	2.4 (1.8, 3.0)	0.3 (−0.7, 1.3)	0.2 (−0.8, 1.1)	− 0.1 (−1.1, 0.8)
4 m - Baseline	1.1 (0.6, 1.7)	2.2 (1.7, 2.8)	2.1 (1.5, 2.7)	**1.1 (0.4, 1.9)**	**1.0 (0.2, 1.8)**	−0.1 (− 0.9, 0.7)
10 m - Baseline	3.8 (3.1, 4.6)	4.3 (3.0, 5.5)	4.2 (3.2, 5.1)	0.4 (−1.0, 1.9)	0.3 (0.8, 1.5)	−0.1 (− 1.6, 1.5)
Folic acid (µg)						
Baseline	26.0 (13.4, 38.7)	27.7 (17.4, 38.1)	30.4 (22.8, 38.0)	1.7 (−14.6, 18.0)	4.4 (− 10.4, 19.2)	2.7 (− 10.1, 15.5)
4 m - Baseline	25.3 (13.1, 37.4)	36.1 (17.6, 54.7)	17.7 (7.6, 27.8)	10.9 (− 11.3, 33.1)	7.6 (23.4, 8.2)	− 18.5 (− 39.6, 2.7)
10 m - Baseline	55.4 (38.6, 72.1)	71.3 (50.1, 92.4)	50.1 (37.3, 63.0)	15.9 (− 11.1, 42.8)	−5.2 (−26.4, 15.9)	− 21.1 (−45.9, 3.6)

Fortified food (FF), Micronutrient powder (MNP), and Syrup (Syrup)
Obtained from a quantile regression with standard errors adjusted for data dependencies within communities; 95% confidence intervals are presented in parentheses
In boldface are the significant differences in differences

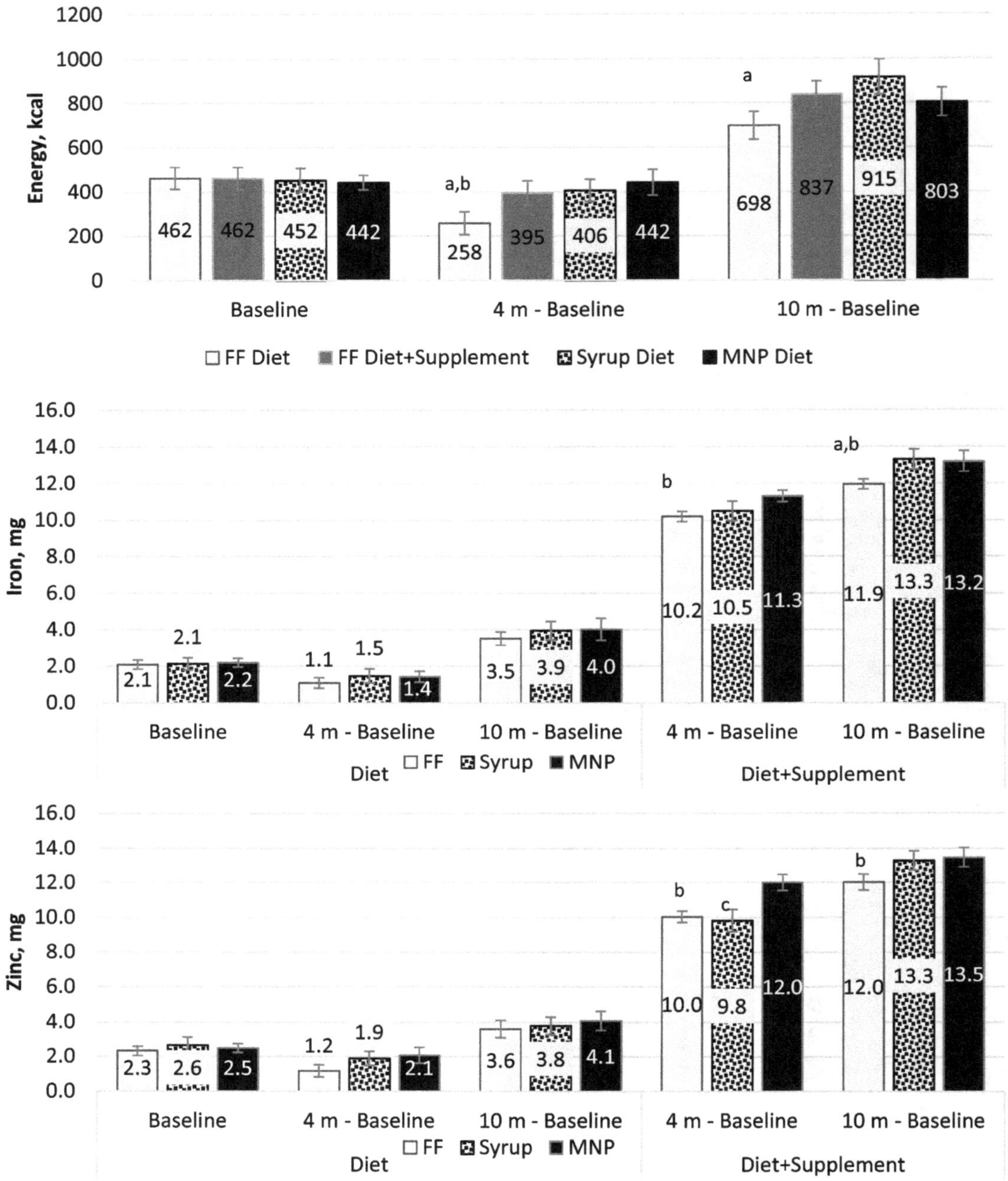

Fortified Food (FF), Micronutrient Powder (MNP) and Syrup (Syrup)

Error bars represent standard errors. Estimates obtained from a quantile regression with standard errors adjusted for data dependencies within communities. Changes were adjusted for baseline characteristics (socioeconomic status and age) and for the first dose of supplement consumption. For more details see Appendix Table B.

a $p<0.05$ FF vs Syrup

b $p<0.05$ FF vs MNP

c $p<0.05$ Syrup vs MNP

Fig. 2 Covariate-adjusted median intake of energy, iron and zinc from diet and diet+supplement at baseline and changes from baseline to follow-up stages by study group

Table 4 Median intake of energy, protein, iron, zinc and folic acid; from diet+supplement at baseline, and changes from baseline, to follow-up stages by supplementation group

Stage study	FF	Syrup	MNP	Syrup vs FF	MNP vs FF	MNP vs Syrup
	Diet + supplement					
Energy (kcal)						
Baseline	372.7 (257.2, 488.3)	463.1 (364.1, 562.1)	438.9 (333.6, 544.2)	90.4 (− 61.8, 242.5)	66.1 (− 90.2, 222.5)	− 24.2 (− 168.7, 120.3)
4 m - Baseline	426.6 (325.0, 528.1)	446.1 (353.9, 538.4)	352.2 (253.4, 451.1)	19.6 (− 117.6, 156.8)	− 74.3 (− 216.0, 67.4)	−93.9 (− 229.1, 41.3)
10 m - Baseline	956.9 (848.6, 1065.1)	955.4 (803.4, 1107.4)	831.9 (701.4, 962.4)	−1.4 (− 188.0, 185.2)	−125.0 (− 294.5, 44.6)	−123.6 (− 323.9, 76.8)
Protein (g)						
Baseline	10.1 (7.0, 13.2)	11.8 (8.6, 14.9)	12.8 (9.7, 15.9)	1.7 (−2.7, 6.1)	2.7 (−1.6, 7.0)	1.0 (− 3.4, 5.4)
4 m - Baseline	14.8 (11.5, 18.2)	16.3 (14.1, 18.6)	13.9 (11.2, 16.6)	1.5 (−2.5, 5.5)	− 0.9 (− 5.2, 3.4)	−2.4 (− 5.9, 1.1)
10 m - Baseline	33.5 (29.8, 37.2)	32.5 (26.9, 38.1)	28.9 (24.9, 32.8)	− 1.0 (− 7.7, 5.7)	−4.6 (− 10.1, 0.8)	−3.6 (− 10.4, 3.2)
Iron (mg)						
Baseline	1.9 (1.1, 2.6)	2.0 (1.5, 2.6)	2.2 (1.6, 2.9)	0.2 (− 0.8, 1.1)	0.4 (− 0.6, 1.4)	0.2 (− 0.6, 1.1)
4 m - Baseline	10.4 (9.7, 11.1)	10.7 (9.4, 12.0)	11.1 (10.3, 11.9)	0.3 (− 1.2, 1.7)	0.7 (−0.4, 1.7)	0.4 (− 1.1, 1.9)
10 m - Baseline	12.6 (12.0, 13.1)	13.7 (12.4, 15.0)	13.2 (12.2, 14.3)	1.2 (−0.3, 2.6)	0.7 (−0.5, 1.9)	− 0.5 (− 2.2, 1.2)
Zinc (mg)						
Baseline	2.2 (1.5, 2.9)	2.5 (1.8, 3.3)	2.4 (1.8, 3.0)	0.3 (−0.7, 1.3)	0.2 (−0.8, 1.1)	− 0.1 (−1.1, 0.8)
4 m - Baseline	10.0 (9.3, 10.7)	10.1 (8.9, 11.4)	12.0 (11.4, 12.6)	0.1 (−1.3, 1.6)	**2.0 (1.0, 2.9)**	**1.8 (0.4, 3.3)**
10 m - Baseline	12.6 (11.8, 13.3)	13.6 (12.7, 14.5)	13.5 (12.5, 14.6)	1.0 (− 0.2, 2.2)	1.0 (− 0.3, 2.3)	− 0.0 (− 1.4, 1.4)
Folic acid (μg)						
Baseline	26.0 (13.6, 38.5)	27.7 (16.9, 38.6)	30.4 (22.9, 37.9)	1.7 (−14.8, 18.2)	4.4 (− 10.1, 19.0)	2.7 (− 10.5, 15.9)
4 m - Baseline	62.8 (53.4, 72.1)	79.0 (62.0, 96.1)	65.6 (55.0, 76.2)	16.3 (−3.2, 35.7)	2.8 (− 11.2, 16.9)	− 13.4 (− 33.5, 6.6)
10 m - Baseline	98.8 (83.4, 114.3)	120.1 (92.0, 148.2)	95.2 (82.6, 107.8)	21.3 (− 10.8, 53.3)	−3.6 (− 23.6, 16.3)	− 24.9 (− 55.7, 5.9)

Fortified food (FF), Micronutrient powder (MNP), and Syrup (Syrup)

Obtained from a quantile regression with standard errors adjusted for data dependencies within communities, 95% confidence intervals are presented in parentheses

In boldface are the significant differences in differences

Discussion

The present study explored median differences in dietary intake of key nutrients by children 6 to 12 months old living in urban areas of Mexico and receiving one of three nutritional supplements, with follow-up after 4 and 10 months. This analysis forms part of a research trial designed to inform improvements to the nutrition component of the *PROSPERA* program. Our findings showed that those receiving FF (with energy and protein supplements provided by the program) consumed less energy, protein and micronutrients from their home diet than those receiving MNP or syrup.

Our study indicates that consumption of FF likely led to displacement of some home foods, resulting in no net contribution to dietary energy and protein intake. Although the supplements themselves were developed with equal micronutrient contents and all three groups showed compliance higher than 80%, the FF group showed lower compliance than the other groups. This observation is likely due to differences in adherence, particularly with regard to the proportion of each dose that was regularly consumed. If adherence in the FF group had been greater, we would expect a greater displacement of the home diet. This finding is consistent with those of several other published studies [28–32].

In the context of urban Mexico, it is likely that energy and protein are not limiting factors in the diets of children. In this setting, the displacement of home foods is desirable to avoid any excess increase in dietary energy. All three supplements provided important contributions to the total intake of several micronutrients that are known to be deficient in the diets of children who are beneficiaries of PROSPERA [25, 33, 34].

Iron supplementation may be indicated for children and women to reduce the occurrence of anemia due to a lack of iron, even in the presence of some known limitations, such as side effects affecting compliance and distribution problems [35]. Providing MNP increases availability and enhances the intake of nutritional supplements. However, granting access to this supplement in the actual setting of program operation is crucial.

A large-scale pilot study was performed in Vietnam, with the purpose of promoting locally produced MNP distribution and making MNP available through sales from the public healthcare system, and the study included training about adequate practices for feeding infants and young children. This type of intervention demonstrated a promising and innovative model for promoting the acquisition and intake of MNP, with the aim of improving nutritional status in a population of children < 5 years old [36]. Other authors demonstrated that children invariably have a more positive response to MNP than to syrup [37, 38]. In a study in Bangladesh in which an MNP intervention was assessed, 60% of mothers stated that they "liked it a lot", 30% "liked it" and the remaining 10% "somewhat liked it", particularly because it was easy to prepare, acceptable and could be added to complementary foods [39].

Similarly, with the purpose of increasing MNP compliance and intake, strategies for supplementation programs must be further researched. In this context, a study was performed in Nepal that documented predictors for obtaining high compliance with MNP intake. These predictors included perceived positive effects on health and nutrition in children < 24 months old among caregivers after MNP intake, as well as having specific materials for promoting the adequate intake of supplements. Such predictors should be considered when MNP supplementation programs are designed and applied with the purpose of increasing supplement intake adherence [40]. The use of MNP has been a novel approach for large-scale public healthcare interventions, with percentages of the prescribed MNP packets consumed during the intervention period as high as 98% [41, 42]. Comparatively, a study demonstrated that the dietary energetic density of babies consuming FF was less than that of babies not consuming FF (1.2 kcal/g vs 1.5 kcal/g). These findings can be explained by the fact that the caregivers may not have prepared the supplement according to the recommendations and may have diluted the papilla in an effort to make the supplement last longer [43]. This observation reveals that when MNP is used, there is greater adherence; and among its advantages, the single daily dose of MNP can be added to food that children can eat at any time; thus, greater supplement intake can be achieved.

There are few studies on the effectiveness of food fortification programs [44]. Supplement acceptance, the vehicle used (e.g., papilla preparations) and ease of preparation are key aspects to consider to ensure adoption of a supplement by the target population [45].

It has been documented that protein requirements among children aged 6–23 months are already covered by normal dietary intake, while requirements for energy and other nutrients (e.g., iron, zinc, and calcium) are not met without supplementation [46–48]. Therefore, accurate and effective strategies that contribute to increasing the intake of several nutrients to adequate levels through supplementation are needed. Teaching mothers how to improve feeding with natural food that is readily available in their places of residence has shown important results. However, some key nutrients fail to be covered in this manner, which can have detrimental effects on the weight and height of the child [47, 49, 50]. Therefore, the use of specific micronutrient supplements to cover infants' daily requirements is essential. In the case of anemia due to a lack of iron, for example, supplements covering iron requirements must be given to children.

According to the sustainable development objectives from the World Health Organization, maternal health is one of the main objectives for supporting healthy lives and promoting lifelong wellbeing. Suggested strategies to prevent maternal-infant malnutrition and nutritional deficiencies during the first thousand days of life (pregnancy and the first two years of life) include the use of prenatal supplements, the promotion of maternal breastfeeding, adequate weaning, the prevention of diseases (such as diarrhea and flu) and specific nutritional interventions with a focus on communities with no food security [47, 51, 52].

Our study has several limitations. The use of an FFQ instrument to assess dietary intake may have led to over-reporting of energy and nutrient consumption. Therefore, it is possible that the absolute nutrient intake levels may be overestimated for our sample. However, the ability to compare dietary intake patterns across the three supplementation groups is not compromised by this general estimation bias. Large proportions (36%) of children were still breastfed after ten months of supplementation. We have no evidence that this feeding influences comparative analyses across supplementation groups. Finally, given the implementation of the study in urban areas and the assessment of dietary intake until only 10 months after the initiation of supplementation, the results cannot be extrapolated to rural areas or to longer supplementation periods. An important strength of the study was the rigorous and continual monitoring of supplement consumption at the household level by highly trained field staff.

Conclusion

Our study among *PROSPERA* beneficiaries in urban Mexico showed that the consumption of FF led to the displacement of home foods in the diets of children 6 to 24 months of age. These results suggest that diets are generally adequate in terms of food quantity (i.e., energy and protein). All three supplements used in the trial were considered highly acceptable by caregivers [53]. Compliance was higher than 80% in the three supplementation groups, with the MNP and syrup groups showing higher compliance than the FF group during the week before the dietary interview after 10 months of follow-up. Our results suggest that alternative supplements, particularly MNPs or syrups, are more cost effective than FFs in increasing the dietary intake of key micronutrients in the studied population. To determine the implications for PROSPERA, however, these results must also be interpreted in conjunction with the

Appendix

Table 5 Covariate-adjusted* median intake of energy, protein, iron, zinc and folic acid from diet and diet+supplement at baseline and changes from baseline to follow-up stages by supplementation group

Stage study	FF	Syrup	MNP	Syrup vs FF	MNP vs FF	MNP vs Syrup	FF	Syrup	MNP	Syrup vs FF	MNP vs FF	MNP vs Syrup
	Diet						Diet + supplement					
Energy (kcal)												
Baseline	462.0 (365.6, 558.4)	451.9 (348.0, 555.7)	442.0 (376.6, 507.4)	−10.1 (− 151.8, 131.6)	− 20.0 (− 136.5, 96.5)	−9.9 (− 132.6, 112.9)	462.0 (365.9, 558.0)	451.9 (348.4, 555.4)	442.0 (376.8, 507.2)	−10.1 (− 151.3, 131.1)	− 20.0 (− 136.1, 96.1)	−9.9 (− 132.2, 112.5)
4 m - Baseline	257.8 (155.9, 359.8)	405.9 (308.2, 503.5)	442.0 (328.9, 555.1)	**148.0 (6.9, 289.2)**	**184.1 (31.9, 336.4)**	36.1 (− 113.3, 185.6)	394.9 (287.4, 502.4)	405.9 (308.4, 503.3)	442.0 (328.1, 555.9)	11.0 (− 134.1, 156.1)	47.1 (− 109.5, 203.7)	36.1 (− 113.8, 186.0)
10 m - Baseline	697.6 (574.9, 820.2)	915.5 (760.6, 1070.3)	802.8 (678.0, 927.5)	**217.9 (20.4, 415.4)**	105.2 (−69.8, 280.2)	− 112.7 (− 311.5, 86.1)	837.3 (718.9, 955.8)	915.5 (761.2, 1069.7)	802.8 (678.4, 927.1)	78.1 (−116.4, 272.6)	− 34.5 (− 206.3, 137.2)	− 112.7 (− 310.8, 85.5)
Protein (g)												
Baseline	13.1 (10.0, 16.3)	14.2 (10.6, 17.8)	14.6 (11.2, 18.1)	1.1 (−3.7, 5.8)	1.5 (− 3.2, 6.2)	0.4 (− 4.5, 5.4)	13.1 (10.1, 16.2)	12.8 (0.3, 25.2)	11.8 (2.1, 21.5)	−0.4 (− 12.0, 11.2)	−1.3 (−9.9, 7.3)	−0.9 (− 12.0, 10.2)
4 m - Baseline	8.0 (2.7, 13.4)	13.0 (9.2, 16.8)	14.0 (10.1, 17.9)	5.0 (−1.6, 11.5)	6.0 (−0.6, 12.6)	1.0 (− 4.4, 6.5)	21.3 (9.9, 32.7)	22.1 (4.7, 39.5)	15.0 (6.5, 23.6)	0.8 (−20.0, 21.6)	−6.3 (− 20.5, 8.0)	−7.1 (− 26.5, 12.3)
10 m - Baseline	25.3 (18.2, 32.4)	29.8 (24.8, 34.8)	26.9 (22.4, 31.4)	4.5 (−4.1, 13.2)	1.6 (− 6.8, 10.0)	− 2.9 (−9.6, 3.8)	51.7 (25.1, 78.4)	46.8 (26.7, 67.0)	49.6 (37.1, 62.0)	− 4.9 (− 38.3, 28.5)	− 2.2 (− 31.6, 27.2)	2.7 (− 21.0, 26.4)
Iron (mg)												
Baseline	2.1 (1.6, 2.6)	2.1 (1.5, 2.8)	2.2 (1.7, 2.7)	0.0 (−0.8, 0.8)	0.1 (− 0.6, 0.8)	0.1 (− 0.7, 0.9)	2.1 (1.6, 2.6)	2.1 (1.5, 2.8)	2.2 (1.8, 2.6)	0.0 (−0.8, 0.9)	0.1 (− 0.5, 0.8)	0.1 (− 0.7, 0.9)
4 m - Baseline	1.1 (0.5, 1.7)	1.5 (0.7, 2.2)	1.4 (0.9, 2.0)	0.4 (−0.6, 1.3)	0.3 (−0.5, 1.1)	− 0.0 (−1.0, 0.9)	10.2 (9.6, 10.7)	10.5 (9.5, 11.5)	11.3 (10.7, 11.9)	0.3 (−0.9, 1.5)	**1.1 (0.3, 1.9)**	0.8 (−0.4, 2.0)
10 m - Baseline	3.5 (2.8, 4.2)	3.9 (2.9, 4.9)	4.0 (2.8, 5.2)	0.4 (−0.8, 1.7)	0.5 (−0.9, 1.9)	0.1 (−1.5, 1.6)	11.9 (11.4, 12.5)	13.3 (12.2, 14.4)	13.2 (12.1, 14.3)	**1.4 (0.1, 2.6)**	**1.2 (0.0, 2.5)**	−0.1 (−1.7, 1.4)
Zinc (mg)												
Baseline	2.3 (1.8, 2.9)	2.6 (1.7, 3.6)	2.5 (2.0, 3.0)	0.3 (−0.8, 1.4)	0.2 (−0.6, 0.9)	− 0.2 (−1.2, 0.9)	2.3 (1.8, 2.9)	2.6 (1.7, 3.6)	2.5 (2.0, 3.0)	0.3 (−0.8, 1.5)	0.2 (− 0.6, 0.9)	−0.2 (−1.3, 0.9)
4 m - Baseline	1.2 (0.5, 1.8)	1.9 (1.1, 2.7)	2.1 (1.2, 3.0)	0.7 (−0.3, 1.7)	0.9 (−0.2, 2.0)	0.2 (−1.0, 1.4)	10.0 (9.4, 10.7)	9.8 (8.6, 11.1)	12.0 (11.1, 12.9)	−0.2 (−1.6, 1.2)	**2.0 (0.9, 3.1)**	**2.2 (0.7, 3.7)**
10 m - Baseline	3.6 (2.6, 4.6)	3.8 (2.8, 4.7)	4.1 (3.0, 5.1)	0.2 (−1.2, 1.5)	0.5 (−1.0, 1.9)	0.3 (− 1.1, 1.7)	12.0 (11.1, 13.0)	13.3 (12.2, 14.4)	13.5 (12.4, 14.6)	1.3 (−0.2, 2.7)	**1.4 (0.0, 2.9)**	0.2 (−1.3, 1.7)
Folic acid (μg)												
Baseline	29.6 (22.4, 36.9)	28.3 (19.9, 36.7)	33.5 (25.1, 41.9)	−1.3 (−12.4, 9.8)	3.9 (−7.2, 15.0)	5.2 (−6.6, 17.1)	29.6 (22.3, 37.0)	28.3 (19.7, 36.9)	33.5 (25.3, 41.8)	−1.3 (− 12.6, 10.0)	3.9 (−7.1, 14.9)	5.2 (− 6.7, 17.1)
4 m - Baseline	15.0 (5.0, 25.0)	29.9 (17.7, 42.2)	12.2 (0.4, 24.1)	14.9 (−0.9, 30.7)	−2.8 (−18.3, 12.7)	**− 17.7 (−34.7, − 0.7)**	56.5 (45.3, 67.8)	70.3 (59.4, 81.2)	60.1 (47.9, 72.2)	13.8 (− 1.9, 29.4)	3.6 (− 13.0, 20.1)	−10.2 (− 26.5, 6.1)
10 m - Baseline	54.6 (44.6, 64.6)	70.7 (49.9, 91.5)	44.6 (29.5, 59.8)	16.1 (−7.0, 39.2)	−10.0 (−28.1, 8.1)	**− 26.1 (− 51.8, − 0.4)**	99.2 (86.7, 111.7)	116.8 (96.9, 136.8)	91.4 (75.1, 107.8)	17.6 (− 5.9, 41.2)	− 7.7 (− 28.3, 12.9)	−25.4 (− 51.2, 0.4)

Fortified food (FF), Micronutrient powder (MNP), and Syrup (Syrup)
Obtained from a quantile regression with age at the onset of supplementation and socioeconomic level as adjustment covariates and standard errors adjusted for data dependencies within communities. *Age at the onset of supplementation and socioeconomic status level
In boldface are the significant differences in differences

impact of the supplements on nutritional outcomes (results forthcoming).

Abbreviations

ENSANUT: (according to its Spanish acronym): National Health and Nutrition Survey; FF: Fortified food; FFQ: Food frequency questionnaire; INSP : (according to its Spanish acronym): National Institute of Public Health, Mexico; Kcals: Kilocalories; MNP: Micronutrient powder; PROGRESA: Education, Health and Alimentation Program; SES: Socioeconomic status

Funding

The results presented here were part of a study financed by the Secretary of Social Development of Mexico, through the National Coordination of the Oportunidades Human Development Program and by the Secretary of Health of Mexico, through the National Commission for Social Protection in Health, who hold the rights to the components financed by each program.

Authors' contributions

All authors certify that they participated sufficiently in manuscript preparation and that they accept its overall validity and take public responsibility for its contents. LMN designed the study and directed its implementation, including quality control. AG-G and the corresponding author of this article helped supervise the field activities and designed the study's analytical strategy. All authors helped conduct the literature review and actively participated in the writing of the materials, methods, and discussion sections of the text. A summary of this work was presented in poster form at the 2008 FASEB Conference (Dietary intake in children consuming three supplements with identical micronutrient content FASEB J March 2008 22:677.4). This manuscript is not currently under review by any other journal, and no portion of the manuscript other than the abstract has been published or posted on the internet. All authors read and approved the final manuscript.

Competing interests

The authors declare that they have no competing interests.

Author details

[1]Instituto Nacional de Salud Publica (INSP), Cuernavaca, Morelos, Mexico. [2]Autonomous University of the State of Morelos, Cuernavaca, Morelos, Mexico. [3]Global Alliance for Improved Nutrition, Geneva, Switzerland. [4]Center for Nutrition and Health Research, INSP, Avenida Universidad 655, Colonia Santa María Ahuacatitlán, Cuernavaca, Morelos, Mexico. [5]Center for Evaluation and Surveys Research, National Institute of Public Health, INSP, Cuernavaca, Morelos, Mexico.

References

1. Micronutrient Initiative, Flour fortification initiative, USAID, GAIN, WHO, the World Bank, UNICEF. Investing in the future: a united call to action on vitamin and mineral deficiencies: global report 2009. Ottawa: The Micronutrient Initiative; 2009.
2. UNICEF. Investing in the future. A united call to action on vitamin and mineral deficiencies. 2009. http://www.unitedcalltoaction.org/documents/Investing_in_the_future.pdf of subordinate document. Accesed 14 Oct 2016.
3. Adu-Afarwuah S, Lartey A, Brown K, et al. Randomized comparison of 3 types of micronutrient supplements for home fortification of complementary foods in Ghana: effects on growth and motor development. Am J Clin Nutr. 2007;86:412–20.
4. Stein A, Barnhart H, Hickey M, Ramakrishnan U, et al. Prospective study of protein-energy supplementation early in life and of growth in the subsequent generation in Guatemala. Am J Clin Nutr. 2003;78:162–7.
5. Ramakrishnan U, Neufeld L, Flores R, Rivera J, Martorell R. Multiple micronutrient supplementation during early childhood increases child size at 2 y of age only among high compliers. Am J Clin Nutr. 2009;89:1125–31.
6. Brown K, Sánchez-Griñan M, Pérez F, et al. Effects of dietary energy density and feeding frequency on total daily energy intakes of recovering malnourished children. Am J Clin Nutr. 1995;62:13–8.
7. Ramakrishnan U, Nguyen P, Martorell R. Effects of micronutrients on growth of children under 5 y of age: meta-analyses of single and multiple nutrient interventions. Am J Clin Nutr. 2009;89:191–203.
8. Galloway R, McGuire J. Determinants of compliance with iron supplementation: supplies, side effects, or psychology? Soc Sci Med. 1994;39:381–90.
9. Ramakrishnan U, Goldenberg T, Allen L. Do multiple micronutrient interventions improve child health, growth, and development? J Nutr. 2011;141:2066–75.
10. Shamah-Levy T, Villalpando S, Jáuregui A, Rivera JA. Overview of the nutritional status of selected micronutrients in Mexican children in 2006. Salud Publica Mex. 2012;54:146–15.
11. Gutiérrez JP, Rivera-Dommarco J, Shamah-Levy T, Villalpando-Hernández S, Franco A, Cuevas-Nasu L, Romero-Martínez M, Hernández-Ávila M. Encuesta Nacional de Salud y Nutrición 2012. Resultados Nacionales. Cuernavaca: Instituto Nacional de Salud Pública; 2012 https://ensanut.insp.mx/informes/ENSANUT2012ResultadosNacionales.pdf. Accessed 19 Oct 2016.
12. Neufeld L, Sotres-Alvarez D, Flores-López L, Tolentino-Mayo L, Jiménez-Ruiz J, Rivera-Dommarco J. Estudio sobre el consumo de los suplementos Nutrisano y Nutrivida en niños y mujeres de zonas urbanas beneficiarios de Oportunidades. Evaluación externa de impacto del Programa Oportunidades 2004. Instituto Nacional de Salud Pública: Cuernavaca; 2005.
13. Secretaria de Desarrollo Social (SEDESOL). Reglas de Operación del Programa de Desarrollo Humano Oportunidades, para el ejercicio fiscal 2012. Diario Oficial, tercera sección 2012. Accessed 14 Oct 2016.
14. Rivera JA, Sotres-Alvarez D, Habicht JP, Shamah T, Villalpando S. Impact of the Mexican program for education, health and nutrition (Progresa) on rates of growth and anemia in infants and young children: a randomized effectiveness study. JAMA. 2004;291:2563–70.
15. Neufeld LM, Steta C, Rivera J, Valle AM, Grados R, Uriega S, López VH. Evaluation for program decision making: a case study of the Oportunidades program in Mexico. J Nutr. 2011;141(11):2076–83.
16. Leroy J, Vermandere H, Neufeld L, Bertozzi S. Improving enrollment and utilization of the Oportunidades program in Mexico could increase its effectiveness. J Nutr. 2008;138(3):638–41.
17. García-Guerra A, Neufeld L, Domínguez-Islas CP, García Feregrino R, HernándezCabrera A. Effect of three supplements with identical micronutrient content on anemia in Mexican children. FASEB J. 2008;22:677.5.
18. García-Guerra A, Rivera-Dommarco J, Neufeld LM, Domínguez-Islas CP. Effect of three supplements with equal micronutrient content on serum zinc concentrations in Mexican children. FASEB J. 2009;23:917.13.
19. Hernández AM, Romieu I, Parra S, Hernández JA, Madrigal H, Willet W. Validity and reproducibility of a food frequency questionnaire to assess dietary intake of women living in Mexico City. Salud Publica Mex. 1998;40: 133–40.
20. Safdie M, Barquera S, Porcayo M, et al., Inventors. Bases de datos del valor nutritivo de los alimentos. Compilación del Instituto Nacional de Salud Pública 2004.
21. Rodrıguez-Ramırez S, Mundo-Rosas V, Jimenez-Aguilar A, Shamah-Levy T. Methodology for the analysis of dietary data from the Mexican National Health and nutrition survey 2006. Salud Publica de Mexico. 2009;51(suppl 4): S523–9.
22. Food and Nutrition Board IOM. Dietary Refrence Intake for Vitamin A, Vitamina K, Arsenic, Boron, Chromium, Copper, Iodine, Iron, Manganese, Milybdenum, Nickel, Silicon, Vanadium and Zinc. Washington, D.C: National Academy Press; 2001.
23. Food and Nutrition Board IOM. Dietary Refrence Intake for Energy,Carbohydrate, Fiber, Fat, Fatty Acids, Cholesterol, Protein and Amino Acids. Washington, D.C: National Academy Press; 2005.
24. Morales-Ruán M, Del C, Villalpando S, García-Guerra A, Shamah-Levy T, Robledo-Pérez R, Avila-Arcos MA, Rivera JA. Iron, zinc, copper and magnesium nutritional status in Mexican children aged 1 to 11 years. Salud Publica Mex. 2012;54(2):125–34.
25. Cuevas-Nasu L, Mundo-Rosas V, Shamah-Levy T, Méndez-Gómez Humaran I, Avila-Arcos MA, Rebollar-Campos Mdel R, Villalpando S. Prevalence of folate and vitamin B12 deficiency in Mexican children aged 1 to 6 years in a population-based survey. Salud Publica Mex. 2012;54(2):116–24.

26. Lohr SL. Complex surveys in: Lohr SL. Sampling: design and analysis. 2nd ed. Boston: Brooks/Cole; 2009.
27. Parente PMDC, Santos Silva JMC. Quantile regression with clustered data. J of Eco Meth. 2016;5(1):1–15.
28. Islam MM, Khatun M, Peerson JM, Ahmed T, Mollah MA, Dewey KG, Brown KH. Effects of energy density and feeding frequency of complementary foods on total daily energy intakes and consumption of breast milk by healthy breastfed Bangladeshi children. Am J Clin Nutr. 2008;88:84–94.
29. Diana A, Mallard SR, Haszard JJ, Purnamasari DM, Nurulazmi I, Herliani PD, et al. Consumption of fortified infant foods reduces dietary diversity but has a positive effect on subsequent growth in infants from Sumedang district, Indonesia. PLoS ONE. 2017;12(4):e0175952. https://doi.org/10.1371/journal.pone.0175952
30. Campbell RK, Hurley KM, Shamim AA, Shaikh S, Chowdhury ZT, Mehra S, de Pee S, Ahmed T, West KP, Christian P. Effect of complementary food supplementation on breastfeeding and home diet in rural Bangladeshi children. Am J Clin Nutr. 2016;104(5):1450–8. https://doi.org/10.3945/ajcn.116.135509
31. Maleta K, Kuittinen J, Duggan MB, Briend A, Manary M, Wales J, Kulmala T, Ashorn P. Supplementary feeding of underweight, stunted Malawian children with a ready-to-use food. J Pediatr Gastroenterol Nutr. 2004;38:152–8.
32. Thakwalakwa CM, Ashorn P, Phuka JC, Cheung YB, Briend A, Maleta KM. Impact of lipid-based nutrient supplements and corn-soy blend on energy and nutrient intake among moderately underweight 8-18-month-old children participating in a clinical trial. Matern Child Nutr. 2015;11(Suppl 4):144–50.
33. Ramírez-Silva I, Rivera J, Leroy J, Neufeld L. The Oportunidades programs fortified food supplement, but not improvements in the home diet, increased the intake of key micronutrients in rural Mexican children aged 12–59 months. J Nutr. 2013;143:656–63.
34. Villalpando S, de la Cruz V, Shamah-Levy T, Rebollar R, Contreras-Manzano A. Nutritional status of iron, vitamin B12, folate, retinol and anemia in children 1 to 11 years old. Results of the Ensanut 2012. Salud Publica Mex. 2015;57:372–84.
35. Mora JO. Iron supplementation: overcoming technical and practical barriers. J Nutr. 2002;132(4 Suppl):853S–5S.
36. Nguyen M, Poonawala A, Leyvraz M, Berger J, Schofield D, Nga TT, Van TK, do TB H, Wieringa FT. A Delivery Model for Home Fortification of Complementary Foods with Micronutrient Powders: Innovation in the Context of Vietnamese Health System Strengthening. Nutrients. 2016;8(5):E259. https://doi.org/10.3390/nu8050259.
37. Zlotkin SH, Arthur P, Antwi KY, Yeung G. Treatment of anemia with microencapsulated ferrous fumarate plus ascorbic acid supplied as 'sprinkles' to complementary (weaning) foods. Am J Clin Nutr. 2001;74:791–5.
38. Zlotkin SH, Schauer C, Christofides A, Sharieff W, Tondeur MC, et al. Micronutrient Sprinkles to Control Childhood Anaemia. Micronutrient Sprinkles to Control Childhood Anaemia. PLOS Medicine. 2005;2(1). https://doi.org/10.1371/journal.pmed.0020001.
39. Hyder SMZ, Zlotkin SH, Haseen F, Zeng L. Efficacy of daily vs. weekly home fortification of weaning foods with Sprinkles among infants and young children in Dhaka, Bangladesh. In: Workshop proceedings from the National Workshop on Home Fortification of Weaning Food with Sprinkles: A new strategy to control iron deficiency anemia among infants and young children; 2004. Dhaka: Bangladesh rural advancement committee. p 1–24 http://research.brac.net/reports/2004_sprinkles_efficacy_report.pdf. Accessed 21 May 2018.
40. Mirkovic KR, Perrine CG, Subedi GR, Mebrahtu S, Dahal P, Staatz C, Jefferds ME. Predictors of micronutrient powder intake adherence in a pilot programme in Nepal. Public Health Nutr. 2016;19(10):1768–76.
41. Ciomarten T, Nanu R, Iorgulascu D, Moldovanue F, Popa S, Palicari G. Iron supplement trial in Romania. In: Nestel P, editor. Proceedings, Iron Interventions for Child Survival. London: USAID and ICH; 1995. p. 89–98.
42. Nestel P, Alnwick D (1997) Iron/multi-micronutrient supplements for young children. Summary and conclusions of consultation. UNICEF, Copenhagen, August 19–20, 1996. Washington, DC: International Life Sciences Institute.
43. Ip H, Hyder S, Haseen F, Rahman M, Zlotkin S. Improved adherence and anaemia cure rates with flexible administration of micronutrient sprinkles: a new public health approach to anaemia control. Eur J Clin Nutr. 2009;63:165–72.
44. Martorell R, de Romaña DL. Components of successful staple food fortification programs: lessons from Latin America. Food Nutr Bull. 2017;38(3):384–404.
45. Neufeld LM, Baker S, Garrett GS, Haddad L. Coverage and utilization in food fortification programs: critical and neglected areas of evaluation. J Nutr. 2017;147(5):1015S–9S.
46. Diana A, Mallard SR, Haszard JJ Purnamasari DM, Nurulazmi I, Herliani PD, et al. Consumption of fortified infant foods reduces dietary diversity but has a positive effect on subsequent growth in infants from Sumedang district, Indonesia. PLoS ONE 2017;12(4):e0175952.
47. Dewey KG. The challenge of meeting nutrient needs of infants and young children during the period of complementary feeding: an evolutionary perspective. J Nutr. 2013 Dec;143(12):2050–4.
48. Osendarp SJ, Broersen B, van Liere MJ, De-Regil LM, Bahirathan L, Klassen E, Neufeld LM. Complementary feeding diets made of local foods can be optimized, but additional interventions will be needed to meet Iron and zinc requirements in 6- to 23-month-old children in low- and middle-income countries. Food Nutr Bull. 2016;37(4):544–70.
49. Vossenaar M, Solomons NW. The concept of "critical nutrient density" in complementary feeding: the demands on the "family foods" for the nutrient adequacy of young Guatemalan children with continued breastfeeding. Am J Clin Nutr. 2012;95(4):859–66.
50. Dewey KG. Reducing stunting by improving maternal, infant and young child nutrition in regions such as South Asia: evidence, challenges and opportunities. Matern Child Nutr. 2016;12(Suppl 1):27–38.
51. Bhutta ZA, Ahmed T, Black RE, Cousens S, Dewey K, Giugliani E, Haider BA, Kirkwood B, Morris SS, Sachdev HPS, Shekar M. Maternal and Child Undernutrition Study Group. What works? Interventions for maternal and child undernutrition and survival. Lancet. 2008;371:417–40.
52. Miller S, Abalos E, Chamillard M, Ciapponi A, Colaci D, Comandé D, Diaz V, Geller S, Hanson C, Langer A, Manuelli V, Millar K, Morhason-Bello I, Castro CP, Pileggi VN, Robinson N, Skaer M, Souza JP, Vogel JP, Althabe F. Beyond too little, too late and too much, too soon: a pathway towards evidence-based, respectful maternity care worldwide. Lancet. 2016;388(10056):2176–92.
53. Flores L, Théodore F, Bonvecchio A, Blanco I, Neufeld LM. Acceptability of three supplements with identical micronutrient content in Mexican children. FASEB J. 2008;22:677.2.

9

Efficacy of high zinc biofortified wheat in improvement of micronutrient status, and prevention of morbidity among preschool children and women

Sunil Sazawal[1,2,3*], Usha Dhingra[1], Pratibha Dhingra[1], Arup Dutta[1], Saikat Deb[1], Jitendra Kumar[1], Prabhabati Devi[1] and Ashish Prakash[3]

Abstract

Background: Biofortification of staple food crops with zinc (Zn) can be one of the cost-effective and sustainable strategies to combat zinc deficiency and prevent morbidity among the target population. Agronomic approaches such as application of Zn fertilizers to soil and/or foliar spray seem to be a practical tool for Zn biofortification of wheat. However, there is a need to evaluate its efficacy from randomized controlled trials. This study aimed to evaluate the efficacy of zinc biofortified wheat flour on zinc status and its impact on morbidity among children aged 4–6 years and non-pregnant non lactating woman of child bearing age (WCBA) in Delhi, India.

Methods: In a community based, double-masked randomized controlled trial, 6005 participants (WCBA and child pairs) were enrolled and randomly allocated to receive either high zinc biofortified wheat flour (HZn, 30 ppm zinc daily) or low zinc biofortified wheat flour (LZn, 20 ppm zinc daily) for 6 months (WCBA @ 360 g/day and children @ 120 g/day). Baseline and endline blood samples were obtained for assessing hematological markers; zinc status and data on compliance and morbidity were collected.

Results: Compliance rates were high; ~ 88% of the WCBAs in both the groups consumed 50% or more of recommended amount of biofortfied wheat flour during the follow up. Similarly 86.9% children in HZn and 87.5% in LZn consumed 50% or more of recommended wheat flour intake. There was no significant difference in mean zinc levels between the groups at end study. This observation might be due to a marginal difference in zinc content (10 ppm) between the HZn and LZn wheat flour, and a short intervention period. However a positive impact of biofortification on self-reported morbidity was observed. Compared to children in LZn group, children in HZn group had 17% (95% CI: 6 to 31%, $p = 0.05$) and 40% (95% CI: 16 to 57%; $p = 0.0019$) reduction in days with pneumonia and vomiting respectively. WCBA in the HZn group also showed a statistically significant 9% fewer days with fever compared to LZn group.

(Continued on next page)

* Correspondence: ssazawal@jhu.edu
[1]Center for Public Health Kinetics, 214A, Vinoba Puri, Lajpat Nagar-II, New Delhi 110024, India
[2]Department of International Health, Johns Hopkins Bloomberg School of Public Health, Baltimore, MD, USA
Full list of author information is available at the end of the article

(Continued from previous page)

Conclusions: Biofortified wheat flour had a good compliance among children and WCBAs. Significant improvement on some of the self-reported morbidity indicators suggests that evaluating longer-term effects of biofortification with higher grain zinc content would be more appropriate.

Keywords: Zinc, Biofortification, Children, Woman of child-bearing age, Morbidity, Plasma zinc, India

Background

Micronutrient malnutrition has been recognized as a huge and rapidly growing public health problem around the globe [1, 2]. More than two billion people worldwide suffer from micronutrient deficiency (especially of zinc and iron) and zinc ranks fifth in the leading risk factors for illness and disease in developing countries with high mortality [3]. Estimates indicate that approximately 20.5% of the world's population might be at risk of zinc deficiency [4]. In India, estimated 25.9% population is at risk of inadequate zinc intake, and is considered to be high-risk category [3]. Risk factors include insufficient dietary intake due to poverty, food taboos and vegetarian diets that are high in phytate and fiber, poor utilization due to environmental factors such as poor hygiene that lead to increased infections and infestations, adverse zinc iron interaction [5] and genetic causes [6].The dietary intake of preschool children in the urban slums of India is no better than those of rural population of India [7].Women of reproductive age (WRA) are also vulnerable to nutritional deficiencies, including that of zinc [8]. Poor maternal zinc status has been associated with negative pregnancy outcomes [9], including spontaneous abortion, congenital malformation, low birth weight, and preterm delivery [10, 11].

Micronutrient deficiencies can be alleviated by direct (nutrition-specific) and indirect (nutrition-sensitive) interventions [12]. Direct interventions focus on consumption behavior and include dietary diversification, micronutrient supplementation, modification of food choices and fortification. Nutrition-sensitive interventions address the underlying determinants of malnutrition and include biofortification. Biofortification is the process of increasing the content and/or bioavailability of essential nutrients in crops during plant growth through genetic and agronomic pathways [13]. Genetic biofortification involves either genetic engineering or classical breeding [14]. Agronomic biofortification is achieved through micronutrient fertilizer application to the soil and/or foliar application directly to the leaves of the crop. Even though this approach seems simple and inexpensive, this strategy has been successful in only limited cases and in particular geographical locations due to the limitations of fertilizer and soil chemistry, together with the added complications of nutrient mobility and storage within the plant.

Although zinc supplementation has been proven to be cost effective strategy in reducing morbidity and improving growth, giving zinc supplementation daily is not feasible as a program [15] thus, other sustainable methods such as food based intervention to increase zinc intakes need to be explored and evaluated. Plant breeding of staple crops, such as wheat or rice, to increase the zinc concentration can be a promising approach to increase zinc intakes of populations in developing countries [16, 17]. In northern India, although the consumption of cereals has declined in the past few decades, wheat consumption has shown no significant change and has the highest dietary share; contributing more than 50% calories to the diet [18], which is similar to consumption in many developing countries [19]. Thus, biofortification of wheat can be one of the novel food based approaches, which can provide higher levels of micronutrients directly into key staple foods [19–21].

Recently, Harvest Plus and its partners have developed wheat lines that can achieve zinc concentration of 60–70 ppm when adequately fertilized with zinc, adding ~ 20–25 ppm of zinc in the daily diet of children (aged 4–6 years) and women of reproductive age. However, there is lack of scientific evidence from randomized controlled trials for its efficacy in improving zinc nutritional status and related health outcomes in the target population groups. Therefore, we evaluated the efficacy of high zinc biofortified wheat flour on zinc status, prevention of morbidity and growth among children aged 4–6 years and non pregnant non lactating women aged 15–49 years compared to group that received low zinc biofortified wheat flour.

Methods

Study population and setting

This study was carried out in Sangam Vihar, a resettlement colony in outskirts of south Delhi; and Harsh Vihar, a semi-urban locality in North East District, Delhi, India. Entire study area at both field sites has been digitized and all the households are geo referenced and numbered. Both sites have similar demographic profile. Most of the inhabitants are migrants from eastern Uttar Pradesh, Bihar and Rajasthan. Literacy rates are low with 50% of the women being illiterate. About 80% of the men work as daily wage laborers or in factories, while 95% of women are housewives. Average family income is below US$600/year. Community has minimal access to sewage, drinking water and paved roads. Diarrhea and respiratory illnesses are common causes of childhood mortality and morbidity. Field sites are representative of wheat eating population of India.

Ethics

The human research and ethical review committees at the Johns Hopkins University, USA; Annamalai University, Tamil Nadu, India and Subharti Medical College, Meerut, UP, India approved the study protocol. The purpose of the study was explained to the participants/parents (in case of children) in the local language, and a written informed consent was obtained.

Sample size

Sample size calculations were based on prevalence of zinc deficiency of 70% (assessed by plasma zinc levels) in previously conducted studies in the same population [22]. A sample size of 3000 (1500 in each of the intervention and placebo groups) each for WCBA and children was sufficient to detect a clinically important difference of 25% between a group 1 proportion, of 0.400 and a group 2 proportion, of 0.455 (odds ratio of 1.250), using a two-sided χ^2test with 80% power, at 5% significance level and assuming 10% attrition rate.

Consent and enrollment

Eligibility criteria

Preschool children Between 4 and 6 years of age, not severely malnourished requiring rehabilitation; parental permission to participate; likely to live in the study area for at least 6 months, wheat as a staple diet.

Women of child-bearing age Between 15 and 49 years of age (non-lactating and non pregnant), not having any severe illnesses requiring hospitalization; consent to participate; permanent residents or staying in the study area for next six months, wheat as a staple diet.

The study area was divided into small working areas (grids) and all the households in the grid were allocated to a study worker. The study worker visited every household in the grid allocated to him/her to identify the mother-child pairs eligible to participate in the study. After identification of potential participants, the study supervisor visited the household and explained the study purpose to the participants/caregivers (in case of child). All potential participants were requested to come to the clinic for formal consent and enrollment into the study. In the clinic, study physician examined the participant (WCBA and child) for eligibility criteria and if successful, the study supervisor obtained the formal consent from the participant/spouse (in case of woman) or parents (in case of children) and enrolled the participants into the study.

Masking and randomization

Households with eligible mother and child pairs were randomly allocated to receive either high zinc biofortified wheat or low zinc biofortified wheat. For masking purposes, wheat bags were labeled with alphanumeric codes. Eight codes (4 for each intervention group) were used. Each of these 8 codes had a letter i.e. A through H in the beginning. These codes were only known to the manufacturer or person doing the packaging of the interventions and to the data safety and monitoring board (DSMB) members. These codes were maintained in a sealed envelope till the study was over. A computerized randomization schedule with permuted block length of 16 was generated for 6050 participants.

Intervention

Harvest Plus provided high zinc biofortified and low zinc biofortified wheat flour free of charge for the entire duration of the project. The wheat variety used for control and intervention groups was a commercial variety (PBW 550) developed and released by Punjab Agricultural University in 2007. Standard farming techniques as prescribed in the package and practices recommended by Punjab Agricultural University, Ludhiana were followed during the entire growing period. Low zinc biofortified wheat was grown in agro-ecological conditions that limit the uptake of soil zinc by plants and received no additional zinc fertilization. The wheat (HZn) for the intervention group was grown in agro-ecological conditions and additional foliar spraying of 0.5% zinc sulphate fertilizer that foster the zinc uptake by the plant and its deposit in the growing seeds was done. PBW 550 is not a genetically modified organism (GMO) and was grown at farmers' fields in Punjab (districts Kapurthala and Bathinda), India. The wheat was milled and packaged by Arti Roller Flour Industries Ltd.- an ISO 22000:2005 certified company.

Intervention delivery and follow up

Participants were provided wheat flour ration every 25 days based on the dietary intake data available from the previously conducted studies and the qualitative data collected on wheat consumption patterns during the preparatory phase of the study. They were clearly explained and demonstrated that they could use the biofortified wheat flour for making chapattis, puris, porridge etc. as with regular wheat flour. The cooked preparation (e.g. *chapatti/tortilia or puri*) could be consumed as such or could be eaten with any lentil or vegetable. Participants were encouraged to take normal home diet ad libitum. During the follow-up, a designated ration (based on the findings from the preparatory phase) was supplied to the enrolled participants by the study staff with an advice to consume 120 g (aged 4–6 years) or 360 g (aged 15–49 years) of assigned wheat flour daily. To prevent sharing of ration with other family members, additional 200 g wheat flour daily per household was provided to the family in both the groups. Wheat flour for family members was same as was given to the participant (HZn or LZn). Participants were followed up on a weekly basis by the study worker for collection of compliance, morbidity information and medication/supplement use. On each visit, the compliance (adherence with the intervention) was assessed by collecting the information on reported intake of biofortified wheat flour in terms of number of days it was being offered and consumed, portion size consumed and unused quantity recovered. The participant/parent of the child was given a pictorial diary card and was asked to record the quantity of wheat flour preparation consumed on a daily basis. Study worker reviewed the diary card on each visit, collected the filled diary card and left a new card for recording information.

If a participant was found to be sick during follow-up, he or she was referred to the study clinic for a detailed morbidity assessment by the study physician. They had been counselled to visit the clinic anytime to seek care for illnesses. The participant was provided treatment by the study physician. During the study, spot checks were carried out to assess the food availability at home. During the follow up, on a sub-sample of participants, dietary data were collected using an interactive 24-h dietary recall method [23] to estimate the macro- or micro-nutrient intake with special emphasis on zinc, iron and vitamin A and antinutrient (phytic acid) content by the trained nutritionist at home.

Data collection

Socio-demographic data collection

Socioeconomic status, demographic details, illness information in the last two weeks was recorded in a pre-designed data-recording sheet at the clinic for baseline data collection.

Baseline assessment

After obtaining the informal consent, participants were asked to visit the clinic on a scheduled date for baseline assessments.

Medical examination The study physician conducted a physical examination and collected information on the medical history of the participant for the last two weeks including history of hospitalizations/blood transfusions in the last 6 months.

Anthropometry measurements Two independent observers measured weight to the nearest 10 g with an electronic scale (ATCO weighing solutions, India) and height to the nearest 0.1 cm using locally improvised height board. In addition, waist of the WRA was measured with a tape measure one inch above the navel while standing and values reported to the nearest quarter inch.

Blood sampling, plasma separation and laboratory procedures A venous blood sample (5 ml) was collected in trace element-free syringe by trained technician. Approximately half ml of blood was transferred to an EDTA tube for hemogram and the remaining blood was transferred to a tube containing zinc free heparin, for separation of plasma. Approx 100 μL of EDTA whole blood was used to determine haemoglobin, RDW, MCV, MCH by a KX21 automated haematological analyzer (Sysmex tech, Japan).

Plasma zinc Plasma was separated within 15 min of blood collection and aliquots transferred into trace element-free Eppendorf plastic tubes for storage at −20 °C until analysis.

Endline assessment

Blood sample and anthropometry assessments were repeated at the end of 6 months of follow up.

Laboratory analysis

Plasma samples were analyzed for zinc status using an atomic absorption spectrometer (AAS 400-Perkin Elmer, USA) at the micronutrient research lab in Subharti Medical College, Meerut. For quality assurance, we ran three in house pooled plasma controls (low, medium and high) after every 10 batch of samples.

Zinc and phytate analysis of wheat flour samples

Biochemical analysis was carried out on all 18 batches of wheat flour received for zinc and phytate content (Additional file 1: Table S1 and Table S2). From batch-9 onwards, zinc analysis was undertaken in one additional lab, in order to ensure the reliability of the test results of wheat flour samples. The zinc content of high zinc biofortified wheat flour was 30 ppm and of low zinc biofortified wheat flour was 20 ppm.

Statistical analyses

We used in house data management system with stringent range and logical checks for data entry and management. Study team used netbooks to enter real time data. The analyses were performed in STATA 13.0 (Stata Corp., College Station, Texas, USA) and SPSS 23 (SPSS Inc., Chicago, Illinois, USA). Intent-to-treat analysis was performed and all participants were included in analysis irrespective of compliance to intervention. For the primary analysis the authors used alphabetical codes for the groups as they were still blinded to the real group identity. The groups were assessed for comparability at baseline. The statistical significance for the group differences of continuous variables was established using a Student's t-test, and of categorical variables by chi-square test. Significance was considered as p-values < 0.05. Participants were considered zinc deficient if their plasma zinc levels were below 70 μg/dL. They were further classified into 3 categories; improved: if they were zinc deficient at baseline but became zinc sufficient at endline; worsened: if sufficient at baseline but became deficient at endline, and no change: if there was no change in status. Risk estimates and confidence intervals were calculated for morbidity indicators for each participant; days with morbidity were considered as numerator while days' informant available was considered as denominator.

Results

Participants

Between April 14, 2014 and February 23, 2015, a total of 6162 participants were screened, 157 failed eligibility criteria and a total of 6005 participants were enrolled. The enrolled participants were randomly allocated to receive either high zinc biofortified (HZn) wheat flour ($n = 2997$) or the low zinc biofortified (LZn) wheat flour ($n = 3008$) (Fig. 1).

Baseline data

Both groups had comparable socio-economic, and demographic profile (Table 1). Mean age at enrollment for WCBA was 29.8 (SD: 5.9) years in HZn and 29.8 (SD: 6.0) in LZn group. Children at enrollment had mean age of 5.0 (SD: 0.8) years in HZn and 5.1 (SD: 0.8) years in LZn group.

Compliance

Compliance was high in both groups. Women in both groups consumed >= 50% of recommended amount of biofortified wheat flour (360 g) on 88% of the follow up days (HZn: 88.1%; LZn: 88.7%). Similarly 86.9% children in HZn and 87.5% in LZn consumed >= 50% of recommended amount of biofortified wheat flour (120 g) during follow up (Table 2).

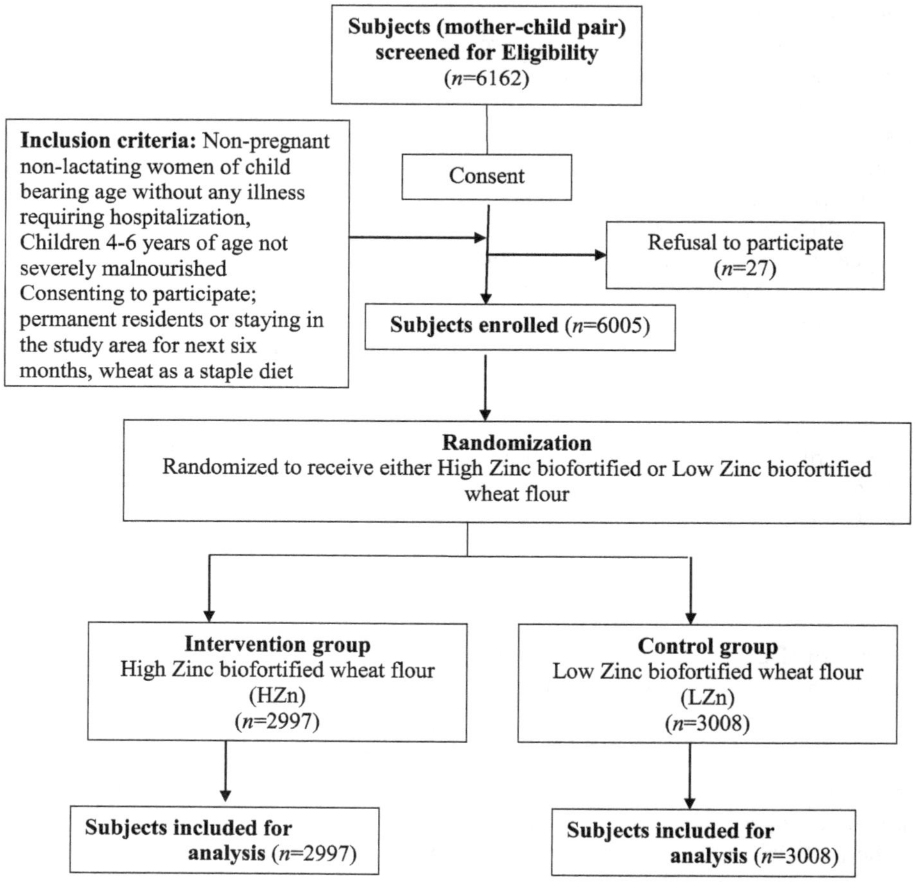

Fig. 1 Study participants flow diagram

Table 1 Baseline characteristics of the study population

	HZn	LZn
Age (years)		
WCBA	29.8 ± 5.9	29.8 ± 6.0
Children	5.0 ± 0.8	5.1 ± 0.8
Type of family		
Nuclear	83.1%	80.9%
Type of household		
Pucca	27.8%	26.2%
Kuccha-Pucca	71.3%	73.3%
Kuccha	0.9%	0.5%
Own house	52.9%	56.3%
Tube well/bore water	86.0%	84.7%

Effect on hematological markers

At baseline 18.0% children in HZn and 16.8% in LZn group were moderately anemic (70–100 g/L); while among WCBA's 19.6% in HZn and 21% in LZn were moderately anemic. At the end of 6 months of follow up, children in HZn and LZn group had mean hemoglobin levels (g/L) of 114.0 ± 15.7 and 114.6 ± 16.1 respectively; 13.5% in HZn and 11.9% in LZn remained moderately anemic at endline sampling. At endline, HZn WCBA's had mean hemoglobin levels (g/L) of 114.1 ± 19.8 while LZn WCBA's had 113.2 ± 19.9. There was a statistically significant difference in RDW between HZn and LZn children at endline but this seems to be by chance since RDW without anemia has no predictive value for iron deficiency anemia [24]. Comparison of hematological markers between the two groups at baseline and after 6 months of intervention is presented in Tables 3 and 4.

Effect on plasma zinc status

At baseline 85.8% of children in HZn and 84.7% in LZn had zinc levels below 70 μg/dL. After 6 months of follow up, 27.2% children in HZn and 26.7% children in LZn showed improvement (Zinc levels above 70 μg/dL) (OR: 0.98; 95% CI 0.81–1.17).There was change in plasma zinc levels from baseline to endline in both the groups (Diff in means (μg/dL):1.08; 95% CI -0.54-2.69). Among WCBAs, 85.5% in HZn group and 87.5% in LZn group were zinc deficient at baseline. Of these 21% WCBAs in HZn and 22.4% in LZn group became zinc sufficient after 6 months of intervention (OR:1.08; 95% CI 0.90–1.31) (Tables 5 and 6).

Effect on morbidity

Based on self-reported morbidity information, HZn children experienced 17% lower days with pneumonia compared to children in LZn group. There was a statistically significant 39% lower risk of days with vomiting in HZn group compared to LZn group children. Days with ear discharge were 17% lower in HZn group compared to LZn group. WCBAs in HZn group had statistically significant 9% reduction in days with fever compared to WCBAs in LZn group (Tables 7 and 8).

Discussion

This study, reports the first large randomized controlled trial, evaluating efficacy of zinc biofortified wheat consumption in improvement of micronutrient status, and prevention of morbidity among preschool children (aged 4–6 years) and non pregnant non lactating women of child bearing age. The study was conducted in a low resource setting in India with high levels of zinc deficiency among children and women of child bearing age.

Table 2 Compliance of biofortified wheat flour among WCBA and children

WCBA	HZn (*n* = 287,514)	LZn (*n* = 286,605)
Days consumed >= 50% of recommended wheat flour	253,254 (88.1)	254,100 (88.7)
Days consumed full (360 g daily)	159,569 (55.5)	161,579 (56.4)
Days consumed more than half	79,432 (27.6)	76,200 (26.6)
Days consumed half	14,253 (5.0)	16,321 (5.7)
Days consumed 1/4th	1087 (0.4)	1051 (0.4)
Days did not consume	33,173 (11.5)	31,454 (11.0)
Children	HZn (*n* = 288,903)	LZn (n = 286,901)
Days consumed >= 50% of recommended wheat flour	251,214 (86.9)	250,981 (87.5)
Days consumed full (120 g daily)	157,547 (54.5)	155,076 (54.1)
Days consumed more than half	71,891 (24.9)	73,714 (25.7)
Days consumed half	21,776 (7.5)	22,191 (7.7)
Days consumed 1/4th	2257(0.8)	2274 (0.8)
Days did not consume	35,432 (12.3)	33,646 (11.7)

Table 3 Baseline and endline hematological parameters among WCBA (HZn vs. LZn)

	HZn	LZn	Difference of means (95% CI)	*p* value
Baseline	(*n* = 1400)	(*n* = 1388)		
Hb (g/L)	113.1 ± 20.6	112.8 ± 20.8	0.6 (−0.9 to 2.1)	0.5
Hct (%)	35.5 ± 5.8	35.4 ± 5.8	0.1 (− 0.3 to 0.5)	0.6
MCH (pg)	27.9 ± 3.8	27.7 ± 4.0	0.2 (−0.07 to 0.5)	0.1
MCV (fl)	87.6 ± 9.7	87.1 ± 10.2	0.5 (−0.2 to 1.3)	0.2
RDW (%)	15.8 ± 2.1	16.0 ± 2.3	−0.1 (− 0.3 to 0.03)	0.1
Endline	(*n* = 1316)	(*n* = 1324)		
Hb (g/L)	114.1 ± 19.8	113.3 ± 19.8	0.8 (−0.7to 2.3)	0.3
Hct (%)	34.8 ± 5.5	34.7 ± 5.5	0.1 (−0.2to 0.5)	0.4
MCH (pg)	28.0 ± 3.8	27.9 ± 3.9	0.1 (−0.2 to 0.4)	0.4
MCV (fl)	85.7 ± 9.7	85.5 ± 9.9	0.2 (−0.6 to 0.9)	0.6
RDW (%)	15.5 ± 2.3	15.6 ± 2.2	−0.1 (− 0.2 to 0.1)	0.6

Hb Hemoglobin, *HCT* Hematocrit, *MCH* Mean corpuscular hemoglobin, *MCV* Mean corpuscular volume, *RDW* Red blood cell distribution width

In our study, consumption of high zinc biofortified wheat flour for 6 months compared to low zinc biofortified wheat resulted in statistically significant reduction in days with pneumonia and vomiting among children and days with fever among women of reproductive age. Similar findings have been reported by earlier zinc supplementation randomized controlled trials showing an effect of zinc supplementation in decreasing morbidity and mortality in children due to gastrointestinal and respiratory infections [25]. Participants in all the zinc supplementation studies were supplemented with zinc daily, over and above regular dietary intake and dose of zinc supplementation ranged from 10 mg to 20 mg and duration from 4.6 to 18 months.

There is limited evidence available on the efficacy of zinc biofortified crops. Rosado et al. [26] carried out a trial among 27 women who consumed 300 g of 95% or 80% extracted wheat flour of tortillas for 2 consecutive days using either biofortified (41 mg Zn/g) or control (24 mg Zn/g) wheat. Zn intake from the biofortified wheat was higher at 80% extraction compared with the corresponding control wheat ($p = 0.007$). In India, Kodkany et al. [27] provided zinc and iron biofortified pearl millet flour to children under 2 years and concluded that quantities of zinc absorbed from biofortified pearl millet as the major food staple is more than adequate to meet the physiological requirements of these nutrients. Study from Zambia [28] indicated that feeding biofortified

Table 4 Baseline and endline hematological parameters among children (HZn vs. LZn)

	HZn	LZn	Difference of means (95% CI)	*p* value
Baseline	(*n* = 1383)	(*n* = 1364)		
Hb (g/L)	112.1 ± 17.1	111.7 ± 16.4	0.4 (−0.9 to 1.6)	0.6
Hct (%)	34.2 ± 4.8	34.2 ± 4.6	0.1 (−0.2 to 0.5)	0.5
MCH (pg)	25.2 ± 3.0	25.2 ± 2.8	0.0 (−0.2 to 0.2)	0.9
MCV (fl)	77.0 ± 7.6	77.0 ± 7.2	0.0 (−0.6 to 0.6)	0.9
RDW (%)	15.4 ± 2.1	15.3 ± 1.9	0.1 (−0.02 to 0.3)	0.1
Endline	(*n* = 1269)	(*n* = 1265)		
Hb (g/L)	114.0 ± 15.7	114.6 ± 16.1	−0.6 (−1.9 to 0.6)	0.3
Hct (%)	33.9 ± 4.3	34.1 ± 4.4	−0.2 (− 0.5 to 0.2)	0.3
MCH (pg)	25.6 ± 2.8	25.5 ± 2.6	0.1 (−0.2 to 0.3)	0.6
MCV (fl)	76.2 ± 7.4	76.1 ± 6.7	0.1 (−0.4 to 0.7)	0.6
RDW (%)	15.1 ± 2.3	14.9 ± 2.0	0.2 (0.05 to 0.4)	0.0

Hb Hemoglobin, *HCT* Hematocrit, *MCH* Mean corpuscular hemoglobin, *MCV* Mean corpuscular volume, *RDW* Red blood cell distribution width

Table 5 Comparison of plasma zinc levels (μg/dL) among children at baseline and endline

	HZn	LZn	
Baseline	(*n* = 1448)	(*n* = 1445)	
Mean ± SD	55.9 ± 14.5	56.9 ± 13.9	
Median	55.5	57.4	
Zinc deficient	1242 (85.8)	1224 (84.7)	
Endline	(*n* = 1239)	(*n* = 1234)	
Mean ± SD	63.0 ± 15.6	63.1 ± 15.7	
Median	61.6	63.4	
Zinc deficient	862 (69.6)	855 (69.3)	
Change in Zinc Status			
Change in mean Zinc levels	7.22 ± 20.3	6.14 ± 20.4	1.08 (−0.54 to 2.69)
Improvement in zinc status	322 (27.2)	312 (26.7)	0.98 (0.81 to 1.17)

maize could meet zinc requirements and provide an effective dietary alternative to regular maize. In contrast the grain zinc concentrations levels achieved using the agronomic Zn foliar sprays/fertilizers in our study were very low. In our study the high zinc biofortified wheat would have at best delivered 3.6 mg/d of zinc to children and 10.8 mg/d to women if they had consumed 100% of recommended intake; in comparison the control group (low zinc biofortified wheat) would have delivered 2.4 mg/d to children and 7.8 mg/d to women. The daily Zn requirement is 15 mg for both adults and children that are 4 and older [29]. To meet this allowance wheat grains should contain 40–60 mg kg^{-1}Zn. Although there was an improvement in zinc status (plasma zinc levels> 70 μg/dL) within each group but given the adjuvant used to enhance zinc absorption through the leaves was not optimal and the minimum expected increase of 20 ppm over the low biofortified wheat was not achieved, this improvement was similar between the groups. This study does indicate the potential for use of biofortification as a means of improving zinc nutrition with a caveat to improve the biofortification process such that wheat grains contain 40–60 mg kg^{-1}Zn to meet the recommended dietary allowance of Zn.

Table 6 Comparison of plasma zinc levels (μg/dL) among WCBAs at baseline and endline

	HZn	LZn	
Baseline	(*n* = 1472)	(*n* = 1476)	
Mean ± SD	55.4 ± 14.0	54.9 ± 14.4	
Median	55.1	55.4	
Zinc Deficient	1258 (85.5)	1292 (87.5)	
Endline	(*n* = 1312)	(*n* = 1317)	
Mean ± SD	60.9 ± 14.7	60.7 ± 14.8	
Median	61.6	59.9	
Zinc Deficient	994 (75.8)	989 (75.1)	
Change in zinc status			
Change in Mean Zinc levels	5.49 ± 19.8	5.91 ± 19.5	−0.42 (−1.92 to 1.08)
Improvement in zinc status	265 (21.0)	285 (22.4)	1.08 (0.90 to 1.31)

Table 7 Effect of consumption of wheat flour (HZn vs. LZn) on morbidity among children

	HZn	LZn	RR	95% CI
Days with diarrhea	126	119	1.05	0.82 to 1.35
Days with pneumonia	203	244	0.82	0.68 to 0.99
Days with fever	934	960	0.96	0.88 to 1.06
Days with vomiting	60	99	0.60	0.44 to 0.83
Days with ear discharge	72	87	0.82	0.60 to 1.12

Zinc bioavailability pilot trial designed to estimate the amount of zinc absorbed from zinc rice compared to conventional rice using the triple stable isotope tracer ratio technique, failed to produce detectable differences in absorbed zinc [30]. High phytate and lower-than-expected zinc in the biofortified zinc variety was suggested as a cause for no significant difference in absorption between groups. Zinc uptake by wheat and translocation into the grains is affected by genetic-environment interactions and evidently by the efficiency of the foliar application of the fertilizer. In our study, the adjuvant used to enhance zinc absorption through the leaves was not optimal and could not produce the HZn variety with expected Zn content.

There is sufficient evidence from previous studies undertaken in 7 countries over different seasons [31] that foliar zinc fertilization can increase both yields and nutritional quality of crops. In these studies there was an average increase of 77% over controls (from 29 ppm to 48 ppm). This efficacy trial affirms importance of zinc biofortification with adequate levels of Zn concentration. The data suggests that there was no bioavailability issue as the plasma zinc levels in both groups did improve substantially between baseline and endline. There has to be a significant differential between the two groups in terms of grain Zn content to be able to show the

Table 8 Effect of consumption of wheat flour (HZn vs. LZn) on morbidity and physical activity among WCBA

	HZn	LZn	RR	95% CI
Days with fever	976	1089	0.90	0.82 to 0.98
Days with usual physical activity	250,313	250,914	1.00	0.99 to1.01
Days with usual activity performance	252,133	252,091	1.00	0.99 to1.01

difference between the groups. The study results indicate that both children and WCBAs consumed a full ration of 120 g/360 g daily only on 55% to 60% of the days, although consumption of 50% or more of recommended intake was close to 90% which further outlines the importance of achieving higher grain Zn concentrations and continuous consumption for longer duration.

Limitation of the study

One main limitation of the study was that the differential zinc content between HZn and LZn was marginal. The study was designed with 40 ppm difference between HZn and LZn but the wheat flour provided for the study had only 10 ppm differential between the two groups. The results of the study need to be inferred in this context. The shorter duration of the study (6 months) could be another limitation for finding meaningful differences between the groups.

Conclusions

Biofortified wheat flour had a good compliance among children and women suggesting agronomic approaches such as application of Zn-containing fertilizers could be a good delivery mechanism. Significant improvement on some of the morbidity indicators suggests that evaluating longer term effects of biofortification with higher zinc content would be more appropriate. Research programs are needed to develop and improve Zn application methods in terms of form, dose, and application time of Zn fertilizers.The drive for higher yields is usually accompanied by a dilution effect of minerals due to the additional grain starch accumulation. The scientists and breeders need to work together to achieve required grain Zn contents.

Abbreviations

AAS: Atomic absorption spectroscopy; CI: Confidence interval; DSMB: Data and safety monitoring board; EAR: Estimated average requirements; EDTA: Ethylenediaminetetraacetic acid; GMO: Genetically modified organism; HZn: High zinc biofortified wheat flour; ISO: International organization for standardization; LZn: Low zinc biofortified wheat flour; MCH: Mean corpuscular hemoglobin; MCV: Mean corpuscular volume; RDW: Red cell distribution width; RR: Relative risk; SD: Standard deviation; SPSS: Statistical package for the social sciences; UP: Uttar Pradesh; WCBA: Woman of child bearing age; WRA: Women of reproductive age; Zn: Zinc; χ^2: Chi Square

Acknowledgements

We are thankful to enrolled women/parents of enrolled children for their time and efforts to participate in the study. We would like to thank the people of Sangam Vihar and Harsh Vihar for their support in the implementation of this trial. We acknowledge the contribution of Subharti Medical College, as a collaborating institution, for providing administrative support. We duly acknowledge the contribution of Arti Rollers Pvt. Ltd. for providing wheat flour on time.

Funding

This study was supported by a grant from the Harvest Plus. It was coordinated by the International Center for Tropical Agriculture (CIAT) and the International Food Policy Research Institute (IFPRI). The funder however did not have any role in study design, data collection, data analysis and interpretation, decision to publish or preparation of the manuscript.

Authors' contributions

SS conceptualized and designed the study, provided oversight for implementation, directed the analysis, helped interpret results and prepare the manuscript. UD contributed to the study design, participated in the literature review, conducted data analysis, interpreted results and prepared the first draft. PD coordinated and supervised data collection, was involved in data analysis, participated in the literature review, and helped to prepare the manuscript. AD designed the data management software, helped with data analysis, reviewed and revised the manuscript. SD was involved in laboratory analysis and quality control, critically reviewed and revised the manuscript. JK and PBD were involved in field implementation of the project, quality control and preparation of manuscript. AP helped with study design and manuscript writing. All authors read and approved the final manuscript.

Competing interests

None of the authors have any competing interest.

Author details

[1]Center for Public Health Kinetics, 214A, Vinoba Puri, Lajpat Nagar-II, New Delhi 110024, India. [2]Department of International Health, Johns Hopkins Bloomberg School of Public Health, Baltimore, MD, USA. [3]Department of Pediatrics, Subharti Medical College, Meerut, Uttar Pradesh, India.

References

1. Sharma A, Patni B, Shankhdhar D, Shankhdhar SC. Zinc – an indispensable micronutrient. Physiol Mol Biol Plants. 2013;19:11–20.
2. Jorge EM, Wolfgang HP, Peter B. Biofortified crops to alleviate micronutrient malnutrition. Curr Opin Plant Biol. 2008;11:166–70. https://doi.org/10.1016/j.pbi.2008.01.007.
3. International Zinc Nutrition Consultative Group (IZiNCG). Technical document #1. Assessment of the risk of zinc deficiency in populations and options for its control. The United Nations University. Food Nutr Bull. 2004; 25(1) Suppl 2):S94–S203.
4. Wuehler SE, Peerson JM, Brown KH. Use of national food balance data to estimate the adequacy of zinc in national food supplies: methodology and regional estimates. Public Health Nutr. 2005;8:812–9.
5. Sandström B, Bügel S, McGaw BA, Price J, Reid MD. A high oat-bran intake does not impair zinc absorption in humans when added to a low-fiber animal protein-based diet. J Nutr. 2000;130:594–9.
6. Seshadri S. Nutritional anaemia in South Asia. In: Gillespie SK, editor. *Malnutrition in South Asia: a regional profile*. UNICEF Regional Office for South Asia. 1997. p. 75–124.
7. Ghosh S, Shah D. Nutritional problems in urban slum children. Indian Pediatr. 2004;41:682–96.
8. Chandyo RK, Strand TA, Mathisen M, Ulak M, Adhikari RK, Bolann BJ, et al. Zinc deficiency is common among healthy women of reproductive age in Bhaktapur, Nepal. Nutr. 2009;139:594–7.
9. Osendarp SJ, West CE, Black RE. The need for maternal zinc supplementation in developing countries: an unresolved issue. J Nutr. 2003;133:S817–27.
10. Prasad AS. Zinc deficiency in women, infants and children. J Am Coll Nutr. 1996;15:113–20.
11. Seshadri S. Prevalence of micronutrient deficiency particularly of iron, zinc and folic acid in pregnant women in South East Asia. Br J Nutr. 2001; 85(Suppl 2):S87–92.
12. Ruel MT, Alderman H. Nutrition-sensitive interventions and programmes: how can they help to accelerate progress in improving maternal and child nutrition? (and the maternal and child nutrition study group). Lancet. 2013; 382:536–51.

13. Bouis HE, Hotz C, McClafferty B, Meenakshi JV, Pfeiffer WH. Biofortification: a new tool to reduce micronutrient malnutrition. FoodNutr Bull. 2011;32:31–40.
14. Saltzman A, Birol E, Bouis HE, Boy E, De MFF, Islam Y, Pfeiffer WH. Biofortification: progress toward a more nourishing future. Glob Food Secur. 2013;2:9–17.
15. Jones G, Steketee RW, Black RE, Bhutta ZA, Morris SS. Bellagio child survival study group. How many child deaths can we prevent this year? Lancet. 2003;362:65–71.
16. Chattha MU, Hassan MU, Khan I, Chattha MB, Mahmood A, Chattha MU, Nawaz M, Subhani MN, Kharal M, Khan S. Biofortification of wheat cultivars to combat zinc deficiency. Front Plant Sci. 2017;14(8):281. https://doi.org/10.3389/fpls.2017.00281.
17. Hotz C. The potential to improve zinc status through biofortification of staple food crops with zinc. IZiNCG Technical Document no 2. Food Nutr Bull. 2009;30(Suppl 1):S172–8.
18. Transition in food consumption patterns. http://nutritionfoundationofindia.res.in/pdfpublication/Nutrition%20Transition%20in%20india1947-2007/6.%20Consumption%20expenditure.pdf. Accessed 21 Apr 2017.
19. Cakmak I. Enrichment of cereal grains with zinc: agronomic or genetic biofortification? Plant Soil. 2008;302:1–17. https://doi.org/10.1007/s11104-007-9466-3.
20. Zhao FJ, McGrath SP. Biofortification and phytoremediation. Curr Opin Plant Biol. 2009;12:373–80. https://doi.org/10.1016/j.pbi.2009.04.005.
21. Bouis HE, Hotz C, McClafferty B, Meenakshi JV, Pfeiffer WH. Biofortification: a new tool to reduce micronutrient malnutrition. Food Nutr Bull. 2011; 32(Suppl 1):S31–40. https://doi.org/10.1177/15648265110321S105.
22. Sazawal S, Dhingra U, Dhingra P, Hiremath G, Sarkar A, Dutta A, Menon VP, Black RE. Micronutrient fortified milk improves iron status, anemia and growth among children 1-4 years: a double masked, randomized, controlled trial. PLoS One. 2010;5(8):e12167.
23. Gibson RS, Ferguson EL. An interactive 24-hour recall for assessing the adequacy of iron and zinc intakes in developing countries. Harvest Plus Technical Monograph 8. Washington (DC) and Cali (Colombia): International Food Policy Research Institute, and International Center for Tropical Agriculture; 2008. p. 1-160.
24. Sazawal S, Black RE, Dhingra U, Dutta A, Deb S, Dhingra P, et al. Identifying iron deficiency anemia in developing country community settings: red cell distribution width with hemoglobin as an investigative tool in public health. J Pediatr Child Nutr. 2015;1(1):100104.
25. Aggarwal R, Sentz J, Miller MA. Role of zinc administration in prevention of childhood diarrhea and respiratory illnesses: a meta-analysis. Pediatrics. 2007;119:1120–30.
26. Rosado JL, Hambidge KM, Miller LV, Garcia OP, Westcott J, Gonzalez K, et al. Quantity of zinc absorbed from wheat in adult women is enhanced by biofortification. J Nutr. 2009;139:1920–5.
27. Kodkany BS, Bellad RM, Mahantshetti NS, Westcott JE, Krebs NF, Kemp JF, et al. Biofortification of pearl millet with iron and zinc in a randomized controlled trial increases absorption of these minerals above physiologic requirements in young children. J Nutr. 2013;143:1489–93.
28. Chomba E, Westcott CM, Westcott JE, Mpabalwani EM, Krebs NF, Patinkin ZW, et al. Zinc absorption from biofortified maize meets the requirements of young rural Zambian children. J Nutr. 2015;145(3):514–9.
29. Lu K, Li L, Zheng X, Zhang Z, Mou T, Hu Z. Quantitative trait loci controlling Cu, Ca, Zn, Mn and Fe content in rice grains. J Genet. 2008;87:305–10.
30. Islam MM, Woodhouse LR, Hossain MB, Ahmed T, Huda MN, Ahmed T, et al. Total zinc absorption from a diet containing either conventional rice or higher-zinc rice does not differ among Bangladeshi preschool children. J Nutr. 2013;143:519–25.
31. Zou CQ, Zhang YQ, Rashid A, Ram H, Savasli E, Arisoy RZ, et al. Biofortification of wheat with zinc through zinc fertilization in seven countries. Plant Soil. 2012;361:119–30.

10

Insights into infancy weight gain patterns for term small-for-gestational-age babies

Huiqing Shi[1†], Xiaodong Yang[1†], Dan Wu[1], Xiulian Wang[1], Tingting Li[1], Honghua Liu[2], Chong Guo[3], Jian Wang[4], Xiangying Hu[4], Guangjun Yu[1*] and Jinjin Chen[1*]

Abstract

Background: Too fast or slow weight gain in infancy is bad for health in later life. In this study, we aim to investigate the optimal weight gain pattern during the first 2 y of life for term small-for-gestational-age (SGA) infants.

Method: We employed data from a longitudinal, community-based cohort study on the growth and development of SGAs collected between 2004 and 2010 in Shanghai, China.

Latent class growth analysis (LCGA) was applied to identify weight gain patterns among 3004 SGAs. BMI curves for each latent class from 1 mo to 5 y were produced through mixed-effects regression analysis. Multivariable regression was performed to examine the association between various classes and adverse outcomes (overweight/ obesity/ malnutrition) during 2–5 y.

Result: Five weight gain patterns aged 0–2 y of 3004 term SGAs were identified and labeled as follows--class 1: excessively rapid catch-up growth (10.7%); class 2: rapid catch-up growth (19.7%); class 3: appropriate catch-up growth (55.7%); class 4: slow catch-up growth (10.2%); class 5: almost no catch-up growth (3.7%). A decreasing age at adiposity rebound (AR) and an increasing BMI value were observed from class 5 to 1. Class 1 and 2 showed an early appearance of AR (< 4 y). SGAs in class 1 and 2 had a higher BMI in 2–5 y of life. After adjustment for potential confounding variables, class 1 and 2 were found to have an increased risk of being overweight/ obese. At the same time, we found the risk of malnutrition was especially prominent among SGAs in classes 4 and 5.

Conclusion: Our results suggest that for term SGA infants, catch-up growth that crossing two centile levels, that is, from < 10th to the interval between 25th and 50th (ΔWAZ> 1.28) in the first several months, along with on track growth and maintenance at a median level by age 2 may be the optimal catch-up growth trajectory, minimizing risk of childhood adverse health outcomes.

Background

Small-for-gestational-age (SGA) refers to newborns with birth weight (BW) below the 10th percentile of gender- and gestational age (GA)-specific reference (INTERGROWTH-21st Project [1]). Most term SGA babies showed significantly rapid weight gain or catch-up growth (CUG) compensating for intrauterine restraint within the first two years of life [2]. Nevertheless, overweight and premature appearance of adiposity rebound (AR), which was reported to be a predictive marker of obesity and other metabolic syndromes in adulthood [3–5], can be observed in early childhood of SGA as well [6]. Growing evidences have suggested an increased long-term risk of excessive adiposity and the accompanying comorbidities across the life among infants who have been found to be with intrauterine growth restriction followed by rapid weight gain in infancy [7–9].

On the other hand, poor growth has also been associated with a variety of adverse health outcomes in later life [10–12]. Rapid weight gain has been shown to be strongly predictive of differences in stature [13]. Therefore, interventions for preventing slow growth and methods for promoting recovery from suboptimal growth have constantly been highly considered to be clinical priorities [14]. Both the WHO and CDC depict

* Correspondence: gjyu2016@163.com; jjvoo@163.com
†Huiqing Shi and Xiaodong Yang contributed equally to this work.
[1]Shanghai Children's Hospital, Shanghai Jiao Tong University, Luding Road 355, Putuo district, Shanghai 200062, China
Full list of author information is available at the end of the article

parallel growth charts for normal infants during the first two years of life, but babies who are in need of CUG ought to attain a higher weight gain rate during the same period [15].

Of equal importance to clinical intervention is appropriate growth monitoring, especially considering that excessive catch-up growth could lead to adverse outcomes in later life [16]. Pediatricians have been an indispensable part of the obesity prevention effort [17]. Yet, most only monitor infancy catch-up weight intensively when development is arrested, generally advising increases in energy intake for infants born with low weight [18]. Recommendations available concerning appropriate growth pattern for infants mostly do not account for the long-term health outcomes of these increased energy intakes. Current recommendations with respect to the time for starting overweight/obesity screening in childhood have generally not included infants: The U.S. Preventive Services Task Force (USPSTF), for example, recommends a screening window by the age of 6 y [19] and the WHO Experts Committee recommends screening by 2 y of age [20]. There is limited study available about the optimal growth trajectory for SGA catch-up growth, a need this work tries to address.

Through a retrospective longitudinal cohort study enriched with term SGA births, we sought to 1) identify common weight growth patterns during the first 2 y of life for term SGA young population; 2) investigate BMI growth patterns for SGA children in each trajectory class from 1 mo to 5 y of age and examine illustrative essential node (BMI value and age at AR) to assess the possibility of forward metabolic disorder; 3) test the association between the potential CUG trends and adverse outcomes in later life, revealing the pattern that has the lowest risk of obesity/overweight or malnutrition by preschool age.

Methodology

Study design

We employed data from a longitudinal, community-based cohort study on child growth of 32,307 SGA infants born between August, 2004 and July, 2010 in Shanghai, China. Anonymous GA, BW, gender and residence information were collected at birth and child anthropometric measurements were retrospectively extracted from health records of the Shanghai Center Disease Control Network. BWs were measured in birth hospitals or maternal healthcare centers and obtained according to maternal self-report during the infants' first visit to the child health care center. Anthropometric measurements of weight, length/height were serially collected during the first 5 y through routine physical examination using standard anthropometric methods.

Subjects

In this study, newborns with BW below the 10th percentile for each corresponding GA were defined as SGA [1]. GA was assessed based on the last menstrual period and confirmed by early ultrasound pregnancy prior to 20 wk. of gestation. Among 32,307 SGAs, preterm (GA < 37 weeks, $N = 9097$) and post-term (GA > 42 weeks, $N = 54$) births were excluded from analysis because WHO growth trajectories are inapplicable to these infants [21]. Individual measurements with unreasonable data such as height-for-age Z-score (HAZ) < − 6 or HAZ > 6, weight-for-age Z-score (WAZ) < − 6 or WAZ > 5, weight-for-length Z-score (WHZ) < − 5 or WHZ > 5, BMI-for-age Z-score (BAZ) < − 5 or BAZ > 5 were excluded ($N = 571$) in the case of possible data-entry error [21]. Only data from infants with anthropometric measurements for both weight and height at each of following age points were used in this analysis: 4 mo (12–16 wk), 8 mo (5–9 mo), 1 y (10–14 mo), and 2 y (22–26 mo). This was done to obtain a more robust growth curve assessment at similar measurement dataset with comparable time points of the identified to generate weight-trajectory patterns. Of these data, only those with at least one follow-up evaluation during the period of 2–5 y were used. In total, 3004 SGAs were included in the final analysis (Fig. 1).

Growth trajectory and profiling

Groupings of SGA growth patterns were identified according to the weight during the first 2 y of life. To find subgroups of children who shared similar linear growth profiles, we used a latent class growth analysis (LCGA), a technique employed to categorize individuals into distinct groups [22]. We used the 2006 WHO growth charts as a reference to calculate gender- and age-specific weight distributions prior to 2 y of age [23]. The weight-for-age Z-score (WAZ) in each time point was used for LCGA modeling. The WAZs was classified into 5 groups (<− 1.28, − 1.28 to (− 0.67), − 0.67 to 0.67, 0.67 to 1.28 and > 1.28, parallel with 10th, 25th, 75th and 90th percentile). The optimum number of growth profiles (latent classes) was selected on the basis of Bayesian information criterion (BIC) in order to possess the maximum likelihood of distribution into a specific latent class. Smaller value implied a better fit.

Deviations from normal physical growth were expressed as the prevalence of malnutrition such as children with Z-score < − 2 for height, weight, weight for height were defined as stunting, underweight, wasting, respectively. For the overnourished, overweight implied BAZ > 1 but < 2, while BAZ ≥ 2 was defined as obesity. Weight gain velocity between two target time points was indicated by different ΔWAZ degrees: first (ΔWAZ <− 0.67), second (− 0.67 ≤ ΔWAZ ≤0.67), third (ΔWAZ > 0.67 to 1.28), and fourth (ΔWAZ > 1.28). These categories are parallel to

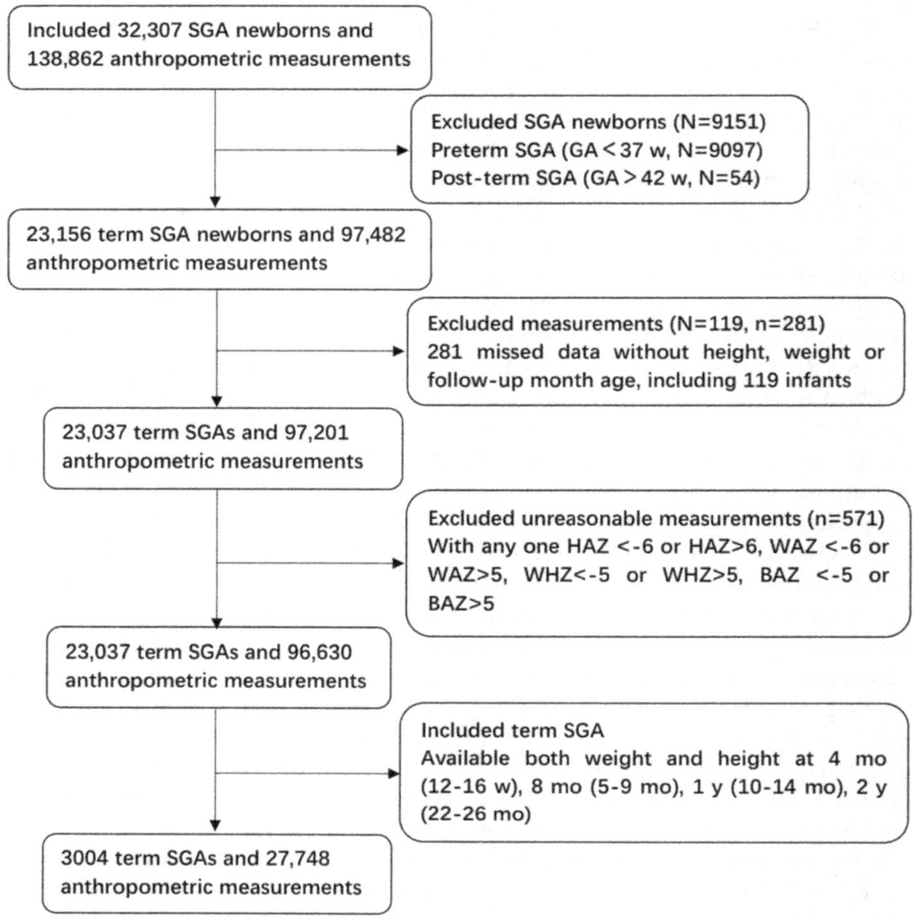

Fig. 1 Flow chart for the study

"crossing down one or more", "no crossing", "crossing up one" and "crossing up two or more" of the main weight centile on the WHO growth chart, respectively.

Statistical analysis

Using LME4 in R, mixed-effects regression model was conducted to establish the 1 mo to 5 y BMI profiles for all five weight growth classes. All 3004 infants in our sample were eligible for growth modeling, because each had a minimum of three serial measurements, as described above. Age and BMI at AR were expressed as Amin and BMImin, respectively, and generated for each class to illustrate the group influence on BMI growth patterns. In addition, with the intention of identifying the independent effects of various growth patterns on adverse growth outcome (malnutrition /overweight /obesity), multiple linear regressions were adopted with adjustment for the following characteristics: gender, BW ($2.5Kg \le BW < 3.0Kg$, $BW < 2.5Kg$), GA (late term $40 \le GA<42$ wk., early term $37 \le GA<40$ wk.) [24], residence (urban, rural).

Results

Table 1 shows the difference between SGAs included and excluded from our study. Most demographic characteristics were not significantly different among groups. By LCGA, the BIC values were 27,258.75,25,684.60,25,387.26,25,327.85, and 25,330.18 when the population was divided into 2–6 categories, of which five were optimal grouping number for the minimum BIC.

Figure 2 presents the trajectories of different classes modeled via LCGA. The identified weight gain trajectory class 1, termed "excessively rapid catch-up growth", accounted for 10.7% of the infants in our sample. This trajectory class possessed the characteristic of accelerating weight gain in the first 4 mo of life and persistence beyond risk level ($WAZ \ge 1$) within the initial 2 y of life ($WAZ = -1.6$, 1.2, 1.3 at birth, 4 mo and 2y, respectively). The weight gain class 2, named "rapid catch-up growth", accounted for 19.7% of the subjects. During the first four months, these infants experienced excessively rapid growth but not as fast as class 1 and remained in the range between standard and risk level ($0 \le WAZ \le 1$)

Table 1 Comparison of included and excluded term SGA of the study

	Term SGA included	Term SGA excluded	*P*-value	Total
Number of children [n (%)]	3004(12.9)	20,206(87.1)	–	23,210 (100.0)
Gender [n (%)]				
Male	1188(39.5)	8343(41.3)	0.07	9531(41.1)
Female	1816(60.5)	11,863(58.7)		13,679(58.9)
Gestational age (GA, wk.)	39.02(1.1)	39.13(1.1)	0.02	39.12(1.1)
GA categories [n (%)]				
Late term (40 wk. ≤ GA<42 wk.)	929(30.9)	5914(29.3)	0.09	6843(29.5)
Early term (37 wk. ≤ GA<40 wk.)	2075(69.1)	14,292(70.7)		16,367(70.5)
Birthweight (BW, Kg)	2.54(0.2)	2.51(0.2)	0.06	2.52(0.2)
BW (Z-score)	−1.70(0.5)	− 1.78(0.6)	< 0.01	− 1.77(0.5)
BW categories [n (%)]				
2.5Kg ≤ BW<3.0 Kg	2156(71.8)	14,233(70.4)	0.13	16,389(70.6)
BW<2.5Kg	848(28.2)	5973(29.6)		6821(29.4)
Residence [n (%)]				
Urban	486(16.2)	3425(16.9)	0.29	3911(16.8)
Rural	2518(83.8)	16,781(83.1)		19,299(83.2)

Continuous variables (gestational age, birthweight, BW (Z-score)) are shown in mean (SD)

while under 2 y of age (WAZ = – 1.6, 0.7, 0.6 at birth, 4 mo and 2y, respectively). Trajectory class 3, termed "appropriate catch-up growth", occupied over half of the infants (55.7%), also crossed centile rapidly in the four months while maintaining around median growth level thereafter (WAZ = – 1.7, – 0.1, 0.0 at birth, 4 mo and 2y, respectively). Trajectory class 4, termed "slow catch-up growth", comprised 10.2% of the sample, featuring rapid growth at first and then leveling off modestly in the range between normal and lower limit (– 1 ≤ WAZ ≤ 0) afterwards (WAZ = – 2.0, – 1.0, – 0.6 at birth, 4 mo and 2 y, respectively). The representation of infants in the last trajectory class was 3.7%. This group exhibited "almost no catch growth" although there was rapid weight

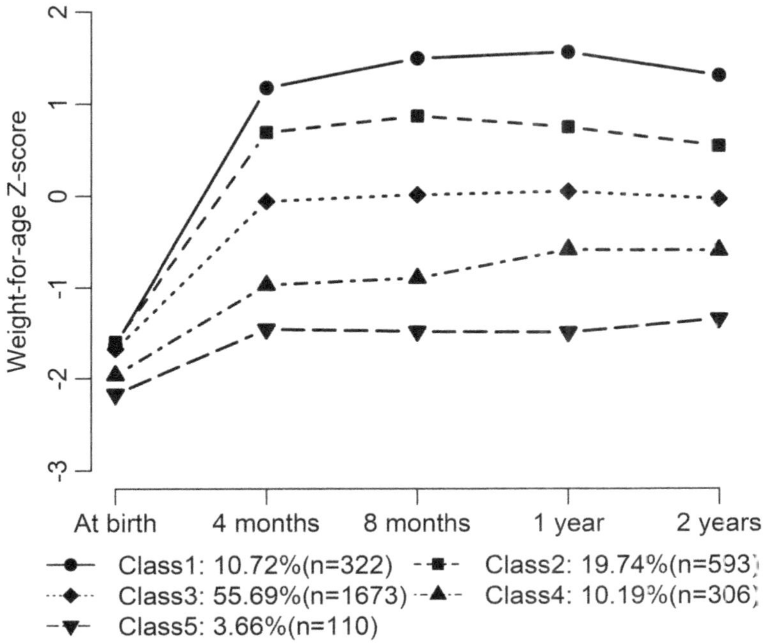

Fig. 2 Trajectories of weight gain grouping classes in term SGA obtained by LCGA

gain during the first four months. This gain did not sufficiently escalated above underweight risk levels (approximately − 2 to − 1 unit off median value), indicating suboptimal weight gain in accordance with WHO children growth standards (WAZ = − 2.2, − 1.5, − 1.3 at birth, 4 mo and 2 y, respectively).

Differences between the classes were observed for some characteristics. Heterogeneity of characteristics was accounted for by adjusting for some potential confounding factors. We further performed several analyses to detect the weight gain of infants in the first 4 mo of life (Table 2). Mean weight gain Z-score decreased by 2.1 unit across class 1 to 5 ($P < 0.01$). Infants from class 1–3 had a higher percentage of fourth (ΔWAZ > 1.28) and third weight gain degree (ΔWAZ > 0.67 to 1.28) than the other two classes during the first 4 mo of life. Most infants in class 4 and 5 were concentrated on the second (ΔWAZ from − 0.67 to 0.67) or third weight gain interval (WAZ < − 0.67).

By using mixed-effects models, distance curves of BMI for each class were generated (Fig. 3). BMI commonly reaches the summit over the first year of life and descends afterward, to the lowest point around 5~ 7 y of age [25]. In this study, different classes showed different appearances of AR before 5 y of age (47, 46, 48, 53, 56 mo across class 1 to 5, respectively). Conversely, an increasing BMI was observed from class 5 to 1(13.6, 14.4, 14.3, 15.1, 15.3).

Weight gain classes in the first 2 y of life were associated with BMI z-score (Fig. 4) and rates of overweight/obesity (Table 3) during age 2–5 y. Table 3 shows when comparing with the class 3 (appropriate catch-up growth), SGAs in class 1 and 2 have a higher BMI age- and gender-specific Z-score during 2–5 y. The corresponding multivariate β value (95%CI) were 1.1 (1.0 to 1.2) for class 1 and 0.4 (0.4 to 0.5) for class 2, respectively, after adjustment for potential confounders. Extremely rapid weight gain (class 1) and rapid weight gain (class 2) in infancy increased the risk of overweight/obesity by 11 times (OR = 11.6; 95CI% from 8.8 to15.3) and 2 times (OR = 2.3; 95CI% from 1.8 to 3.0), respectively. An increased risk of malnutrition appeared to be particularly prominent among SGAs who were in class 4 and 5. After adjusting for other factors, the

Table 2 The baseline characteristics of the SGA by weight gain class

	Class 1 Excessively rapid catch-up growth	Class 2 Rapid catch-up growth	Class 3 Appropriate catch-up growth	Class 4 Slow catch-up growth	Class 5 Almost no catch growth	P for trend
Number of children [n (%)]	322(10.7)	593(19.7)	1673(55.6)	306(10.1)	110(3.6)	–
Gender [n (%)]						
Male	117(36.3)	201(33.8)	659(39.3)	145(47.3)	66(60.0)	< 0.01
Female	205(63.6)	392(66.1)	1014(60.6)	161(52.6)	44(40.0)	
Gestational age (GA, wk.)	39.06(1.1)	39.13(1.0)	39.06(1.0)	38.70(1.1)	38.70(1.2)	< 0.01
GA categories [n (%)]						
Late term (40 wk. ≤ GA<42 wk.)	102(31.6)	159(26.8)	490(29.2)	126(41.1)	52(47.2)	< 0.01
Early term (37 wk. ≤ GA<40 wk.)	220(68.3)	434(73.1)	1183 (70.7)	180(58.8)	58(52.7)	< 0.01
Birthweight (BW, Kg)	2.57(0.1)	2.58(0.1)	2.55(0.1)	2.45(0.2)	2.37(0.2)	< 0.01
BW (Z-score)	−1.63(0.4)	−1.60(0.4)	−1.68(0.4)	−1.96(0.6)	−2.17(0.6)	< 0.01
BW categories [n (%)]						
2.5Kg ≤ BW<3.0Kg	248 (77.0)	466(78.5)	1255(73.8)	165(53.9)	42(38.1)	< 0.01
BW<2.5Kg	74(22.9)	127(21.4)	438(26.1)	141(46.0)	68(61.8)	
Residence [n (%)]						
Urban	65 (20.1)	100(16.8)	249 (14.8)	56 (18.3)	16(14.5)	0.12
Rural	257(79.8)	493(83.1)	1424(85.1)	250(81.7)	94(85.4)	
ΔWeight-for-age Z-score degrees between 4 mo and birth[n (%)]	2.81(0.6)	2.29(0.6)	1.62(0.5)	0.99(0.6)	0.71(0.6)	< 0.01
First (ΔWAZ <−0.67)	0(0.0)	0(0.0)	1(0.0)	2(0.65)	1(0.91)	
Second (−0.67 < ΔWAZ< 0.67)	0(0.0)	4(0.6)	75(4.4)	99(32.35)	52(47.27)	
Third(0.67 < ΔWAZ<1.28)	6(1.8)	27(4.5)	403(24.0)	116(37.91)	40(36.36)	
Fourth (ΔWAZ> 1.28)	316(98.1)	56(94.7)	1194(71.3)	89(29.08)	17(15.45)	

Chi-square (categorical variables) or ANOVA (continuous variables) for linear trend, including all children ($n = 3004$); Data are expressed as mean ± SDS or No. (%).The Z-scores were calculated relative to age- and gender-specific WHO children growth standards. Continuous variables (gestational age, birthweight, BW (Z-score)) are shown in mean (SD)

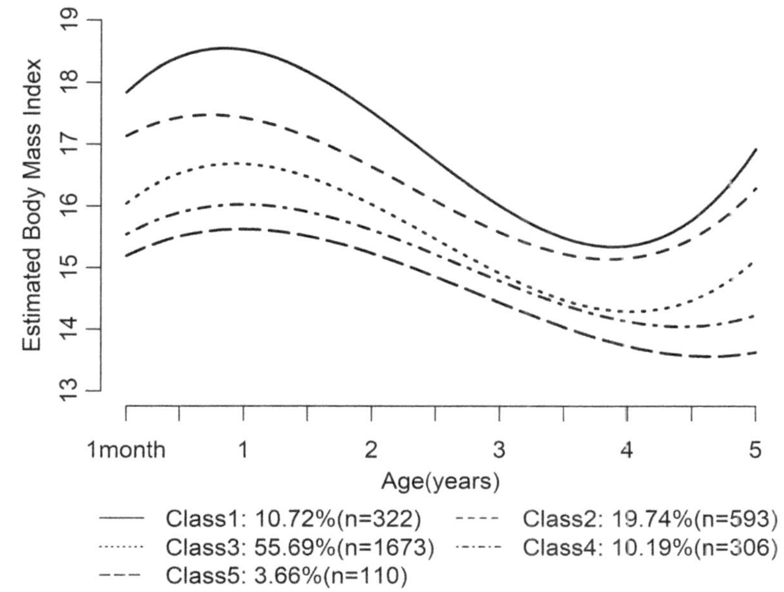

Fig. 3 BMI growth trajectories age 1 mo to 5 y for each weight gain class

corresponding ORs (95%CI) were 4.4 (2.7 to 7.1) and 21.2 (12.6 to 35.6).

Discussion

Small-for-gestational-age births affect approximately 1 in 10 newborns worldwide. Several studies have been performed to demonstrate that rapid postnatal weight gain early in life is related to obesity later [26–29]. However, we are not aware of any work suggesting optimal growth patterns in infancy for reducing the risk of SGA obesity. The present study establishes the optimal postnatal weight gain pattern in the first two years of life by employing data from a large cohort study. Our study suggests that for term SGA infants, catch-up growth crossing two centile levels, that is, from < 10th to the interval between 25th and 50th ($\Delta WAZ > 1.28$) in the

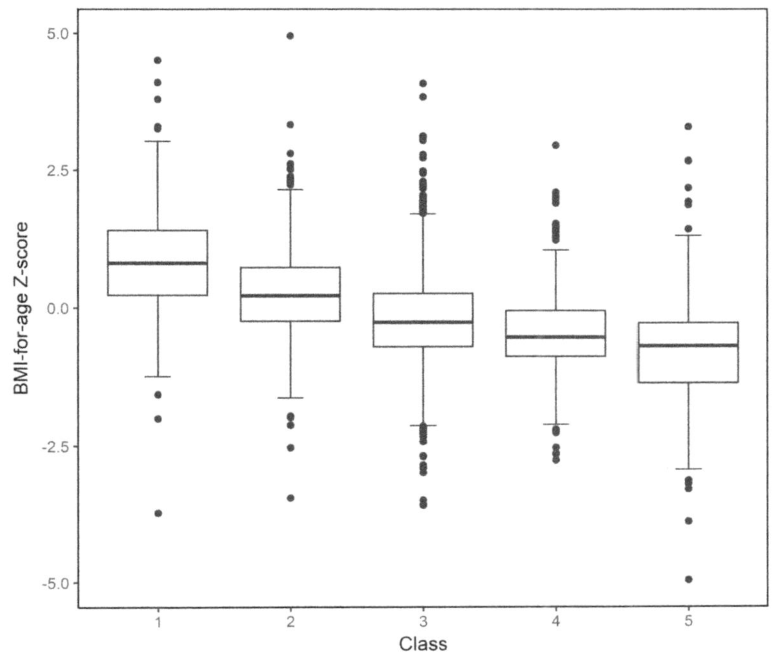

Fig. 4 BMI Z-score when aged 2–5 y stratified by weight gain classes in the first 2 y

Table 3 BMI z-score and risks of adverse growth outcomes at age 2–5 y in each weight gain class

Trajectories classes	BMI-for-age Z-score	Overweight/obesity		Malnutrition	
	β (95CI %)	*N* (%)	OR (95CI %)	*N* (%)	OR (95CI %)
Class 1 Excessively rapid catch-up growth					
Unadjusted	1.1(1.0,1.2)§	174 (54.0)	10.6(8.1,13.9)§	6(1.9)	0.7(0.3,1.6)
Adjusted	1.1(1.0,1.2)§		11.6(8.8,15.3)§		0.7(0.3,1.6)
Class 2 rapid catch-up growth					
Unadjusted	0.4(0.4,0.5)§	118 (19.9)	2.2(1.7,2.9)§	2(0.3)	0.1(0.0,0.5)‡
Adjusted	0.4(0.4,0.5)§		2.3(1.8,3.0)§		0.1(0.0,0.5)‡
Class 3 Appropriate catch-up growth (referent)	1.0	167 (10.0)	1.0	45(2.7)	1.0
Class 4 Slow catch-up growth					
Unadjusted	−0.3(−0.4,-0.2)§	16 (5.2)	0.5(0.3,0.8)‡	34(11.1)	4.5 (2.8,7.2)§
Adjusted	−0.3(− 0.4,-0.2)§		0.5(0.3,0.8)‡		4.4(2.7,7.1)§
Class 5 Almost no catch-up growth					
Unadjusted	−0.7(−0.8,-0.5)§	5 (4.5)	0.4(0.2,1.1)§	42(38.2)	22.3(13.8,36.3)§
Adjusted	−0.7(− 0.8,-0.5)§		0.4(0.2,1.0)§		21.2(12.6,35.6)§

Adjusted for gender, birthweight (2.5Kg ≤ BW<3.0Kg, BW<2.5Kg), gestational age (late term 40 ≤ GA<42 wk., early term 37 ≤ GA<40 wk.), residence (urban, rural)
CI confidence interval, *OR* odds ratio
‡*P*<0.01; §*P*<0.001

first several months and maintaining on track growth at median level by two years of age is the optimal catch-up growth trajectory that presents the lowest risk of adverse health outcomes. Moreover, both inadequate and excessive catch-up growth patterns were found to be associated with poor outcomes. Our study demonstrated a significant difference in weight gain patterns in the early period of life, implicating the importance of early monitoring for SGAs.

As illustrated by DOHaD, low birth weight or SGAs have been reported to be associated with obesity and non-communicable diseases (NCD) [30, 31]. The emergence of AR at a younger age has been recognized as a predictor for obesity, NCD, and metabolic syndrome [4–6, 32]. Therefore, we characterized the timing of AR appearance in the different growth trajectory classes we modeled. Other researchers have presented early AR as the emergence of ascending BMI at ages under four [33]. In our work, both BMI and age of AR were found to be correlated with growth trajectory class. Earlier ARs and higher BMIs were observed in class 1 and 2: 2 and 1 mo earlier and 1.06 and 0.86 units higher than SGA children in class 3 (AR at 48 mo, BMI 14.28). The typical AR is the lowest BMI followed by an increased BMI after the rebound. Subsequent to the nadir in BMI growth trajectory, SGAs in each class showed accelerated BMI growth. The slope for this growth increased across classes (from class 5 to 1), which implicates a faster BMI growth for SGA children in school age. According to reports in previous literature, the BMI of SGA children with no infancy catch-up growth was low at 4 y [34], as depicted in class 5, confronting the challenge of malnourishment.

We also found that weight gain in the first two years was related to BMI-for-age Z-score, overweight/obesity, as well as malnutrition at preschool age in a dose-dependent pattern over all trajectories classes, even after adjustment for potential confounders. Overweight/obesity at preschool age was less prevalent in SGA class 4 and 5 than those (class 1, 2, 3) with faster weight gain growth in the same period. Excessive growth in early life appeared to be linked with less incidence of malnutrition at preschool age compared to class 4 and 5. However, it is essential to identify an optimal growth pattern to obtain balance between the requirement for ensuring sufficient intake versus the need to prevent childhood obesity and other associated health risks.

Our findings can be of real significance in clinical practice. Previous studies have reported that most SGA infants exhibit catch-up weight during early childhood [35, 36]. Sufficient infancy weight gain in SGAs appears to help prevent poor growth outcomes and may benefit neurodevelopment [25, 37]. Nevertheless, in spite of catch-up growth being beneficial, this study demonstrates that exceedingly fast weight gain in the first several months and a high weight later in infancy are both risk factors for overweight/obesity, necessitating appropriate weight gain control with cooperation between health workers and caregivers [38].

One of the limitations in this study is that the growth of a child is influenced by feeding status, nevertheless, it was not confirmed whether all SGAs consumed similar calories complying with feeding guideline of WHO. Secondly, the genetic potential (presented as the parental heights and weights) was unknown. The third is the lack of information about fetal life, such as maternal malnutrition, placenta origin, and genetic or chromosomal condition. Thus we were unable to detect the fetal origin of growth restrictions. It is quite likely the growth trajectories we obtained will vary considerably depending on different fetal growth histories. A fourth limitation is the limited information about health outcomes. In this study, we only possessed data about overweight/obesity and malnutrition. There are some other health indicators and biomarkers such as leptin and adiponectin that we were unable to assess, limiting the range of outcomes we could analyze. We also had a small number of babies with malnutrition, the result could be uncertain with wide confidence intervals. Despite the limitation, it is a large sample of community-based study covering complete ranges of age till 5 y. Furthermore, we conducted longitudinal analysis and evaluated growth by employing an effective and easy-to-fill screening method.

Conclusion

In conclusion, suboptimal infant growth patterns of term SGAs are associated with adverse health outcomes during 2 to 5 years of age. Catch-up growth in SGA children is of great significance to erase the deficit at birth but should not extend to overgrowth or misbalanced growth. Monitoring and ensuring optimal catch-up growth starting from birth could be the first step towards prevention of childhood adverse outcomes.

Abbreviations

AR: Adiposity rebound; BAZ: BMI-for-age Z-score; BMI: Body mass index; BW: Birth weight; CI: Confidence intervals; CUG: Catch-up growth; GA: Gestational age; HAZ: Height-for-age Z-score; LCGA: Latent Class Growth Analysis; OR: Odds ratios; SGA: Small-for-gestational-age; WAZ: Weight-for-age Z-score; WHZ: Weight-for-height Z-score

Funding

National Natural Science Foundation of China, 81670810; Science and Technology Commission of Shanghai Municipality Medical Guiding Project, 14411965200; Shanghai Hospital Development Center Clinical Research Innovation Project, SHDC12015305; Shanghai Hospital Development Center Clinical Popularization and Application of Appropriate Technology, 16CR4016A; Shanghai Children's Health Service capacity Building Project GDEK201710; Education Commission Gaofeng Clinical Medicine Grant, 20161432.

Authors' contributions

HS and XY contributed equally to this manuscript and considered to be co-first authors. HS conducted the statistical analysis and drafted the manuscript; HL, DW, HW, TL, CG provided advice on the statistical analysis and helped to collect data; JW, XH provide the community data; JC, GY both contributed equally to design, guide of the study, review and edition of the manuscript, they considered to be co-corresponding authors.

Competing interests

The authors declare that they have no competing interests.

Author details

[1]Shanghai Children's Hospital, Shanghai Jiao Tong University, Luding Road 355, Putuo district, Shanghai 200062, China. [2]Dongying People's Hospital, Dongcheng South First Road 317, Dongying 257091, China. [3]Maternal and Children Hospital, Daoshan Road 18, Gulou District, Fuzhou 350001, China. [4]Jing'an District Maternal and Child Healthcare Center of Shanghai, 1297 Kangding Road, Shanghai 200072, China.

References

1. Villar J, et al. Postnatal growth standards for preterm infants: the preterm postnatal follow-up study of the INTERGROWTH-21(st) project. Lancet Glob Heal. 2015;3(11):e681.
2. Karlberg J, Albertsson-Wikland K. Growth in full-term small-for-gestational-age infants: from birth to final height. Pediatr Res. 1995;38(5):733.
3. Marakaki C, Karapanou O, Gryparis A, et al. Early adiposity rebound and premature Adrenarche. J Pediatr. 2017;186:72.
4. Koyama S, Ichikawa G. Kojima M, Shimura N, Sairenchi T, Arisaka O. Adiposity rebound and the development of metabolic syndrome. Pediatrics. 2014;133(1):e114.
5. Suchomlinov A, Tutkuviene J. The relationship between birth weight, adiposity rebound and overweight at the age of 17 years (results of the Lithuanian longitudinal growth study, 1990 - 2008). Anthr Anz. 2014; 71(4):329–46.
6. Maeyama K, et al. Gestational age-dependency of height and body mass index trajectories during the first 3 years in Japanese small-for-gestational age children. Sci Rep. 2016;6:38659.
7. Singhal A. Long-term adverse effects of early growth acceleration or catch-up growth. Ann Nutr Metab. 2017;70(3).
8. Mortaz M, Fewtrell M, Cole T, Lucas A. Birth weight, subsequent growth, and cholesterol metabolism inchildren 8-12 years old born preterm. Arch Dis Child. 2001;84(3):212–7.
9. Cho WK, Suh BK. Catch-up growth and catch-up fat in children born small for gestational age. Korean J Pediatr. 2016;59(1):1–7.
10. Prado EL, Dewey KG. Nutrition and brain development in early life. Nutr Rev. 2014;72(4):267–84.
11. Gatyablonski G, Phillip M. Nutritionally-induced catch-up growth. Nutrients. 2015;7(1):517–51.
12. Raaijmakers A, Allegaert K. Catch-up growth in former preterm neonates: no time to waste. Nutrients. 2016;8(12):817.
13. Wright CM, Marie CK, Andrea S, Maria FV, Pearce MS, Adamson AJ. To what extent do weight gain and eating avidity during infancy predict later adiposity? Public Health Nutr. 2012;15(4):656–62.
14. Norris S. The relationship of rapid weight gain in infancy to obesity and skeletal maturity in childhood. Obesity. 2003;11(3):457–60.
15. Oregon Pediatric Nutrition Practice Group. Nutrition Practice Care Guidelines for Preterm Infants in the Community. Available: http://www.oregon.gov/oha/.
16. Okada T, Takahashi S, Nagano N, Yoshikawa K, Usukura Y, Hosono S. Early postnatal alteration of body composition in preterm and small-for-gestational-age infants: implications of catch-up fat. Pediatr Res. 2015; 77(1-2):136.
17. Daniels SR, Hassink SG, Nutrition CO. The role of the pediatrician in primary prevention of obesity. Pediatrics. 2015;136(1):275–92.
18. Wang G, Sara J, Gong Y, et al. Weight gain in infancy and overweight or obesity in childhood across the gestational Spectrum: a prospective birth cohort study. Sci Rep. 2016;6:29867.
19. Barton M. Screening for obesity in children and adolescents: US preventive services task force recommendation statement. Pediatrics. 2015, 125(125):361–7.
20. Bowdoin JJ. Appendix: expert committee recommendations on the assessment, prevention, and treatment of child and adolescent overweight and obesity. Pediatrics. 2008;121(4):833–4.
21. WHO AnthroPlus for personal computers Manual: Software for assessing growth of the world's children and adolescents. Geneva: WHO, 2009 (http://www.who.int/growthref/tools/en/).

22. W. M. G. R. S. group: WHO child growth standards based on length/height, weight and age. Acta Paediatr Suppl. 2006;95(S450):76–85.
23. Berlin KS, Williams NA, Parra GR. An introduction to latent variable mixture modeling (part 1): overview and cross-sectional latent class and latent profile analyses. J Pediatr Psychol. 2014;39(2):174.
24. A. C. O. Obstetriciansgynecologists, ACOG committee opinion no. 560. Medically indicated late-preterm and early-term deliveries. Obstet Gynecol. 2013;121(4):908–10.
25. M. F. Rollandcachera, M. Deheeger, M. Maillot, and F. Bellisle: Early adiposity rebound: causes and consequences for obesity in children and adults. Int J Obes 2006, 30 Suppl 4(12):11.
26. Longo S, Bollani L, Decembrino L, et al. Short-term and long-term sequelae in intrauterine growth retardation (IUGR). The journal of maternal-fetal & neonatal medicine : the official journal of the European Association of Perinatal Medicine, the Federation of Asia and Oceania Perinatal Societies, the International Society of Perinatal Obstetricians. 2013;26(3):222–5.
27. Ong KK, et al. Postnatal growth in preterm infants and later health outcomes: a systematic review. Acta Paediatr. 2015;104(10):974–86.
28. Woo Baidal JA, Locks LM, Cheng ER, Blake-Lamb TL, Perkins ME, Taveras EM. Risk factors for childhood obesity in the first 1,000 days. A Systematic Review Am J Prev Med. 2016;50(6):761–79.
29. Souza LG, et al. Predictors of overweight/obesity in a Brazilian cohort after 13 years of follow-up. Nutr J. 2018;17(1):10.
30. Barker DJ, Osmond C. Infant mortality, childhood nutrition, and ischaemic heart disease in England and wales. Lancet. 1986;327(8489):1077–81.
31. Barker DJ, Osmond C, Forsén TJ, Kajantie E, Eriksson JG. Trajectories of growth among children who have coronary events as adults. N Engl J Med. 2005;353(17):1802–9.
32. Wadsworth M, Butterworth S, Marmot M, Ecob R, Hardy R. Early growth and type 2 diabetes: evidence from the 1946 British birth cohort. Diabetologia. 2005;48(12):2505–10.
33. Eriksson JG. Epidemiology, genes and the environment: lessons learned from the Helsinki birth cohort study. J Intern Med. 2007;261(5):418–25.
34. Taal HR, Vd Heijden AJ, Steegers EA, Hofman A, Jaddoe VW. Small and large size for gestational age at birth, infant growth, and childhood overweight. Obesity. 2013;21(6):1261–8.
35. Leger J, Levy-Marchal C, Bloch J, et al. Reduced final height and indications for insulin resistance in 20 year olds born small for gestational age: regional cohort study. Bmj British Medical Journal. 1997;315(7104):341–7.
36. Hokkenkoelega ACS, Ridder MAJD, Lemmen RJ, et al. Children born small for gestational age: do they catch up[quest]. Pediatr Res. 1995;38(2):267.
37. Varella MH, Moss WJ. Early growth patterns are associated with intelligence quotient scores in children born small-for-gestational age. Early Hum Dev. 2015;91(8):491–7.
38. Sunguya BF, et al. Effectiveness of nutrition training of health workers toward improving caregivers feeding practices for children aged six months to two years: a systematic review. Nutr Journal. 2013;12(1):66.

11

Maternal fruit and vegetable or vitamin C consumption during pregnancy is associated with fetal growth and infant growth up to 6 months: results from the Korean Mothers and Children's Environmental Health (MOCEH) cohort study

Won Jang[1†], Hyesook Kim[1†], Bo-Eun Lee[2] and Namsoo Chang[1*]

Abstract

Background: Based on data obtained from pregnant women who participated in the Mothers and Children's Environmental Health (MOCEH) study in South Korea, we aimed to determine whether maternal intake of fruits and vegetables or vitamin C is associated with fetal and infant growth.

Methods: A total of 1138 Korean pregnant women at 12–28 weeks gestation with their infants were recruited as study participants for the MOCEH. Intake of fruits and vegetables or vitamin C during pregnancy was assessed by a 1-day 24-h recall method. Fetal biometry was determined by ultrasonography at late pregnancy. Infant weight and length were measured at birth and 6 months.

Results: A multiple regression analysis after adjusting for covariates showed that maternal intake of fruits and vegetables was positively associated with the biparietal diameter of the fetus and infant's weight from birth to 6 months. Also, maternal vitamin C intake was positively associated with the abdominal circumference of the fetus and infant birth length. In addition, there was a significant inverse relationship between consumption of fruits and vegetables (below the median compared to above the median of ≥519 g/d) and the risk of low growth (<25th percentile) of biparietal diameter (odds ratio (OR): 2.220; 95% confidence interval (CI): 1.153–4.274) and birth weight (OR: 1.434; 95% CI: 1.001–2.056). A significant inverse relationship also existed between vitamin C consumption (below vs above the estimated average requirement (EAR) of ≥85 mg/d) and the risk of low growth (<25th percentile) of birth weight (OR: 1.470; 95% CI: 1.011–2.139), weight from birth to 6 months (OR: 1.520; 95% CI: 1.066–2.165), and length at birth (OR: 1.579; 95% CI: 1.104–2.258).

Conclusions: An increased intake of fruits and vegetables or vitamin C at mid-pregnancy is associated with increased fetal growth and infant growth up to 6 months of age.

Keywords: Fruits, Vegetables, Vitamin C, Birth weight, Birth length, Fetal growth, Infant growth

* Correspondence: nschang@ewha.ac.kr
†Won Jang and Hyesook Kim contributed equally to this work.
[1]Department of Nutritional Science and Food Management, Ewha Womans University, Seoul, South Korea
Full list of author information is available at the end of the article

Background

Vitamin C, also known as ascorbic acid, acts as an antioxidant by scavenging reactive oxygen and nitrogen species in an aqueous environment [1] and plays a major role in defense against increased oxidative stress during pregnancy [2]. The human body cannot produce or adequately store vitamin C and, consequently, it must regularly be obtained through the diet. Vitamin C levels decrease during pregnancy, due to inadequate intake [3] and physiological changes in pregnancy, leading to hemodilution [4, 5].

The increased consumption of fruit and vegetables, an excellent source of vitamin C, during pregnancy has been shown to be positively associated with birth weight [6, 7]. In contrast, inadequate dietary intake of vitamin C may result in adverse outcomes, such as low birth weight (below 5% standard birth weight for gestational age) [8] and preterm delivery (birth that occurs before the 37th week of pregnancy) [9]. Two prospective cohort studies, one in the UK [10] and the other in India [6], reported a positive association between maternal vitamin C intake during pregnancy and birth weight.

To the best of our knowledge, only two studies have examined the association between maternal vitamin C status and birth outcomes in South Korea. One of these prospective cohort studies ($n = 239$) [11] indicated that maternal serum vitamin C levels during the second trimester were positively correlated with birth weight and length in full-term babies. In the other survey ($n = 383$) [12], a high maternal concentration of vitamin C was significantly linked to increased infant weight and head circumference during the first 3 years of life. However, both these studies involved a small sample size and neither determined growth measurements (such as fetal biometry) before the baby was born. These two studies focused mostly on the relationship between vitamin C status during pregnancy, especially blood concentration of vitamin C and infant growth.

The easiest way to raise the blood levels of vitamin C is to consume vitamin C through fruits and vegetables. A previous observation identified dietary vitamin C intake as the variable with the greatest influence on plasma vitamin C concentrations [13]. Measuring vitamin C concentrations in the body has more advantages than dietary intake, but dietary intake data represent significant measures of habitual vitamin C consumption. Therefore, it is also necessary to consider the relevance of infant growth based on the intake of fruits and vegetables, and vitamin C, regarding the practical application. Many studies [6–10] have reported an association between the consumption of either fruits and vegetables or vitamin C with infant growth, but there have been no in-depth studies of Korean women in this regard. Therefore, this research investigated whether maternal intake of vitamin C, based on a diet abundant in fruit and vegetables, is associated with fetal and infant growth, namely birth length and weight, in pregnant Korean women.

Methods

Study subjects and data collection

This study was based on data obtained by the Mothers and Children's Environmental Health study (MOCEH), which is an ongoing multi-center (Seoul, metropolitan city; Ulsan, industrial region; and Cheonan, medium-sized urban area), prospective cohort study in South Korea. Detailed information about the MOCEH study has been reported elsewhere [14]. The study protocol was attentively reviewed and authorized by the Institutional Review Boards at Ewha Womans University School of Medicine, Dankook University Hospital, and Ulsan University Hospital, respectively, and the informed consent for participation was acquired from all subjects. The study subject selection process is outlined in Fig. 1. The MOCEH study population consists of 1751 pregnant women at 12–28 weeks of gestation and their infants after birth. The subjects were recruited between August 2006 and December 2010. Of these 1751 subjects, 31 women carrying twins, 23 who suffered spontaneous abortions, 3 who had an intrauterine growth restriction, and 12 whose fetus had a congenital anomaly were excluded. Of the remaining 1682 subjects, 329 whose pregnancy outcome data were not available due to drop out from the study, 60 whose pregnancy lasted less than 37 or more than 42 weeks, and 34 who had pregnancy complications (hypertension or/and diabetes) were excluded. From the 1259 subjects left, 116 whose dietary intake data were not collected, and 5 whose total energy consumption was < 500 kcal/d or > 4000 kcal/d were also excluded. Thus, 1138 women and their babies were finally included in the analysis. Among these subjects, babies with data related to fetal biometric measurements, such as biparietal diameter ($n = 703$), abdominal circumference ($n = 589$) and femur length ($n = 689$) at late pregnancy (between 29 and 42 weeks gestation) were analyzed. We were only able to follow-up 741 infants from birth to 6 months (Fig. 1).

Dietary assessment

Maternal dietary intake data during mid-pregnancy were collected for one 24-h recall for intake on the day before the participant's visit to the center. The 24-h dietary recall was administered by experienced, well-trained dietary interviewers, who instructed the respondents to recall and describe all foods and beverages, including nutritional supplements, they had consumed over the past 24 h. The dietary information was processed using a computerized nutrient intake assessment program (CAN-Pro 4.0, Korean Nutrition Society, Seoul, Korea).

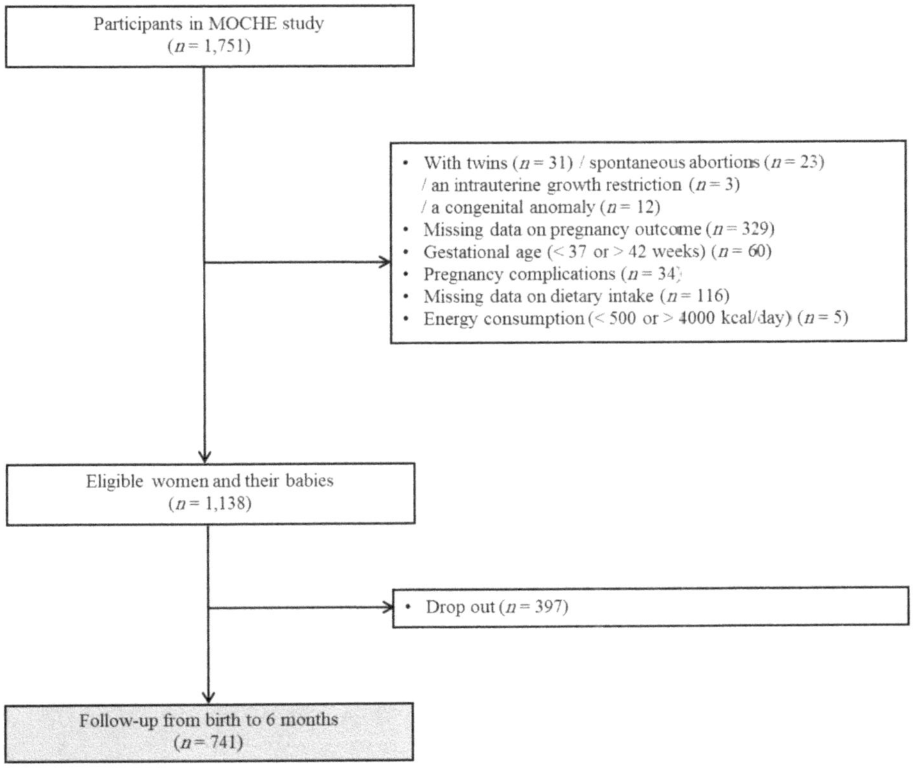

Fig. 1 Flow chart of the subject inclusion and exclusion criteria in the study

General characteristics and pregnancy outcomes

The method used to survey the general characteristics of the subjects has been described in detail elsewhere [15]. Information on demographic and socioeconomic status and health-related behaviors [maternal age (years), height (cm), and weight (kg) at pre-pregnancy; education status; family income; parity; supplement use; smoking; alcohol consumption] were gathered by well-trained interviewers. Urine samples were collected and stored frozen until they could be delivered to a specialized laboratory for analysis. During pregnancy, maternal oxidative stress status was assessed by measuring the urinary levels of malondialdehyde (MDA; an oxidation product of lipoperoxidation), which is indicated to be a useful biomarker of oxidative stress in pregnant women [16]. The urinary MDA levels were analyzed by high-performance liquid chromatography (HPLC) with fluorescence detection. The urinary level of cotinine (a reliable biomarker of nicotine exposure) was measured by HPLC-isotope dilution tandem mass spectrometry (Agilent 6410 Triple Quad LCMS, Agilent Technologies, Santa Clara, CA, USA). The data were adjusted relative to the urinary creatinine level, to correct for urine volume. As indices for fetal biometry, the biparietal diameter, abdominal circumference, and femur length were assessed by ultrasonography at late pregnancy, by a certified ultrasonographer at Ewha Womans University Hospital. The gestational age, determined by ultrasound measurement, was obtained from medical records. Neonatal gender, gestational age at delivery (weeks), birth weight (kg), and birth length (cm) data were also retrieved from medical records. Gestational age at delivery was inferred by subjects' self-reports of the last menstrual period and was also estimated via ultrasonography. Weight (±0.1 kg) and length (±0.1 cm) at 6 months were measured using a DS-B02 infantometer (Dong Sahn Jenix Co. Ltd., Seoul, Korea), by laying each infant in the center of the scale. When participants visited the hospital after birth, mothers were asked to complete questionnaires that pertained to information about breastfeeding status, as well as any change in demographic characteristics, family disease history, and environmental conditions, since the previous visit.

Statistical analysis

A descriptive analysis was conducted to present general characteristics, health-related behaviors, dietary intakes, and growth measurements, including pregnancy outcomes, of the study population. Continuous variables were expressed as mean ± standard deviation (SD), and the categorical variables were indicated as frequency and percentage. The food and nutrient intake data, and urinary cotinine levels were log-transformed to normalize their distributions. A multiple regression analysis was conducted to investigate the relationship between maternal fruit and vegetable/vitamin C intake and fetal growth. For estimating the difference in fetal growth, according to maternal fruit and vegetable/vitamin C intake level, the subjects were divided into two groups [fruits and vegetables, below/above the median value of 519 g/d] [vitamin C, below/above the estimated average requirement (EAR) of 85 mg/d] and the data then analyzed by a generalized linear model test, after controlling for confounding factors. The adjusted odds ratios (ORs) (with 95% confidence interval, CI) for the prevalence of low growth (<25th percentile) in infants of mothers with low fruit and vegetable/vitamin C intake levels were calculated by logistic regression analysis. Variables that were considered to be confounding factors (having the potential to influence the relationship between maternal vitamin C intake and weight and length at birth, observed from the univariate analysis of these data or reported from other literature) were included as covariates. These covariates included maternal age (years), pre-pregnancy BMI (kg/m^2), log-transformed urinary cotinine level (μg/g creatinine), neonatal gender (male or female), gestational age at delivery (weeks), and the use of supplements (yes or no), residential area (metropolitan area, industrial area, urban area), parity (0 or ≥ 1), father's height (cm), and log-transformed intakes of energy (kcal), vitamin E (mg alpha-tocopherol equivalents, α-TE), and β-carotene (μg). The infant's growth at 6 months was additionally adjusted for breastfeeding status (exclusive breastfeeding or formula-feeding or combined) at 6 months. For repeated measures analyses from birth to 6 months, mixed models (for continuous dependent variables) and general estimating equation models (for categorical dependent variables) were used. SAS 9.3 (SAS Institute, Cary, NC, USA) was used for all data analyses, and the level of significance was set at $P < 0.05$.

Results

Characteristics of the study population

The participants had a mean age of 30.2 ± 3.6 years and a pre-pregnancy BMI of 21.3 ± 3.1 kg/m^2. Approximately 55.7% of the subjects took dietary supplements (Table 1).

The average vitamin C intake of the pregnant women was 134.8 ± 99.2 mg/d, and 36.1% did not meet the EAR (85 mg/d) for the Korean Dietary Reference Intake. The average fruit and vegetable consumption of the pregnant women was 594.4 ± 365.4 g/d. Gestational age at the time of ultrasound measurement, fetal biparietal diameter, abdominal circumference, and femur length were 36.4 ± 2.5 weeks, and 8.9 ± 0.1, 32.1 ± 2.5, and 6.9 ± 0.5 cm, respectively. Gestational age at delivery was 39.1 ± 1.1 weeks, birth weight was 3.3 ± 0.4 kg, and birth length was 50.5 ± 2.5 cm. The

Table 1 Characteristics of the pregnant women and infants

	n	Mean ± SD or *n(%)*
General characteristics		
Age, years	1136	30.2 ± 3.6
Pre-pregnancy BMI, kg/m^2	1099	21.3 ± 3.1
Education	1078	
≤ High school		293 (27.2)
≤ University		714 (66.2)
≥ Graduate school		71 (6.7)
Family monthly income, USD	1064	
< 2000		288 (27.1)
2000–4000		596 (53.5)
≥ 4000		207 (19.5)
Parity	967	
0		485 (50.2)
≥ 1		482 (49.8)
Supplement user	1138	634 (55.7)
Urinary cotinine, μg/g creatinine	1057	20.9 ± 159.2
Urinary MDA, μmol/g creatinine	1036	1.8 ± 1.4
Dietary intakes		
Total food intake, g/d	1138	1368.0 ± 450.0
Fruit and vegetables, g/d	1138	594.4 ± 365.4
Energy, kcal/d	1138	1774.6 ± 502.6
Carbohydrates, g/d	1138	276.4 ± 82.0
Protein, g/d	1138	68.7 ± 25.0
Fat, g/d	1138	47.0 ± 24.2
Vitamin C, mg/d	1138	134.8 ± 99.2
Vitamin E, mg α-TE/d	1138	17.1 ± 8.5
β-carotene, μg/d	1138	2703.5 ± 2275.6
Fetal biometry at late pregnancy		
Biparietal diameter, cm	703	8.94 ± 0.56
Abdominal circumference, cm	589	32.13 ± 2.54
Femur length, cm	689	6.85 ± 0.53
Pregnancy outcomes		
Neonatal gender (male)	1132	582 (51.4)
Gestational age at delivery, weeks	1138	39.1 ± 1.1
Birth weight, kg	1138	3.3 ± 0.4
Birth length, cm	1138	50.5 ± 2.5
Breastfeeding status, yes	741	480 (64.8)
Infants characteristics at 6 months		
Weight, kg	741	10.1 ± 1.0
Length, cm	740	76.7 ± 2.5

BMI Body mass index, *MDA* Malondialdehyde, *α-TE* Alpha-tocopherol equivalents general characteristics did not differ significantly between the included and excluded subjects (data not shown).

Correlation between fruit and vegetable/vitamin C intake and urinary MDA levels during pregnancy

According to the correlation analysis (Table 2), maternal intake of fruits and vegetables during pregnancy was positively correlated ($r = 0.727$, $P < 0.0001$) with vitamin C intake. Also, maternal fruit and vegetable ($P < 0.05$) and vitamin C ($P < 0.05$) intakes were both negatively correlated with urinary MDA levels at mid-pregnancy, respectively.

Association of maternal fruit and vegetable/vitamin C intake with fetal growth at late pregnancy

Multiple regression analysis indicated that maternal fruit and vegetable intake during pregnancy was not associated with the biparietal diameter ($\beta = 0.045$, $P = 0.0511$) at late pregnancy. A general linear model adjusted for covariates revealed that biparietal diameter was higher in fetuses whose mothers had a fruit and vegetable consumption above the median value (≥519 g/d) than in fetuses of mothers with a lower fruit and vegetable intake ($p = 0.0245$). Similar analyses for vitamin C intake during pregnancy showed a significant result in the abdominal circumference. Maternal vitamin C intake was positively associated with abdominal circumference ($\beta = 0.279$, $P = 0.0354$) at late pregnancy. Abdominal circumference in fetuses of mothers with intakes of vitamin C above the EAR (≥85 mg/d) was significantly higher compared to fetuses of mothers with intakes below the EAR ($P = 0.0234$). After controlling for confounding factors in the multiple logistic regression analysis, a significant inverse relationship was noted between fruit and vegetable consumption and the risk of low biparietal diameter (<25th percentile). Compared with fetuses whose mothers had a fruit and vegetable consumption above the median value (≥519 g/d), those of mothers with a lower fruit and vegetable intake had a higher risk (OR: 2.220; 95% CI: 1.153–4.274) of low biparietal diameter (<25th percentile) at late pregnancy (Table 3).

Association of maternal fruit and vegetable/vitamin C intake with infant growth at birth and up to 6 months

Fetal biometric measurements, such as biparietal diameter, abdominal circumference, and femur length, were positively correlated ($P < 0.0001$) with infant birth weight and length (data not shown). Based on the multiple regression analysis (Table 4), maternal fruit and vegetable intake during pregnancy was not associated with infant weight and length at birth and 6 months, respectively. However, when we conducted mixed models analysis for repeated measures from birth to 6 months, fruit and vegetable intake was positively associated with infants' weight ($\beta = 0.054$, $P = 0.0184$). Birth weight in neonates born to mothers who consumed above the median fruit and vegetable value (≥519 g/d) was significantly higher than those born to mothers who consumed below the median value ($P = 0.0024$); these results were also observed in mixed models analysis for birth to 6 months ($P = 0.0077$). Maternal vitamin C intake was positively associated with infant birth length ($\beta = 0.314$, $P = 0.0056$). Birth weight ($P = 0.0400$) and length ($P = 0.0010$) in neonates born to mothers who consumed above the EAR (≥85 mg/d) of vitamin C were significantly higher than in neonates born to mothers who consumed below the EAR ($P = 0.0010$). After adjusting for covariates, a significant negative relationship was observed between maternal fruit and vegetable consumption and low infant weight at birth (<25th percentile) [OR (95% CI) for below the median compared to above the median (≥519 g/d): 1.434 (1.001–2.256)]. There was also a significant negative correlation between the vitamin C consumption and low weight at birth (<25th percentile) [OR (95% CI) for below the EAR compared to above the EAR (≥85 mg/d): 1.470 (1.011–2.139)]. A similar trend was revealed between vitamin C intake and low weight from birth to 6 months (<25th percentile) [OR (95% CI) for below the EAR compared to above the EAR (≥85 mg/d): 1.520 (1.066–2.165)] and low length at birth (<25th percentile) [OR (95% CI) for below the EAR compared to above the EAR (≥85 mg/d): 1.579 (1.104–2.258)].

Discussion

In the present large cohort study, we investigated the association of maternal fruit and vegetable and vitamin C intakes during mid-pregnancy with increased fetal growth and infant growth up to 6 months of age, in a Korean population. We found maternal fruit and vegetable intake had a positive association with the biparietal diameter of the fetus and infant weight at birth to 6 months. Also, maternal vitamin C intake was positively associated with the abdominal circumference of the fetus and infant birth length.

Similar results, demonstrating fruit and vegetable consumption during pregnancy favorably influences fetal

Table 2 Coefficients of correlation (*r*) between fruit and vegetable intake, vitamin C intake and urinary malonaldehyde (MDA) concentrations at mid-pregnancy ($n = 1036$)

Intake	Urinary MDA concentration	Fruit and vegetable intake	Vitamin C intake
Fruit and vegetables	−0.064*	1	0.727**
Vitamin C	−0.065*	0.727**	1

Intake data were log-transformed to conform to normal distribution. *$p < 0.05$. **$p < 0.0001$

Table 3 Association of maternal fruit and vegetable/vitamin C intake with fetal growth at late pregnancy

Intake	At late pregnancy								
	Biparietal diameter (cm)			Abdominal circumference (cm)			Femur length (cm)		
	n	β (SE)/ lsmean ± SD	p	*n*	β (SE)/ lsmean ± SD	p	*n*	β (SE)/ lsmean ± SD	p
Fruit and vegetables									
Continues									
Unadjusted	703	0.004 (0.031)	0.8919	589	0·046 (0.161)	0.7743	689	0.032 (0.030)	0.2835
Adjusted[a]	515	0.045 (0.023)	0.0511	433	0·175 (0.135)	0.1964	507	0.001 (0.023)	0.9747
Categorical[a]									
< median (519 g/d)		8.92 ± 0.02	0.0245		32.11 ± 0.12	0.2464		6.88 ± 0.02	0.8144
≥ median (519 g/d)		8.99 ± 0.02			32.30 ± 0.12			6.87 ± 0.02	
Vitamin C									
Continues									
Unadjusted	703	0.006 (0.030)	0.8457	589	0.045 (0.155)	0.7730	689	−0.022 (0.029)	0.4344
Adjusted[b]	515	0.030 (0.023)	0.1898	433	0.279 (0.132)	0.0354	507	0.021 (0.023)	0.3463
Categorical[b]									
< EAR (85 mg/d)		8.94 ± 0.03	0.3342		31.94 ± 0.14	0.0234		6.86 ± 0.02	0.3632
≥ EAR (85 mg/d)		8.97 ± 0.02			32.35 ± 0.11			6.89 ± 0.02	
ORs (95% CI) for low fetal biometry (<25th percentile)									
Fruit and vegetables									
< median (519 g/d)		2.220 (1.153–4.274)	0.0170		1.695 (0.900–3.192)	0.1023		0.772 (0.388–1.537)	0.4613
≥ median (519 g/d)		1 (ref)			1 (ref)			1 (ref)	
Vitamin C									
< EAR (85 mg/d)		1.468 (0.753–2.865)	0.2600		1.682 (0.848–3.335)	0.1367		1.139 (0.535–2.423)	0.7359
≥ EAR (85 mg/d)		1 (ref)			1 (ref)			1 (ref)	

β value is the coefficient from the multiple regression analysis
Least squares means (lsmeans) is a mean estimated from a general linear model
EAR is estimated average requirement
ORs is odds ratios
Intake data were log-transformed for normal distribution
[a]Adjusted for maternal age, pre-pregnancy body mass index (BMI), urinary cotinine level (log-transformed), infant gender, gestational age at the time of ultrasound measurement, use of supplements, residential area, parity, father's height, energy intake (log-transformed)
[b]Adjusted for maternal age, pre-pregnancy BMI, urinary cotinine level (log-transformed), infant gender, gestational age at the time of ultrasound measurement, use of supplements, residential area, parity, father's height, energy intake (log-transformed), vitamin E intake (log-transformed), β-carotene intake (log-transformed)

growth, have been reported by previous investigators. Rao et al. [9] and Mikkelsen et al. [7] documented a significant increase in birth weight with increased fruit and vegetable consumption (as a food group). Ramón et al. [17] observed an increased intake of vegetables, but not fruit, during pregnancy was associated with birth length and weight. Loy et al. [18] noted that vegetable intake was linked to birth length and head circumference, and fruit intake was correlated with birth weight and length, and head circumference.

In our study, the multiple logistic regression analysis revealed a significant inverse relationship between fruit and vegetable consumption and the risk of low growth (<25th percentile) of biparietal diameter and weight at birth. In line with this result, there was a significant inverse relationship between consumption of vitamin C (an abundant nutrient in fruit and vegetables) and the risk of low (<25th percentile) weight at birth, weight from birth to 6 months, and length at birth. Prior research has demonstrated that the vitamin C contained in fruit and vegetables may contribute to both, placental functions and optimal immune system functioning [19], which are paramount for fetal development.

Along with maternal vitamin consumption, we investigated maternal oxidative stress (MDA level), considering that it might be increased under normal pregnancy environments and cause adverse birth outcomes. Although the correlation coefficient value is very low, the maternal fruit and vegetable, and vitamin C intakes were negatively correlated with the oxidant marker (MDA) levels at mid-pregnancy, in agreement with the literature [16]. This factor could partly explain the underlying reason for our findings that women consuming low amounts of fruit and vegetables, and vitamin C had low birth outcomes; with

Table 4 Association of maternal fruit and vegetable/vitamin C intake with infants' weight and length from birth to 6 months

Intake	Weight (kg)									Length (cm)								
	At birth			At 6 months			Birth to 6 months			At birth			At 6 months			Birth to 6 months		
	n	β (SE)/ lsmean ± SD	p	*n*	β (SE)/ lsmean ± SD	p	*n*	β (SE)/ lsmean ± SD	p	*n*	β (SE)/ lsmean ± SD	p	*n*	β (SE)/ lsmean ± SD	p	*n*	β (SE)/ lsmean ± SD	p
Fruit and vegetables																		
Continues																		
Unadjusted	1138	0.014 (0.017)	0.4295	741	−0.058 (0.058)	0.3150	1138	0.013 (0.017)	0.4609	1138	0.116 (0.101)	0.2471	740	0.073 (0.162)	0.6520	1138	0.120 (0.101)	0.2329
Adjusted[a]	816	0.031 (0.020)	0.1182	559	−0.056 (0.064)	0.3848	639	0.054 (0.023)	0.0184	816	0.172 (0.119)	0.1479	558	−0.043 (0.189)	0.8214	639	0.170 (0.133)	0.2032
Categorical[a]																		
< median (519 g/d)		3.22 ± 0.03	0.0024		10.09 ± 0.11	0.6718		3.23 ± 0.04	0.0077		50.44 ± 0.20	0.1620		76.82 ± 0.34	0.5126		50.78 ± 0.22	0.2993
≥ median (519 g/d)		3.29 ± 0.03			10.12 ± 0.11			3.31 ± 0.04			50.65 ± 0.20			76.98 ± 0.32			50.95 ± 0.22	
Vitamin C																		
Continues																		
Unadjusted	1138	0.015 (0.016)	0.3537	741	0.018 (0.053)	0.7344	1138	0.014 (0.016)	0.3941	1138	0.197 (0.092)	0.0333	740	0.231 (0.148)	0.1182	1138	0.202 (0.092)	0.0294
Adjusted[b]	816	0.035 (0.019)	0.0677	559	0.017 (0.060)	0.7803	639	0.037 (0.021)	0.0808	816	0.314 (0.113)	0.0056	558	0.054 (0.178)	0.7624	639	0.289 (0.125)	0.0214
Categorical[b]																		
< EAR (85 mg/d)		3.22 ± 0.04	0.0400		10.07 ± 0.12	0.4290		3.23 ± 0.04	0.0565		50.20 ± 0.21	0.0010		77.00 ± 0.36	0.7231		50.53 ± 0.24	0.0068
≥ EAR (85 mg/d)		3.28 ± 0.03			10.14 ± 0.11			3.29 ± 0.04			50.74 ± 0.19			76.90 ± 0.31			51.02 ± 0.21	
ORs (95% CI) for low birth outcomes and low growth up to 6 months (<25th percentile)																		
Fruit and vegetables																		
< median (519 g/d)		1.434 (1.001–2.056)	0.0494	0.863 (0.627–1.186)	0.3631			1.311 (0.939–1.829)	0.1117		1.316 (0.933–1.857)	0.1178		0.875 (0.636–1.204)	0.4126	1.152 (0.845–1.570)	0.3714	
≥ median (519 g/d)		1 (ref)		1 (ref)				1 (ref)			1 (ref)			1 (ref)		1 (ref)		
Vitamin C																		
< EAR (85 mg/d)		1.470 (1.011–2.139)	0.0439	0.910 (0.645–1.284)	0.5916			1.520 (1.066–2.165)	0.0206		1.579 (1.104–2.258)	0.0124		1.182 (0.837 1.669)	0.3416	1.262 (0.900–1.770)	0.1773	
≥ EAR (85 mg/d)		1 (ref)		1 (ref)				1 (ref)			1 (ref)			1 (ref)		1 (ref)		

β value is the coefficient from the multiple regression analysis
Least squares means (lsmeans) is a mean estimated from a general linear model
EAR is estimated average requirement
ORs is odds ratios
Intake data were log-transformed to follow a normal distribution
For repeated measures analyses from birth to 6 months, mixed models (when the dependent variables are continuous) and general estimating equation models (when dependent variables are categorical) were used
[a]Adjusted for maternal age, pre-pregnancy body mass index (BMI), urinary cotinine level (log-transformed), infant gender, gestational age at delivery, use of supplements, residential area, parity, father's height, energy intake (log-transformed) at birth; additionally, adjusted for breastfeeding status at 6 months
[b]Adjusted for maternal age, pre-pregnancy BMI, urinary cotinine level (log-transformed), infant gender, gestational age at delivery, use of supplements, residential area, parity, father's height, energy intake (log-transformed), vitamin E intake (log-transformed), β-carotene intake (log-transformed) at birth; additionally, adjusted for breastfeeding status at 6 months

the offspring having low growth up to 6 months. Antioxidant defense systems are vital to protecting tissues and cells from damage caused by oxidative stress. Consequently, an imbalance between increased oxidative stress and decreased antioxidant defense can adversely affect pregnancy outcomes, including fetal growth retardation [20]. Increased vitamin C consumption (supplement or via fruits and vegetables) during pregnancy may be advantageous to birth size due to its role in the endogenous antioxidant defense system. In a previous epidemiological study in Spain of 586 newborns, an increase in dietary vitamin C intake during pregnancy was implicated to reduce the association between estimated maternal dietary benzo[a]pyrene (a cigarette smoke carcinogen) intake and infant size at birth [21]. Also, maternal fruit and vegetable intake may modify the association between birth weight and bulky DNA adduct levels, which are purported to be a sensitive biomarker of genotoxic agents [22].

Another possibility is that vitamin C, an essential cofactor for two key enzymes (lysyl and prolyl hydroxylase) in collagen biosynthesis, is beneficial for cartilage and bone development [23]. Some experimental studies have found that vitamin C inadequacy can result in a decreased proliferation of chondrocytes in the growth plate and impaired matrix synthesis [24] in mice, and low bone mineral density and bone length in a scorbutic guinea pig model [25]. However, further investigation is needed to unveil the true effects of vitamin C intake during pregnancy on fetal bone growth and collagen metabolism.

During normal prenatal development, fetal vitamin C concentrations in plasma are higher than maternal levels. One study demonstrated an approximately two-fold higher vitamin C level in newborns at birth than in their mothers [26], implying that a high vitamin C status is of particular importance in the fetus. However, our subjects did not meet the optimal vitamin C range. The mean vitamin C intake in our subjects was 134.3 mg/d, and about 36.2% and 51.2% of pregnant women had vitamin C intakes below the EAR and recommended nutrient intake, respectively (data not shown). The vitamin C intake status in our pregnant women is higher than that reported in China [27], Iran [28], England [29], New Zealand [30], and Brazil [31], but lower than that documented in Thailand [32] and the USA [33].

The main vitamin C sources were fruits (40.3%) and vegetables (46.5%) (data not shown), but the correlation between fruit and vegetable/vitamin C with fetal and infant growth was partly inconsistent. Notably, in the biparietal diameter, a significant inverse relationship between fruit and vegetable intake and a low growth rate (<25th percentile) was observed, whereas mothers with a relatively lower vitamin C intake did not have a higher risk of low biparietal diameter. It may be that fruits and vegetables have played a role in other ways, such as provide unexpected bioactive components that are not vitamin C. The high number of bioactive components are found in fruits and vegetables, such as vitamins, minerals, phytosterols, phenolic compounds [34], carotenoids, and fiber. Also, fruit and vegetable intakes may be a pivotal part of a healthy lifestyle and dietary pattern and may be associated with other health factors besides the variables we have adjusted [35, 36].

Our study had some limitations. First, we did not measure plasma vitamin C concentrations, which are considered to be a more objective means to assess vitamin C status than dietary vitamin C intake reports alone, due to the limited amounts of samples for other measurements (e.g., environmental heavy metals and toxins). Second, the maternal dietary intake data from a single 24-h recall may not be sufficient to determine typical daily intake, due to a probable and considerable intra-individual variability in food and nutritional intake. However, the well-trained dietitians applied standard protocols to assist the subjects' recollection of their daily diet and thereby minimize any potential bias. Regarding intra-individual variability of nutrient intake, as part of the 4th Korean National Health and Nutrition Examination Survey in 2009 [37], the intra-individual variation in nutrient intake measured by a single 24-h dietary recall was compared to an original 1-d dietary interview. Regarding total energy and, particularly, vitamin C intake, comparable values were obtained from each interview. Besides, the seasonality of food can be a problem for 24-h dietary recall. To minimize its undesired effect, the season could be added as a covariate in our analysis. However, there was no difference between fruits and vegetables and vitamin C intake according to the season (data not shown). This observation seems to be because the timing of the pregnant women's recruitment, that is, the period of the dietary survey was evenly distributed. Therefore, we decided that it was not necessary to include the season as a covariate. In addition, a Greek study investigating the impact of seasonality on the mean nutrient intake of children and adolescents reported that the intake of vitamin C and the macronutrient contribution to the total energy intake, estimated by two 24-h recalls of different seasons, were statistically similar between the two periods (spring/summer and autumn/winter) [38]. Evaluation of potential genotypes that can affect oxidative stress metabolism, as well as the enzymatic activity for heterozygotes and assessment of some specific oxidative markers, might also have improved the reliability of our results.

The strengths of our study include the sample size and the research strategy, considering the strictly-controlled prospective birth cohort design of the MOCEH study in

Korea. Also, this research collected reliable data from medical records. Furthermore, an adjustment for crucial confounders having the potential to affect the correlation between maternal vitamin C intake and birth outcomes of newborns were considered, in detail, for more precise analysis.

Fetal growth is an important determinant of health and disease throughout a human's lifetime. Interestingly, a prospective birth cohort study in Brazil noted a positive association of birth length with blood pressure at 11 years of age, whereas birth weight and blood pressure were not associated [39]. It exemplifies the importance of the relationship between maternal vitamin C and infant birth length as modifiers that could affect children later in life.

Conclusion

In conclusion, an increased intake of dietary vitamin C, which is abundant in fruit and vegetables, at mid-pregnancy is associated with increased fetal growth and infant growth up to 6 months of age.

Abbreviations

CI: Confidence interval; DRI: Dietary Reference Intake; EAR: Estimated average requirement; HPLC: High-performance liquid chromatography; IUGR: Intrauterine growth restriction; KNHANES: Korean National Health and Nutrition Examination Survey; MDA: Malondialdehyde; MOCEH: Mothers' and Children's Environmental Health; OR: Odds ratio; RNI: Recommended nutrient intake; SD: Standard deviation

Acknowledgments

Not applicable.

Funding

This research was supported by the Ministry of Environment and by the Basic Science Research Program (NRF-2018R1C1B4A01023629) funded by the Ministry of Science, ICT, and Future Planning, Republic of Korea.

Authors' contributions

NC designed the research; WJ, HK, and BL conducted the research; WJ and HK analyzed the data; WJ, HK, and NC wrote the manuscript, and NC was primarily responsible for the final content. All the authors read and approved the final manuscript.

Competing interests

The authors declare that they have no competing interests.

Author details

[1]Department of Nutritional Science and Food Management, Ewha Womans University, Seoul, South Korea. [2]Environmental Health Research Division, National Institute of Environmental Research, Incheon, South Korea.

References

1. Richter HG, Camm EJ, Modi BN, Naeem F, Cross CM, Cindrova-Davies T, et al. Ascorbate prevents placental oxidative stress and enhances birth weight in hypoxic pregnancy in rats. J Physiol. 2012;590(6):1377–87.
2. Ibrahim BS, Barioni ÉD, Heluany C, Braga TT, Drewes CC, Costa SG, et al. Beneficial effects of vitamin C treatment on pregnant rats exposed to formaldehyde: reversal of immunosuppression in the offspring. Toxicol Appl Pharmacol. 2016;300:77–81.
3. Ugwa EA, Iwasam EA, Nwali MI. Low serum vitamin C status among pregnant women attending antenatal care at general hospital Dawakin kudu, Northwest Nigeria. Int J Prev Med. 2016;7:40.
4. Wang YZ, Ren WH, Liao WQ, Zhang GY. Concentrations of antioxidant vitamins in maternal and cord serum and their effect on birth outcomes. J Nutr Sci Vitaminol (Tokyo). 2009;55(1):1–8.
5. Dejmek J, Ginter E, Solansky I, Podrazilová K, Stávková Z, Benes I, et al. Vitamin C, E and a levels in maternal and fetal blood for Czech and gypsy ethnic groups in the Czech Republic. Int J Vitam Nutr Res. 2002;72(3):183–90.
6. Rao S, Yajnik CS, Kanade A, Fall CHD, Margetts BM, Jackson AA, et al. Intake of micronutrient-rich foods in rural Indian mothers is associated with the size of their babies at birth: Pune maternal nutrition study. J Nutr. 2001; 131(4):1217–24.
7. Mikkelsen TB, Osler M, Orozova-Bekkevold I, Knudsen VK, Olsen SF. Association between fruit and vegetable consumption and birth weight: a prospective study among 43,585 Danish women. Scand J Public Health. 2006;34(6):616–22.
8. Saker M, Mokhtari NS, Merzouk SA, Merzouk H, Belarbi B, Narce M. Oxidant and antioxidant status in mothers and their newborns according to birthweight. Eur J Obstet Gynecol Reprod Biol. 2008;141(2):95–9.
9. Siega-Riz AM, Promislow JH, Savitz DA, Thorp JM Jr, McDonald T. Vitamin C intake and the risk of preterm delivery. Am J Obstet Gynecol. 2003;189(2): 519–25.
10. Mathews F, Yudkin P, Neil A. Influence of maternal nutrition on outcome of pregnancy: prospective cohort study. BMJ. 1999;319(7206):339–43.
11. Lee BE, Hong YC, Lee KH, Kim YJ, Kim WK, Chang NS, et al. Influence of maternal serum levels of vitamins C and E during the second trimester on birth weight and length. Eur J Clin Nutr. 2004;58(10):1365–71.
12. Hong J, Lee HA, Park EA, Kim YJ, Lee H, Park BH, et al. Association of mid-pregnancy antioxidative vitamin and oxidative stress levels with infant growth during the first 3 years of life. Food Nutr Res. 2014;58(1):ID 20207.
13. Dehghan M, Akhtar-Danesh N, McMillan CR, Thabane L. Is plasma vitamin C an appropriate biomarker of vitamin C intake? A systematic review and meta-analysis. Nutr J. 2007;6:41.
14. Kim BM, Ha M, Park HS, Lee BE, Kim YJ, Hong YC, et al. The mothers and Children's environmental health (MOCEH) study. Eur J Epidemiol. 2009;24(9): 573–83.
15. Hur J, Kim H, Ha EH, Park H, Ha M, Kim Y, et al. Birth weight of Korean infants is affected by the interaction of maternal iron intake and GSTM1 polymorphism. J Nutr. 2013;143(1):67–73.
16. Ugwa E, Gwarzo M, Ashimi A. Oxidative stress and antioxidant status of pregnant rural women in north-West Nigeria: prospective cohort study. J Matern Fetal Neonatal Med. 2015;28(5):544–7.
17. Ramón R, Ballester F, Iñiguez C, Rebagliato M, Murcia M, Esplugues A, et al. Vegetable but not fruit intake during pregnancy is associated with newborn anthropometric measures. J Nutr. 2009;139(3):561–7.
18. Loy SL, Marhazlina M, Nor Azwany Y, Hamid Jan JM. Higher intake of fruits and vegetables in pregnancy is associated with birth size. Southeast Asian J Trop Med Public Health. 2011;42(5):1214–23.
19. Ahn YM, Kim YJ, Park H, Park B, Lee H. Prenatal vitamin C status is associated with placental apoptosis in normal-term human pregnancies. Placenta. 2007;28(1):31–8.
20. Al-Gubory KH. Environmental pollutants and lifestyle factors induce oxidative stress and poor prenatal development. Reprod BioMed Online. 2014;29(1):17–31.
21. Duarte-Salles T, Mendez MA, Meltzer HM, Alexander J, Haugen M. Dietary benzo(a)pyrene intake during pregnancy and birth weight: associations modified by vitamin C intakes in the Norwegian mother and child cohort study (MoBa). Environ Int. 2013;60:217–23.
22. Pedersen M, Schoket B, Godschalk RW, Wright J, von Stedingk H, Törnqvist M, et al. Bulky DNA adducts in cord blood, maternal fruit-and-vegetable consumption, and birth weight in a European mother–child study (NewGeneris). Environ Health Perspect. 2013;121(10):1200–6.

23. Temu TM, Wu KY, Gruppuso PA, Phornphutkul C. The mechanism of ascorbic acid-induced differentiation of ATDC5 chondrogenic cells. Am J Physiol Endocrinol Metab. 2010;299(2):E325–34.
24. Wegger I, Palludan B. Vitamin C deficiency causes hematological and skeletal abnormalities during fetal development in swine. J Nutr. 1994; 124(2):241–8.
25. Kipp DE, McElvain M, Kimmel DB, Akhter MP, Robinson RG, Lukert BP. Scurvy results in decreased collagen synthesis and bone density in the Guinea pig animal model. Bone. 1996;18(3):281–8.
26. Jain SK, Wise R, Yanamandra K, Dhanireddy R, Bocchini JA Jr. The effect of maternal and cord-blood vitamin C, vitamin E and lipid peroxide levels on newborn birth weight. Mol Cell Biochem. 2008;309(1–2):217–21.
27. Cheng Y, Dibley MJ, Zhang X, Zeng L, Yan H. Assessment of dietary intake among pregnant women in a rural area of western China. BMC Public Health. 2009;9:222.
28. Kazemian E, Dorosty-Motlagh AR, Sotoudeh G, Eshraghian MR, Ansary S, Omidian M. Nutritional status of women with gestational hypertension compared with normal pregnant women. Hypertens Pregnancy. 2013;32(2): 146–56.
29. Mouratidou T, Ford F, Prountzou F, Fraser R. Dietary assessment of a population of pregnant women in Sheffield, UK. Br J Nutr. 2006;96(5):929–35.
30. Watson PE, McDonald BW. Major influences on nutrient intake in pregnant New Zealand women. Matern Child Health J. 2009;13(5):695.
31. Zentner LEA, Rondo PHC, Duran MC, Oliveira JM. Relationships of blood lead to calcium, iron, and vitamin C intakes in Brazilian pregnant women. Clin Nutr. 2008;27(1):100–4.
32. Sukchan P, Liabsuetrakul T, Chongsuvivatwong V, Songwathana P, Sornsrivichai V, Kuning M. Inadequacy of nutrients intake among pregnant women in the deep south of Thailand. BMC Public Health. 2010;10:572.
33. Litonjua AA, Rifas-Shiman SL, Ly NP, Tantisira KG, Rich-Edwards JW, Camargo CA Jr, et al. Maternal antioxidant intake in pregnancy and wheezing illnesses in children at 2 y of age. Am J Clin Nutr. 2006;84(4):903–11.
34. Liu RH. Health-promoting components of fruits and vegetables in the diet. Adv Nutr. 2013;4(3):384S–92S.
35. Fulton SL, McKinley MC, Young IS, Cardwell CR, Woodside JV. The effect of increasing fruit and vegetable consumption on overall diet: a systematic review and meta-analysis. Crit Rev Food Sci Nutr. 2016;56(5):802–16.
36. Simões-Wüst AP, Moltó-Puigmartí C, van Dongen MC, Dagnelie PC, Thijs C. Organic food consumption during pregnancy is associated with different consumer profiles, food patterns and intake: the KOALA Birth Cohort Study. Public Health Nutr. 2017;20(12):2134–44.
37. Korea Centers for Disease Control and Prevention. Report presentation of the Korea National Health and nutrition examination survey (KNHANES) IV. Seoul: Ministry of Health and Welfare; 2009, 2010.
38. Yannakoulia M, Drichoutis AC, Kontogianni MD, Magkanari F. Season-related variation in dietary recalls used in a paediatric population. J Hum Nutr Diet. 2010;23(5):489–93.
39. Menezes AMB, Hallal PC, Horta BL, Araújo CLP, de Fátima VM, Neutzling M, et al. Size at birth and blood pressure in early adolescence: a prospective birth cohort study. Am J Epidemiol. 2007;165(6):611–6.

12

Vegetables and legumes in new Australasian food launches: how are they being used and are they a healthy choice?

Beth Gilham[1,2]*, Ramon Hall[2] and Julie L. Woods[1]

Abstract

Background: Despite the health benefits of regular vegetable and legume consumption, on average Australians are consuming only half of the recommended daily intake. The reasons for this low consumption are complex, and are particularly driven by societal shifts towards convenient and ready-to-eat meal options. It is currently unknown how legumes and vegetables are being utilised in food products within the Australian context, and the nutritional value or level of processing of these products.

Methods: The Mintel Global New Food Database was used to identify all new products launched between May 2012 and May 2017 in Australasia which at least 0.5 serves of vegetables and/or legumes per recommended serving. Eligible products were coded using the NOVA food classification system and the Healthy Choices guidelines, and were categorized by the researchers based on the type and proportion of vegetable and legume ingredients used.

Results: Overall, 1313 products were identified, which contained a median of 55% vegetable and legume ingredients (IQR = 45%). This translated to approximately 1 (IQR = 1) serves of vegetables and legumes per recommended serving of the products. The product launches were most likely to be classified as an 'amber' choice, and be classified as either 'processed' or 'ultra-processed'. Vegetables and legumes were mainly found in the form of new prepared meals, soups or whole vegetables products, however there were some more innovative uses of these ingredients, such as yoghurts and pastas.

Conclusions: Most of the new products currently released onto the Australian market which contain vegetable and legume ingredients do not provide meaningful amounts of these ingredients, and tend to be highly processed and unhealthier options. A multi-faceted approach is needed to improve vegetable and legume consumption, which includes improving the availability of products which help consumers to meet vegetable and legume consumption recommendations. Future research should consider the acceptability of these products to consumers, and the barriers for food manufacturers in creating products with a higher amount of vegetables and legumes.

Keywords: Food supply, Vegetables, Legumes, Pulses, Packaged foods

Introduction

In a society where poor diet habits are one of the largest contributor to the burden of disease [1], it is vital that we find ways to improve population-level consumption of healthier diets. Vegetables and legumes, such as chickpeas, lentils, lupins and beans, form a key part of a healthy diet, and regular consumption of these foods has been shown to have a positive impact on improving risk factors for a range of non-communicable diseases [2–4]. Despite being the most prominent food group in the Australian Dietary Guidelines, vegetables and legumes are one of the most under-consumed food groups in the Australian diet [5]. On average, most Australians are currently consuming only half of the recommended five serves (1 serve = 75 g) from the vegetable and legumes group per day [5]. This poor consumption has been linked to a range of barriers in the Australian context,

* Correspondence: bethgilham92@gmail.com
[1]Institute for Physical Activity and Nutrition (IPAN), School of Exercise and Nutrition Sciences, Deakin University, Geelong 3220, Australia
[2]Centre for Advanced Sensory Science, School of Exercise and Nutrition Sciences, Deakin University, 221 Burwood Highway, Burwood, VIC 3125, Australia

such as preference for other foods or dislike of vegetables [6, 7], the consumer perspective that they consume more vegetables than they actually do [6] and poor access to, and higher cost of fresh produce, particularly in rural or outer-metropolitan areas [7–10]. Legumes in particular are not well recognised or understood by consumers [11, 12], which has been described as a significant barrier to consumption and led to the creation of the 'International Year of Pulses' campaign in 2016 by the Food and Agricultural Organisation of the United Nations [13].

Societal changes and the globalisation of the food supply have led to a shift in the types of food people eat, as well as the way they are eaten, with consumers increasingly choosing convenient food options that require minimal preparation such as ready-to-eat meals and snack foods [14, 15]. Concurrently, we are consuming more discretionary foods (foods which do not form a key part of the diet, such as chips, chocolate and muesli bars) and products which have been ultra-processed [5, 16]. These products tend to be energy dense and nutrient poor, but are typically considered more convenient and palatable compared to fresh, minimally processed, healthier options [17, 18]. The modern food environment offers many convenient options, however it is unknown whether these products contain healthier ingredients such as vegetables and legumes, and the relative nutritional value of these products.

A recent study by Spiteri et al. found that only 3% of all new products launched onto the Australian market in 2015 were categorized as 'fruit and vegetables'. Of these 'fruit and vegetables' products, were classified as 'green' (ie. the healthiest choice) using the Healthy Choices guidelines [19]. As expected, there was considerable overlap between the products in this study [19] and the current study; however the study by Spiteri et al. was conducted for one year only, and only counted fruit and vegetables categorized in the 'fruit and vegetables' category, not in mixed meals or other product categories. To date, there has been a dearth of information relating to the measurement of the use of vegetables and legumes in new food products in Australia. Likewise, there is no indication of whether these new products, despite containing healthier vegetable and legume ingredients, are a healthy and/or minimally processed option. This information is essential to establish a baseline understanding of the situation and products currently available. It is particularly important for the food industry in order to establish the current use of vegetable and legume ingredients in food products, and to identify new innovations in this area.

The objective of this study was to examine the use of vegetables and legumes in new food and beverage products released in Australia and New Zealand over a 5-year time period based on i) proportion of vegetable and legume ingredients; ii) number of serves of vegetables and legumes; iii) type of food or beverage product; iv) nutritional quality and; v) level of processing.

Materials and methods

Data collection

This study identified new food and beverage launches in Australia between May 2012 and May 2017 using the Mintel Global New Product Database (Mintel GNPD). The Mintel GNPD is a large industry database which catalogues all new packaged food and beverage launches in 60 economies worldwide, including Australia and New Zealand [20]. Each entry provides detailed product information, such as price, ingredients, claims made and nutritional information, as well as photographs of all sides of the packaging. Approximately 33,000 new product launches are added to the entire database per month, and the products available are predicted to represent 75–80% of all new launches in countries where data is collected [20, 21].

New food and beverage products launched between May 2012 and May 2017 in Australia, which contained at least 0.5 serves of vegetables and legumes per recommended serving were included in this study (Table 1). Vegetables are the edible portion of a plant, either in the form of a raw product or processed in a way that retains the bulk of the raw product [22]. In general, vegetables are an excellent source of fibre and a wide range of essential vitamins and minerals. There is a wide variety of different vegetables available in Australia, with the main examples being green leafy vegetables (such as spinach), Brassica vegetables (such as broccoli), gourd vegetables (such as pumpkin), edible plant stems (such as asparagus) and Allium vegetables (such as onion or garlic) [23]. This study also included vegetables such as tomatoes and potatoes, which are not universally classified as vegetables, but are included in the Australian Dietary Guidelines [23]. Vegetable and legume flours and juices were included in addition to raw or whole versions.

Products were excluded if the sole vegetable or legume ingredient did not resemble the nutritional properties of the whole ingredient, such as vegetable oils. While corn was included as a vegetable, corn flour was considered as a grain due to its low fibre and micronutrient content [24], and therefore products containing corn flour as the

Table 1 Inclusion and exclusion criteria

Included	Excluded
• New food and beverage products (May 2012 – May 2017) • < 0.5 approximate serves of vegetables and legumes • Tomatoes, potatoes • Vegetable and legume juices and flours	• Soybeans and peanuts • Vegetable oils • Corn flour

sole vegetable or legume ingredient were excluded. While both soybeans and peanuts are part of the legume family, they are usually considered as oilseeds due to their high lipid content [25], and therefore products where these were the only vegetable or legume ingredient were not included in the analysis. Once calculated, products with less than 0.5 approximate serves of vegetables and legumes were dropped.

The Mintel GNPD search was conducted on 23rd June 2017, using the search parameters listed in Table 2. Additional searches were conducted using the same parameters and specific key words in order to identify products which may not be consistently classified in the vegetable category ('potato', 'pea', 'tomato', 'chickpea', 'kidney', 'lentil'). The results of all searches were exported to Microsoft Excel, where duplicate results and excluded products were dropped.

Foods in Mintel GNPD are classified into 22 main categories, with additional sub-categories: baby food, bakery, breakfast cereal, carbonated soft drinks, chocolate confectionery, dairy, desserts and ice cream, fruits and vegetables, hot beverages, juice drinks, meals and meal centres, other beverages, processed fish, meat and egg products, sauces and seasonings, savoury spreads, side dishes, snacks, soup, sports & energy drinks, sugar & gum confectionery, sweet spreads and water. Some of these categories were excluded from the search as they were inappropriate for this study. This included categories which are considered condiments (such as vinegar, dressings and sugar/sweetener), discretionary foods with small serving sizes (such as chocolate confectionary) and drinks which are not suitable for general consumption (such as alcoholic beverages). Sensitivity analyses including these categories revealed no reportable change to the results.

Categorization based on type and proportion of vegetable and legume ingredients

All products were initially classified as containing 'vegetables-only', 'legumes-only' or 'both legumes and vegetables'. All other variable categories (food category, food sub-category) were directly sourced from Mintel GNPD as described above.

The approximate proportion of vegetable and legume ingredients was determined based on the proportion listed in the ingredients list. Where no percentage was listed for one or all of the legume and vegetable ingredients in the ingredients list, the proportion was estimated based on similar products, and the proportion of other ingredients in the product. This percentage was converted to grams of vegetable and legume ingredients, based on the recommended serving size of the product. The equivalent number of serves from the vegetables and legumes group was then determined, where one serve was equal to 75 g of vegetables and legumes as per the Australian Dietary Guidelines [23]. The number of vegetable and legume serves was rounded down to the closest 0.5 serve to account for potential loss of product through preparation or wastage, and to prevent overestimation of the vegetable and legume content.

Categorization based on nutrition quality and level of processing

The nutritional quality of products was determined using the Victorian Government "Healthy Choices" framework, which classifies products as 'green' (healthiest choice), 'amber' (choose carefully) or 'red' (limit) based on several attributes, such as nutritional profile and serving size [26]. Level of processing was determined using the NOVA food classification system, which classifies products as 'unprocessed or minimally processed foods', 'processed culinary ingredients', 'processed foods' or 'ultra-processed food and drink products' [27].

Initial coding of the products using both classification systems was conducted by one researcher (BG). A random sample of 5% of the total products was cross-checked by the two other researchers (JW, RH), as per similar literature in this area [28]. Where discrepancies were identified, these were discussed as a group to determine the final classification.

Table 2 Search strategy for Mintel Global New Product Database

Search variables	Parameters
Country	Australia
Date published	Between May 2012 and May 2017
Ingredient search	"Vegetables and Vegetable Products and all child ingredients"
Mintel GNPD categories included	'Baby food', 'bakery', 'breakfast cereals', 'dairy', 'desserts & ice cream', 'fruit & vegetables', 'meal & meal centers', 'processed fish/meat/egg products', 'savoury spreads', 'side dishes', 'snacks', 'soup', 'sweet spreads', 'juice drinks', 'other beverages', 'RTDs', 'sports & energy drinks', 'sauces & seasonings' (sub-categories: 'cooking sauces', 'other sauces & seasonings', 'pasta sauces', 'pickled condiments', 'table sauces')
Mintel GNPD categories excluded	'Chocolate confectionary', 'sugar & gum confectionary', 'sweeteners & sugar', 'alcoholic beverages', 'carbonated soft drinks', 'hot beverages', 'water', 'pet food', 'sauces & seasonings' (sub-categories: 'dressings & vinegar', 'mayonnaise', 'oils', 'seasonings', stocks')

Statistical analysis

All analyses were conducted using SPSS 23 (SPSS Inc., Chicago, SPSS for Windows, version 23). Frequency tests were conducted to determine the number of products within each category, and median values with interquartile ranges were calculated to determine the average proportion of vegetable and legume ingredients, and number of vegetable and legumes serves in each product.

Ethics

This study was exempt from ethics approval as the analysis was conducted on food products and did not directly use human or animal data.

Results

Between May 2012 and May 2017, 1313 products were released in Australia which contained greater than 0.5 serves of vegetables or legumes per standard serve. This constituted 6% of the total food and beverage launches in the period (*n* = 21,111). The majority of these products contained vegetables only (*n* = 1013; 77%), while a smaller proportion of products contained legumes only (*n* = 108; 8%) or both vegetables and legumes (*n* = 192; 15%).

Proportion of vegetable and legume ingredients

The proportion of vegetable and legume ingredients in each product varied between 11 and 100%, with a median of 55% (IQR = 45%). Fifty-eight percent of products contained over 50% vegetable and legume ingredients (*n* = 764), and 24% contained greater than 80% vegetable and legume ingredients (*n* = 319).

Number of vegetable and legume serves

New product launches containing vegetable and legume ingredients had a median of 1 (IQR = 1) serve of vegetables and legumes per recommended serving size of the product (Fig. 1). Forty-nine percent (*n* = 915) of products provided between 0.5 and 1 serve of vegetables and legumes per recommended serve of the product, while only 14% (*n* = 178) contained 2 or more serves per recommended serve. One product, a tomato and capsicum soup, provided approximately 5 serves of vegetables per 430-g serve.

Type of food or beverage product

New product launches containing vegetable and legume ingredients were most likely to be from the 'meals and meal centers' category (*n* = 362; 28%), which included ready-to-eat prepacked meals such as curries or lasagnes (Table 3). Other common launch categories containing vegetable and legume ingredients included 'fruit and vegetables' (*n* = 259; 20%), 'soup' (*n* = 238; 18%) and 'side dishes' (*n* = 124; 9%). 'Sauces and seasonings' in large serving sizes, such as pasta sauces, cooking sauces or pickled condiments, made up 11% of the launches (*n* = 138).

Table 3 shows that the highest proportion of products was in the sub-categories 'prepared meals' (*n* = 265; 20%) and 'vegetables' (*n* = 258; 20%). In some food sub-categories, there were only several new launches during the study period, however they were examples of more innovative uses of vegetable and legume ingredients. These included 'spoonable yoghurts' (yoghurt flavoured with sweet potato or pumpkin), 'water-based ice lollies' (frozen apple, carrot and beetroot juice), 'stuffing, polenta and other side dishes' (roasted, ready-to-eat, blended vegetable and legume 'delights'), 'pasta' (pastas made with legume flour) and 'meal replacements and other drinks' (smoothie bases containing broccoli, beetroot and spinach). There were several examples of more convenient products containing vegetables and legumes, including zucchini 'pasta,' pre-cut vegetables, and microwavable rice products.

Additionally, there were some innovations in the 'bean-based snacks' sub-category, in the form of chips made from beans and rice, snacks made from roasted chickpeas, and muesli bars with popped chickpeas. Similarly, creative innovations in the 'vegetable snacks' sub category included crackers made from crushed zucchini. These snacks were not included in the final analysis due to their small serving size, however are worth noting for some potential future uses of vegetables and legumes, if there is some consideration to nutritional value and level of processing.

Nutritional quality and level of processing

Table 4 shows that the highest proportion of products was classified as 'amber' (46%). This included products such as soups, salads, vegetable juices, canned fish with tomato, frozen roasted vegetables (if baked rather than fried) and some ready-to-eat meals such as pastas and risottos. This was followed by 'green' options (the healthiest choices), which made up 28% of the products and included products such as canned baked beans, salads, fresh or frozen mixed vegetables, and several ready-to-eat meals composed primarily of vegetables and lean meat Approximately a quarter of product launches were classified as 'red' (*n* = 339), such as potato crisps, pizzas, some ready-to-eat meals, and soups made with cream and large quantities of salt. The majority of product launches were classified as either 'processed' (45%) or 'ultra-processed' (40%), with only 15% as 'unprocessed or minimally processed'. No products were classified as 'processed culinary ingredients'.

Discussion

Products containing at least 0.5 serves of vegetable and legume ingredients per recommended serving represented

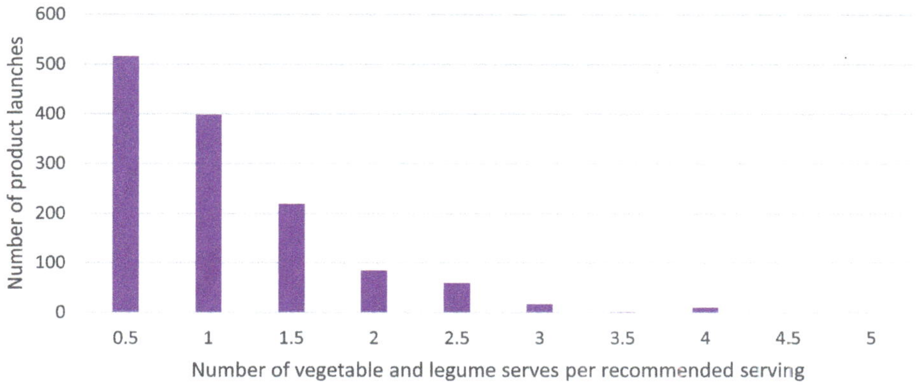

Fig. 1 Number of new product launches by number of vegetable and legume serves

6% of new product launches between May 2012 and May 2017. On average, these products contained approximately 55% vegetable or legume ingredients, however this translated to only 1 serve of vegetable and legumes per recommended serving size. The product launches were most likely to be 'meal and meal centers', or ready-to-eat meals, were an 'amber' choice, and were classified as either 'processed' or 'ultra-processed'.

There are many barriers to consumption of vegetables and legumes, which makes it a complex issue to tackle. Public health campaigns conducted both in Australia and internationally, such as the Western Australia "Go for 2 & 5" campaign, have aimed to increase awareness of the benefits of regular fruit and vegetable consumption and drive this change [29]. While these campaigns have been demonstrated to increase awareness and lead to modest increases in consumption in the short term, the majority have been unable to sustain increased vegetable consumption in the long term [29]. Given the complexity of the issue, a multi-faceted approach is most likely to be successful at driving increased vegetable and legume intake. In addition to improved education and public health campaigns to support the consumption of fresh produce, a food environment with a wide range of products containing vegetables and legumes could help to increase opportunities to meet the 5 serves per day recommendation. While fresh produce should be the main source of vegetables and legumes, processed or pre-packaged options can compliment this action by providing an additional opportunity for consumers to consume meaningful amounts of these healthier ingredients. The current evidence from this study indicates that with 1 serves of vegetables and legumes per serve, the new products currently being introduced onto the market are not yet supporting this.

Only 208 new products launched annually in Australia between 2012 and 2017 had legumes as a main ingredient. Less than 5% of the Australian population report consuming legumes or legume-based products, and the per capita consumption of legumes in Australia (2.9 kg per year) is well below the world average of 5 kg per year [30]. Legumes are unfamiliar to Australian consumers [11, 12, 30, 31], although some legumes, such as chickpeas, are becoming more common in products, such as hummus dip [30]. Food manufacturers in this market have the opportunity to improve consumer knowledge of legumes and how to use them, although this may be difficult if food manufacturers are also unfamiliar with legumes. The International 'Year of Pulses' campaign in 2016 aimed to address this lack of familiarity in all parts of the food supply, including consumers, manufacturers and growers [32]. The effects of this campaign have not yet been fully evaluated, and given that new product development and reformulation can be a lengthy process, it may be several years before more legume-based products appear on the market.

While this study indicates that vegetables and legumes are most commonly used in traditional ways, such as in pre-prepared meals ('meals and meal centers'), soups and sauces, they are beginning to be used in a wider range of foods. These include pastas made from legume flour, yoghurts with pureed sweet potato and zucchini 'pasta'. The incorporation of vegetables and legumes into commonly-eaten foods presents a new opportunity to introduce these ingredients to consumers, and could be included as complementary source of these ingredients to fresh vegetables and legumes. While a range of factors need to be taken into consideration, such as manufacturing methods, loss of key nutrients and chemical properties, healthier products such as pasta with up to one serve of vegetables and legumes per serve are possible [33, 34]. Whether consumers like these products, and consequently purchase and consume the product remains unknown, however it is promising that these types of products are beginning to become more widely available. Future research in this area could explore the acceptability and

Table 3 Number and proportion of product launches in each food category and sub-category

Food category	Food sub-category	# products	% total products	Mean # serves
Baby Food	Baby Fruit Products, Desserts & Yogurts	1	0%	1.5
	Baby Juices & Drinks	1	0%	0.5
	Baby Savoury Meals & Dishes	56	4%	0.9
	Other Baby Food	1	0%	0.5
	Total	59	4%	0.9
Bakery	Baking Ingredients & Mixes	3	0%	0.5
	Bread & Bread Products	1	0%	1.0
	Total	4	0%	0.6
Dairy	Spoonable Yogurt	1	0%	0.5
	Total	1	0%	0.5
Fruit & Vegetables	Fruit	1	0%	1.0
	Vegetables	258	20%	1.1
	Total	259	20%	1.1
Juice Drinks	Juice	53	4%	1.4
	Nectars	14	1%	1.3
	Total	67	5%	1.4
Meals & Meal Centers	Instant Noodles	3	0%	0.8
	Instant Pasta	5	0%	1.0
	Meal Kits	40	3%	1.0
	Pastry Dishes	15	1%	0.5
	Pizzas	5	0%	1.0
	Prepared Meals	265	20%	1.1
	Salads	22	2%	1.0
	Sandwiches/Wraps	7	1%	0.5
	Total	362	28%	1.0
Other Beverages	Meal Replacements & Other Drinks	4	0%	0.6
	Total	4	0%	0.6
Processed Fish, Meat & Egg Products	Fish Products	5	0%	0.5
	Meat Products	3	0%	0.5
	Meat Substitutes	14	1%	0.8
	Poultry Products	2	0%	0.8
	Total	24	2%	0.7
Sauces & Seasonings	Cooking Sauces	36	3%	0.7
	Pasta Sauces	95	7%	1.1
	Pickled Condiments	7	1%	0.6
	Total	138	11%	0.9
Savoury Spreads	Dips	7	1%	0.5
	Savoury Vegetable Pastes/Spreads	1	0%	0.5
	Total	8	1%	0.5
Side Dishes	Pasta	20	2%	0.8
	Potato Products	70	5%	1.1
	Rice	4	0%	0.5
	Stuffing, Polenta & Other Side Dishes	30	2%	0.7
	Total	124	9%	0.9

Table 3 Number and proportion of product launches in each food category and sub-category *(Continued)*

Food category	Food sub-category	# products	% total products	Mean # serves
Snacks	Bean-Based Snacks	1	0%	0.5
	Corn-Based Snacks	1	0%	0.5
	Hors d'oeuvres/Canapes	11	1%	0.7
	Potato Snacks	8	1%	0.5
	Vegetable Snacks	4	0%	0.5
	Total	25	2%	0.6
Soup	Dry Soup	40	3%	1.0
	Wet Soup	198	15%	1.5
	Total	238	18%	1.5
	Total	1313		1.1

consumption of these new products, as well as the viability from a food manufacturing perspective.

The nutritional value of products with healthier ingredients, such as vegetables and legumes, is important. While vegetables and legumes provide a range of health and nutritional benefits in a less processed form, these benefits could be counteracted by adding excessive amounts of oil, salt and sugar during packaging or processing. This study found that the highest proportion of new product launches containing vegetable and legume ingredients were classified as 'amber' options. While these products are not considered the healthiest option, they typically contain less sodium, energy and fat compared to 'red' options, and are recommended to be consumed only occasionally as part of a healthy diet. Conversely, only 28% of launches were for products classified as 'green' options, or the healthiest options, which should make up the majority of the diet. This nutrient-base profiling system is not completely indicative of the value of foods in the diet: for example, a 'red' soup with a large proportion of vegetables may be a better choice compared to an 'amber' soup with less sodium but also less vegetables. However, when considered in conjunction with the other product classification systems used in this study, it can help to identify the general healthiness of new product launches, particularly in relation to products high in sodium and saturated fat, or those with large serving size. These findings indicate that overall, more work needs to be done on developing more healthier 'green' choices containing vegetables and legumes, while continuing to reduce the less healthy 'red' and 'amber' options, as well as promoting fresh vegetables and legumes.

Table 4 Number and proportion of launches in each Healthy Choices or NOVA category

	Number of launches	Proportion of launches
Healthy Choices classification		
'Green'	373	28.4%
'Amber'	601	45.8%
'Red'	339	25.8%
TOTAL	1313	
NOVA food classification		
'Unprocessed or minimally processed'	196	14.9%
'Processed culinary ingredients'	0	0%
'Processed foods'	590	44.9%
'Ultra-processed food and drink products'	527	40.1%
TOTAL	1313	

The findings from this study show that the food market in Australia appears to be geared toward 'ultra-processed' foods, which may pose an issue to public health. 'Ultra-processed' products are industrial formulations with a large number of ingredients and additives designed to enhance hyper-palatability and mimic natural ingredients [27]. Previous literature has identified that 'ultra-processed' foods tend to be energy dense, nutritionally unbalanced and contain fewer beneficial nutrients such as protein and fibre [35, 36]. A focus on increasing the supply of minimally processed foods with legumes and vegetables, such as vegetable juice without additives, raw vegetables which have been peeled and chopped or vacuum-packed vegetables or legumes, is most likely to ensure the products are nutritionally beneficial and are more aligned with the Australian Dietary Guidelines. However, this may not always be possible from a manufacturing perspective. 'Processed foods' may provide a middle-ground, as these products are typically composed of a few core, minimally processed ingredients, with additives used to preserve the product or resist contamination only [27]. Where the use of oil, sugar and salt is minimized, healthier 'processed' products with a higher content of vegetables and legumes may help to address the previously discussed barriers to consumption, such as accessibility to fresh produce, and make these healthier ingredients more accessible to consumers.

Limitations

Some limitations to this study should be noted. The proportion of vegetable and legume ingredients was based on the ingredients list provided, however it is possible that these were not completely accurate, as it is the prerogative of each manufacturer to supply this information. Although, with truth in labelling laws [37], manufacturers must ensure that the ingredient list is accurate and up-to-date. The use of proportion of vegetable and legume ingredients was also limited as it did not always give a true reflection of how the product contributes to overall vegetable and legume consumption. Despite 58% of the products containing greater than 50% vegetable and legume ingredients, when consumed as recommended, the majority of the products contained 1 serve of vegetables and legumes. The estimated number of vegetable and legume serves used the recommended serving size listed on the product, however it is unknown whether consumers adhere to this recommended size and hence consume the calculated vegetable and legume serves. Some product may be lost to wastage, leading to less serves, or conversely, consumers may actually consume more than one recommended serve in an eating occasion. Overall, this study provides a good indication of the new products available on the market, but unless they are purchased by consumers and remain on the market long-term, these products are unlikely to have a significant impact on vegetable and legume intake. Future research could explore the real-world consumption of these products, and identify the key enablers and barriers to the long-term success of these products in the marketplace.

Conclusions

As a core part of a healthy diet, vegetables and legumes need to take more prominence in Australians' diets, as well as the food products they have access to. A multi-faceted approach is needed to improve vegetable and legume consumption, however food manufacturers have a role to play by continuing to innovate and providing a larger variety of healthier options which provide more vegetables and legumes per recommended serving.

Most of the new products currently released onto the Australian market which contain vegetable and legume ingredients do not provide meaningful amounts of these ingredients, and tend to be highly processed and unhealthier options. While consumption of minimally processed foods is preferable from a nutritional perspective, this may not be possible for all people, and therefore there is a place for healthier, processed options containing whole legumes and vegetables to address a range of consumer needs and potentially increase consumption of this poorly consumed food group. This study provides a baseline understanding of the use of vegetables and legumes in the Australian context, which can be used to identify and drive new areas for healthier product development.

Acknowledgements
Not applicable.

Funding
Not applicable.

Authors' contributions
BG led the project, conducted data collection, cleaning, classification and analysis, and was responsible for the write up of preliminary and final drafts. RH contributed to methodological design, critically reviewed manuscript drafts, and cross-checked data classification. JW conceived the concept for the paper, contributed to methodological design, critically reviewed manuscript drafts, and cross-checked data classification.

Competing interests
The authors declares that they have no competing interests.

References
1. Gakidou E, Afshin A, Abajobir AA, Abate KH, Abbafati C, Abbas KM, et al. Global, regional, and national comparative risk assessment of 84 behavioural, environmental and occupational, and metabolic risks or clusters of risks, 1990-2016: a systematic analysis for the global burden of disease study 2016. Lancet. 2017. https://doi.org/10.1016/S0140-6736(17)32366-8.
2. Wang X, Ouyang Y, Liu J, Zhu M, Zhao G, Bao W, et al. Fruit and vegetable consumption and mortality from all causes, cardiovascular disease, and cancer: systematic review and dose-response meta-analysis of prospective cohort studies. BMJ : British Medical Journal. 2014. https://doi.org/10.1136/bmj.g4490.
3. Hu D, Huang J, Wang Y, Zhang D, Qu Y. Fruits and vegetables consumption and risk of stroke: a meta-analysis of prospective cohort studies. Stroke. 2014. https://doi.org/10.1161/strokeaha.114.004836.
4. Rebello CJ, Greenway FL, Finley JW. A review of the nutritional value of legumes and their effects on obesity and its related co-morbidities. Obes Rev. 2014. https://doi.org/10.1111/obr.12144.
5. Australian Bureau of Statistics. Australian Health Survey: consumption of food groups from the Australian Dietary Guidelines 2011–12. Canberra: 2016.
6. Chapman K, Havill M, Watson WL, Wellard L, Hughes C, Bauman A, et al. Time to address continued poor vegetable intake in Australia for prevention of chronic disease. Appetite. 2016. https://doi.org/10.1016/j.appet.2016.08.003.
7. Thurber KA, Banwell C, Neeman T, Dobbins T, Pescud M, Lovett R, et al. Understanding barriers to fruit and vegetable intake in the Australian longitudinal study of indigenous children: a mixed-methods approach. Public Health Nutr. 2017. https://doi.org/10.1017/S1368980016003013.
8. Moayyed H, Kelly B, Feng X, Flood V. Is living near healthier food stores associated with better food intake in regional Australia? Int J environ res public health. 2017.
9. Rossimel A, Han SS, Larsen K, Palermo C. Access and affordability of nutritious food in metropolitan Melbourne. Nutr Diet. 2016. https://doi.org/10.1111/1747-0080.12142.
10. Palermo C, McCartan J, Kleve S, Sinha K, Shiell A. A longitudinal study of the cost of food in Victoria influenced by geography and nutritional quality. Aust N Z J Public Health. 2016. https://doi.org/10.1111/1753-6405.12506.

11. Lea E, Worsley A, Crawford D. Australian adult consumers beliefs about plant foods: a qualitative study. Health Educ Behav. 2005. https://doi.org/10.1177/1090198105277323.
12. Phillips T, Zello GA, Chilibeck PD, Vandenberg A. Perceived benefits and barriers surrounding lentil consumption in families with young children. Can J Diet Pract Res. 2015. https://doi.org/10.3148/cjdpr-2014-025.
13. Global Pulse Confederation. 2016 International Year of Pulses Dubai2016. Available from: http://iyp2016.org/.
14. Spencer S, Kneebone M. FOODmap: an analysis of the Australian food supply chain. Canberra: Department of Agriculture, Fisheries and Forestry; 2012.
15. Benson K, Fond E. FOOD CHATS: Australia's most comprehensive study integrating consumer attitudinal trends with consumption behaviour change. Ipsos Australia, 2015–16.
16. Baker P, Friel S. Food systems transformations, ultra-processed food markets and the nutrition transition in Asia. Glob Health. 2016. https://doi.org/10.1186/s12992-016-0223-3.
17. Poti JM, Mendez MA, Ng SW, Popkin BM. Is the degree of food processing and convenience linked with the nutritional quality of foods purchased by US households? Am J Clin Nutr. 2015;10:3945.
18. Pulker CE, Scott JA, Pollard CM. Ultra-processed family foods in Australia: nutrition claims, health claims and marketing techniques. Public Health Nutr. 2017. https://doi.org/10.1017/S1368980017001148.
19. Spiteri SA, Olstad DL, Woods JL. Nutritional quality of new food products released into the Australian retail food market in 2015 – is the food industry part of the solution? BMC Public Health. 2018. https://doi.org/10.1186/s12889-018-5127-0.
20. GNPD - Global New Products Database: Mintel Group Ltd; 2017 [7/5/2017]. Available from: http://www.mintel.com/global-new-products-database.
21. GNPD help: frequently asked questions: Mintel Group; 2017 [9/8/2017]. Available from: http://www.gnpd.com/sinatra/gnpd/help/all_5.
22. Definition and classification of commodities: 7. Vegetables and derived products Rome: Food and Agricultural Organization of the United Nations; 1994 [2/8/17]. Available from: http://www.fao.org/waicent/faoinfo/economic/faodef/fdef07e.htm.
23. National Health and Medical Research Council. Australian Dietary Guidelines. Canberra: 2013.
24. NUTTAB 2010 Online Searchable Database: flour, cornflour, from maize & wheat starch: Food Standards Australia New Zealand; 2018 [3/08/2018]. Available from: http://www.foodstandards.gov.au/science/monitoringnutrients/nutrientables/nuttab/pages/default.aspx.
25. Codex Alimentarius: Cereals, pulses, legumes and vegetable proteins. Rome: World Health Organization & Food and Agricultural Organization of the United Nations, 2007.
26. Department of Health & Human Services. Healthy choices: food and drink classification guide. Melbourne: Victorian Government; 2016.
27. Monteiro C, Cannon G, Levy R, Moubarac J-C, Jaime P, Martins A, et al. NOVA. The star shines bright. [Food classification. Public health]. World Nutrition. January–March 2016.
28. Dunford EK, Wu JHY, Wellard-Cole L, Watson W, Crino M, Petersen K, et al. A comparison of the Health Star Rating system when used for restaurant fast foods and packaged foods. Appetite. 2017; https://doi.org/10.1016/j.appet.2017.06.005.
29. Rekhy R, McConchie R. Promoting consumption of fruit and vegetables for better health. Have campaigns delivered on the goals? Appetite. 2014; https://doi.org/10.1016/j.appet.2014.04.012.
30. Euromonitor International. Pulses in Australia. Retrived from Euromonitor Passport database. March 2017.
31. Karlsen MC, Ellmore GS, McKeown N. Seeds - health benefits, barriers to incorporation and strategies for practitioners in supporting consumption among consumers. Nutr Today. 2016.
32. Food and Agricultural Organization of the United Nations. About the International Year of Pulses Rome, Italy 2016 [20/6/2017]. Available from: http://www.fao.org/pulses-2016/about/en/.
33. Oliviero T, Fogliano V. Food design strategies to increase vegetable intake: the case of vegetable enriched pasta. Trends Food Sci Technol. 2016. https://doi.org/10.1016/j.tifs.2016.03.008.
34. Foschia M, Horstmann SW, Arendt EK, Zannini E. Legumes as functional ingredients in gluten-free bakery and pasta products. Annu Rev Food Sci Technol. 2017.
35. Martínez Steele E, Popkin BM, Swinburn B, Monteiro CA. The share of ultra-processed foods and the overall nutritional quality of diets in the US: evidence from a nationally representative cross-sectional study. Popul Health Metr. 2017. https://doi.org/10.1186/s12963-017-0119-3.
36. Ultra-processed food and drink products in Latin America: trends, impact on obesity, policy implications. Washington, DC: PAHO, 2015.
37. Food and beverage industry: food descriptors guideline to the Trade Practices Act. Australian Competition & Consumer Commission, November 2006.

Efficacy of a long-term home parenteral nutrition regimen containing fish oil-derived n-3 polyunsaturated fatty acids: a single-centre, randomized, double blind study

Helene Bohnert[1†], Max Maurer[1†], Philip C. Calder[2,3], Johann Pratschke[1], Paul Thul[1^] and Verena Müller[1*]

Abstract

Background: Data on the use of lipid emulsions containing fish-oil (FO) derived n-3 polyunsaturated fatty acids (n-3 PUFAs) in addition to medium- and long-chain triglycerides (MCT/LCT) for long-term home parenteral nutrition (HPN) are limited. This study aimed to compare HPN regimens containing either MCT/LCT/FO-derived n-3 PUFAs (test group) or MCT/LCT (control group) with respect to efficacy and safety during 8 weeks of HPN using a non-inferiority trial design with change of body mass index (BMI) as primary endpoint.

Methods: This prospective, randomized, double-blind study was conducted at the Charité, Berlin, Germany, from 02/2008 until 01/2014. Adult patients ($n = 42$; aged 18 to 80 years) requiring HPN for at least 8 weeks were randomly assigned to the test or control group. Assessments included weight, height, physical examination (cardiovascular system, abdomen, respiratory tract, liver, spleen, kidney, urine tract, skin, mucous membrane, neurology, psyche, musculoskeletal system, lymph nodes), bio impedance analysis, calorimetry, blood samplings (haematology, biochemistry, fatty acid analysis) and quality of life questionnaire.

Results: BMI increased in both groups with 8 weeks of HPN ($\Delta BMI_{(test\ group)} = 1.3 \pm 1.1$ kg/m^2; $\Delta BMI_{(control\ group)} = 0.6 \pm 0.9$ kg/m^2) demonstrating non-inferiority of the test regimen regarding nutritional efficacy. Assessment of secondary efficacy endpoints revealed that after 8 weeks of HPN with the test regimen, the proportion of n-3 PUFAs in serum, platelet and red blood cell phospholipids significantly increased, while the proportion of n-6 PUFAs decreased. The fatty acid pattern in the control group remained mostly stable. No statistically significant differences were detected between groups regarding inflammatory markers or quality of life. Laboratory parameters reflecting the safety endpoints liver function, bone metabolism, renal function, metabolic activity, lipid metabolism, coagulation and haematology were stable in both groups and no group differences were detected regarding (serious) adverse events.

Conclusions: The HPN regimen prepared with MCT/LCT/FO-derived n-3 PUFAs was at least as efficient in maintaining or even improving nutritional status during HPN as the control MCT/LCT regimen. Administration of FO-derived n-3 PUFAs for 8 weeks altered the fatty acid pattern of serum, platelet and red blood cell phospholipids. Both regimens were safe and well tolerated.

(Continued on next page)

* Correspondence: verena.mueller@charite.de
[†]Helene Bohnert and Max Maurer contributed equally to this work.
[^]Deceased
[1]Charité-Universitätsmedizin Berlin, Department of Surgery, Campus Charité Mitte | Campus Virchow-Klinikum, Chariteplatz 1, 10117 Berlin, Germany
Full list of author information is available at the end of the article

(Continued from previous page)

Keywords: Home parenteral nutrition, Lipid emulsion, N-3 polyunsaturated fatty acids, Fish o l

Introduction

Home parenteral nutrition (HPN) was first introduced in the early 1970s and is nowadays an established therapy in the home care setting in western countries, as morbidity and mortality associated with HPN are low [1]. HPN aims to provide adequate amounts of amino acids, glucose, lipids, electrolytes and water in order to prevent malnutrition in patients requiring long-term parenteral nutrition (PN) due to prolonged gastro-intestinal tract failure [1, 2]. As prolonged malnutrition leads to weight loss, reduction of quality of life, increase in morbidity and mortality, and is associated with poor clinical outcome due to slow wound healing or impaired immune response [3–5], HPN intends to improve the patient's clinical prognosis and quality of life.

During the last decade it has been recognized that lipid emulsions administered as part of the PN regimen not only function as a source of energy: lipid emulsions provide physiologically active polyunsaturated fatty acids (PUFAs), namely n-6 PUFAs and n-3 PUFAs. These PUFAs are incorporated into phospholipids of serum and cellular membranes and are metabolized into bioactive mediators [6]. Mediators derived from the n-6 PUFA arachidonic acid (2-series prostaglandins and thromboxanes, 4-series leukotrienes) generally exert pro-inflammatory effects, while n-3 PUFAs are converted into far less inflammatory mediators (3-series prostaglandins and thromboxanes, 5-series leukotrienes) and even to mediators that are anti-inflammatory and inflammation resolving (e.g. resolvins, protectins, maresins) (reviewed in [6–8]). Depending on their content of n-6 PUFAs and n-3 PUFAs, lipid emulsions can thus exert influence on inflammatory and immune functions [9, 10].

Several lipid emulsions are available that differ in terms of lipid composition [11]. Lipid emulsions derived from soya-bean oil deliver long-chain triglycerides (LCT) and are rich in n-6 PUFAs (mainly linoleic acid, the precursor of arachidonic acid). Those based on soya-bean and coconut oil deliver medium- and long-chain triglycerides (MCT/LCT) and have a reduced content of n-6 PUFAs compared with soya-bean oil. Lipid emulsions based on soya-bean oil, coconut oil and oil from cold-water fish (i.e. fish oil; FO) deliver a mixture of MCT, LCT and FO-derived n-3 PUFAs and have a reduced content of n-6 PUFAs while being rich in n-3 PUFAs.

The safety of parenteral administration of FO containing lipid emulsions has been established in several clinical trials and beneficial effects of FO supplementation including modulation of inflammatory markers, reduced length of hospital stay as well as reduced infectious morbidity have been shown for surgical patients [12–19], as reviewed in [20]. Concerns have been raised regarding an increased risk of bleeding due to the administration of n-3 PUFAs, based on early observations in the Greenland Inuit population which indicated a longer bleeding time associated with high consumption of fish [21]. However, clinical trials found no evidence for an increased risk of bleeding upon n-3 PUFA administration [22, 23].

Data on efficacy and safety of FO containing regimens during long-term PN in the home-care setting are limited [1]. Indeed, a recent systematic review [24] identified only one randomised controlled trial of FO-containing HPN in adult patients which indicated that long-term administration of n-3 PUFAs in the setting of HPN was safe for a period of four weeks and led to an increased n-3/n-6 PUFA ratio in plasma and red blood cells [25].

The current clinical trial extended the study duration and for the first time a period of eight weeks of HPN with n-3 PUFAs was assessed. The trial was designed to show non-inferiority of an HPN regimen prepared with a MCT/LCT/FO-derived n-3 PUFA containing lipid emulsion as compared to a conventional HPN regimen without FO-derived n-3 PUFAs with respect to nutritional efficacy (primary endpoint: change of body mass index (BMI) after 8 weeks of HPN). Secondary endpoints of this clinical trial covered safety parameters and assessed potential beneficial effects of such a regimen on quality of life and body composition as compared to a conventional HPN regimen. The aim of this study was to provide evidence that an eight week treatment with HPN containing FO-derived n-3 PUFAs is as efficient and safe as HPN without n-3 PUFAs.

Materials and methods

Study design

This was a prospective randomized, double-blind, single centre Phase-IV-study with two parallel groups. It was conducted at the Department of Surgery at the Charité, Berlin, Germany, from February 2008 until January 2014 in accordance with the principles of the Declaration of Helsinki and requirements of Good Clinical Practice. The conduct of the study was approved by the German Federal Institute for Drug and Medical Devices (BfArM) and approval was provided by the Ethic Committee of Berlin (LAGeSo). Informed consent was obtained from all participating patients prior to any study procedure.

This study was sponsored by B. Braun Melsungen AG, Germany. A populated CONSORT checklist is provided as Additional file 1.

Patient population

Male and female patients aged between 18 and 80 years in need of long-term HPN for at least 8 weeks recruited from the ambulatory nutritional service at the Department of Surgery at the Charité, Berlin, Germany, were considered for study participation. Eligible patients had insufficient absorption capacity not compensable by enteral nutrition (EN), and were mentally and physically capable of adhering to study procedures. Patients with contraindications for parenteral nutrition and infusion therapy were excluded from study participation as well as patients suffering from (severe) sepsis, septic shock, autoimmune disease, hemodynamic failure of any origin, alterations of coagulation, ketoacidosis within 7 days prior to enrolment, renal insufficiency, severe liver dysfunction, lipid disorders, or necrotizing pancreatitis. Further reasons for exclusion were hypersensitivity to egg-, soya-, and fish proteins or any of the ingredients of the test or reference investigational products, pregnancy and lactation, known or suspected drug abuse and participation in another clinical trial.

Nutritional regimen

HPN regimens were either prepared using the test lipid emulsion (MCT/LCT/FO-derived n-3 PUFAs; Lipidem® 20%) or the reference lipid emulsion (MCT/LCT; Lipofundin® MCT 20%). Test and reference lipid emulsions only differed in terms of lipid composition: the test lipid emulsion contained MCT, LCT and FO-derived n-3 PUFAs in a ratio of 5:4:1, while the reference lipid emulation contained MCT and LCT in a 1:1 ratio. The test lipid emulsion contains 3.69 ± 0.14 wt% and 2.53 ± 0.14 wt% of the n-3 PUFAs eicosapentaenoic acid and docosahexaenoic acid. [26]. For regimen preparation, test or reference lipid emulsion (bottles of 500 mL, composition see Table 1) as well as vitamins and trace elements (according to individual needs) were added to a NuTRIflex® plus 2-chamber bag (1500 ml, 1190 kcal, containing amino acids and glucose) via a transfer set. In line with the routine of the investigator, i.e. the treating physician, 44.5% of caloric intake was provided in the form of lipids. HPN-patients were trained in preparing the all-in-one admixture and administered the PN regimen as a continuous infusion overnight via a central venous catheter. Depending on individual caloric requirements (calculated based on the results of indirect calorimetry performed during the baseline visit (BL) or based on estimated needs of about 25 to 35 kcal/kg/day), PN treatment was administered on 4 to 6 nights per week in order to cover at least 70% of caloric needs. Both PN regimens contained sufficient soya-bean oil to cover essential fatty acid requirements [1]. Patients were randomly assigned to either the test group (receiving MCT/LCT/FO-derived n-3 PUFAs) or to the control group (receiving MCT/LCT) in a 1:1 ratio according to a randomisation list (chronological enrolment number corresponding to a random number) prepared by an independent statistician prior study start using a permuted block design with varying block size of 2, 4 and 6. Test and reference lipid emulsions were labelled at the manufacturing site. To assure blinding of study participants, investigators and staff involved in this study, labels displayed only the patient's random number and the content as '20% lipid emulsion'. After a blind data review meeting and subsequent data base lock, data was unblinded for statistical analysis.

Table 1 Composition of test and reference lipid emulsion (per 500 mL)

Substance	Test lipid emulsion (Lipidem® 20%)	Reference lipid emulsion (Lipofundin® MCT 20%)
MCT	50.0 g	50.0 g
LCT (soybean oil)	40.0 g	50.0 g
Fractionated FO	10.0 g	0.0 g
Egg yolk phospholipids	6.0 g	6.0 g
Glycerol	12.5 g	12.5 g
Essential fatty acids		
• Linoleic acid (n-6)	19.2–23.2 g	24.0–29.0 g
• α-Linolenic acid (n-3)	2.0–4.4 g	2.5–5.5 g
• Eicosapentaenoic acid +Docosahexaenoic acid (n-3)	4.3–8.6 g	0.0 g
Energy content	3995 kJ (955 kcal)	3995 kJ (955 kcal)
Osmolality	~ 410 mOsm/l	~ 380 mOsm/l
Titration acidity/–alkalinity (pH 7.4)	< 0.5 mmol/l	< 0.5 mmol/l
pH-value	6.5–8.5	6.5–8.5

Investigations

Study related investigations were performed during a baseline visit (Day 1, BL), 4 weeks ±5 days (V1) and 8 weeks ±5 days (V2) after study start. BMI, used to calculate the primary endpoint ΔBMI, was determined at BL, V1 and V2 based on patient's weight (weighing in underwear with the same scale at all time points) and patient's height (measured according to clinical routine) using the formula: BMI = (weight [kg])/(height [m])^2. In addition, the following secondary efficacy endpoints were determined at BL, V1 and V2: bio impedance analysis (BIA, equipment: Data Input GmbH), fatty acid pattern in erythrocytes, platelets and serum phospholipids, markers for inflammatory state (IL-6, IL-10, TNF-alpha, CRP), and quality of life questionnaire (EORTC QLQ-C-30, Version 3.0; scores calculated according to EORTC scoring guidelines). For organizational reasons (no successor found for the person in charge of blood sample processing on the ward), fatty acid pattern was assessed for a subset of patients only.

Routine laboratory parameters were determined at BL, V1 and V2 to assess the following safety endpoints: liver function (Alanine Transaminase, Aspartate Transaminase, γ-Glutamyl-Transferase, Alkaline Phosphatase and Bilirubin), bone metabolism (Ostase), renal function (Creatinine and Urea), metabolic activity (Albumin, Lactate, Glucose, pH, Sodium, Potassium, Calcium, Magnesium and Chloride), lipid metabolism (Triglycerides, Total cholesterol, HDL cholesterol, LDL cholesterol, Vitamin E), coagulation (activated Partial Thromboplastin Time, Prothrombin Time, platelet count) and haematology (Leukocyte count, Erythrocyte count, Haematocrit, Haemoglobin, Transferrin). Blood samples were collected and processed according to routine procedures at the Charité laboratory. (Serious) adverse events ((S)AEs) were recorded continuously throughout the study.

Furthermore, physical examination of cardiovascular system, abdomen, respiratory tract, liver and spleen, kidney and urine tract, skin and mucous membrane, neurology and psyche, musculoskeletal system and lymph nodes was performed, and vital signs were assessed.

All investigations except fatty acid pattern were part of the routine assessment at the trial site. Fatty acid patterns were determined at the Faculty of Medicine, University of Southampton, according to established methods of fatty acid extraction, fatty acid methyl ester (FAME) formation and FAME separation using gas chromatography (for details see [27, 28]). FAME were detected by flame ionization detection and identified by comparison with run times of authentic standards. Peak areas and the percentage contribution of each peak to the total were calculated.

Statistics

This study was designed to show non-inferiority of the test lipid emulsion regarding the primary endpoint 'difference of BMI between V2 and BL' (ΔBMI). The non-inferiority margin for the treatment difference $\Delta BMI_{test} - \Delta BMI_{control}$ was defined as – 1.1 kg/m^2 based on the following assumptions:

- For patients considered for study participation, cachexia is one of the most life threatening risks and maintenance of BMI ($\Delta BMI_{test} = 0$) is a clinical success.
- Based on routinely generated data in everyday practice at the study site, BMI increase over 8 weeks HPN support in adults was expected to be 1.1 kg/m^2 (i.e. $\Delta BMI_{control} = 1.1$ kg/m^2).

Sample size was initially calculated based on routinely generated data in everyday practice at the study site indicating an average BMI increase over 8 weeks of 1.1 kg/m^2 with a standard deviation σ of 1.57 kg/m^2 (significance level $\alpha = 0.025$, power $1-\beta = 0.80$). Considering a drop out rate of 10%, sample size was determined to be 74, i.e. 37 patients per group. In the course of this study, the standard deviation of BMI increase was adjusted to $\sigma = 1.07$ kg/m^2 based on the evaluation of data originating from the pilot phase [29], and sample size calculation was amended accordingly resulting in 32 completely evaluable subjects. Considering a drop out rate of 30% as experienced in the pilot phase, sample size was determined to be 42, i.e. 21 patients per group. As the Per Protocol population (PP) is the more conservative patient population in non-inferiority trials, the primary endpoint, ΔBMI, was assessed by PP (i.e. all eligible patients without major protocol violations) with a one-sided 97.5% confidence interval (CI) using a parametric one-sided t-test. Non-inferiority was postulated if the lower bound of this confidence interval was above – 1.1 kg/m^2. In addition, analysis of the primary endpoint in the Full-analysis-set (FAS), comprising all patients who got the treatment at least once and a statement regarding the primary endpoint is possible, was planned. In this study, PP and FAS comprised the same patients and PP and FAS were therefore identical.

Demographic and anamnestic parameters were analysed in the Intent-to-treat population (ITT, all patients who received study medication at least once) and in the PP population. Statistical analyses of secondary efficacy parameters were performed by PP and FAS. Safety parameters were assessed in the ITT population only. Depending on the type of variable, Mann-Whitney or Kruskal-Wallis test (ordered categorical counts, non-paired data), Wilcoxon or Friedman test (ordered categorical counts, paired data), exact Fisher test (dichotomous variables), Pearson chi-square test (categorical character with more than two categories), or McNemar test (paired categorical data) were used. Data are presented as mean ± standard deviation (SD). Means were compared via the 2-sample t-test or analysis of variance (ANOVA) as appropriate and the significance level was defined as 5%.

Results

Study population

A total of 43 adult patients requiring HPN for at least 8 weeks, recruited from the ambulatory nutritional service at the University Hospital of the Charité Berlin, were screened for study participation. 42 patients were eligible and randomly assigned to receive either the test lipid emulsion (MCT/LCT/FO-derived n-3 PUFAs as Lipidem®, test group) or the reference lipid emulsion (MCT/LCT as Lipofundin®, control group). A total of nine patients prematurely discontinued the study ($n = 6$ and $n = 3$ in test and control groups, respectively, see Fig. 1 for further details). ITT analyses comprised data of 42 patients ($n = 21$ in each treatment group) while PP analyses were based on data from 33 patients ($n = 15$ and $n = 18$ in the test and control group, respectively). FAS and PP were identical in this study.

Test and control group were homogenous for most demographic and anamnestic parameters; only the proportion of patients that experienced diseases within three months prior to study start was significantly higher in the control group (see Table 2). Most patients had concomitant diseases and required concomitant medication.

Extent of exposure, treatment compliance

During the course of this study, the mean amount of lipid emulsion taken was 36.4 ± 11.4 bottles in the test group and 41.0 ± 10.4 bottles in the control group. As mean study duration was 48.0 ± 16.6 days and 59.1 ± 14.6 days in test and control group, respectively, this corresponded to a daily lipid intake of approximately 76 g in the test and 70 g in the control group. Patients in the test group therefore received about 7.6 g fractionated FO per day.

Treatment compliance, defined as 'number of bottles of lipid emulsions used'/'number of bottles of lipid emulsions prescribed' was good and comparable between groups (90.9 and 94.8% in test and control groups, respectively).

Efficacy of nutritional treatment

BMI increased in both groups after 8 weeks of HPN ($\Delta BMI_{(test\ group)} = 1.3 \pm 1.1\ kg/m^2$ and $\Delta BMI_{(control\ group)} = 0.6 \pm 0.9\ kg/m^2$) and analysis of treatment

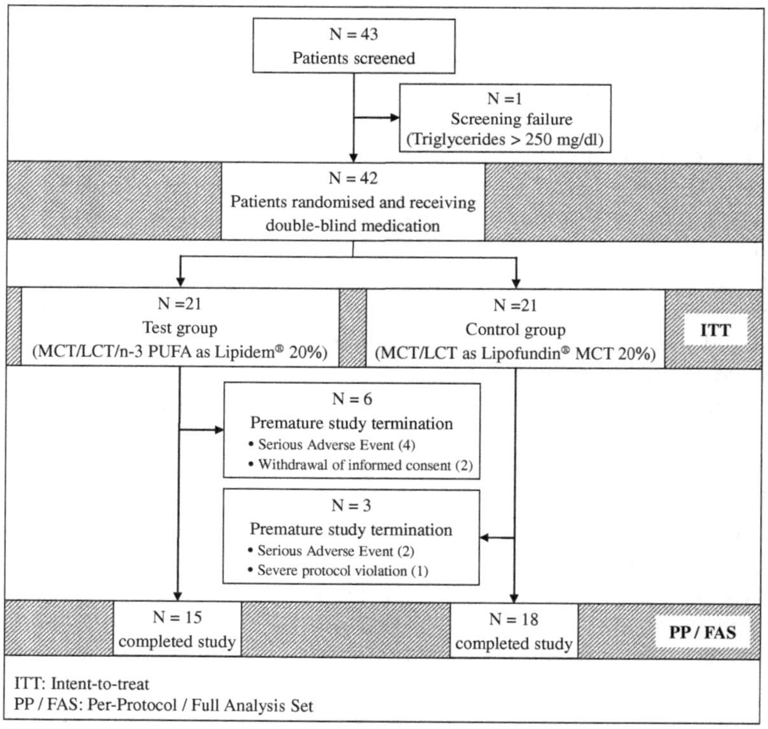

Fig. 1 Flowchart of study patients. Figure displays the number of patients screened, randomised and included for ITT and PP / FAS analyses. Nine patients of the ITT population were excluded from PP analysis because of premature study termination due to severe protocol deviation ($N = 1$), withdrawal of informed consent ($N = 2$) or serious adverse events (SAEs; $N = 6$). SAEs leading to premature study discontinuation were not investigational product related but required discontinuation of study medication due to necessary hospitalisation

Table 2 Baseline demographic and anamnestic parameters (ITT population)

Baseline Parameter	Test group (MCT/LCT/FO-derived n-3 PUFAs) $N = 21$	Control group (MCT/LCT) $N = 21$	*p*-value
Age (years, mean ± SD)	55.8 ± 15.1	58 ± 13.0	0.6160
Male / Female (%)	66.7 / 33.3	57.1 / 42.9	–
Weight (kg, mean ± SD)	62.7 ± 12.3	63.2 ± 10.1	0.9001
Height (cm, mean ± SD)	170.6 ± 9.9	174.1 ± 9.7	0.2523
BMI (kg/m^2, mean ± SD)	21.4 ± 2.6	20.8 ± 2.3	0.4041
Diseases within last 3 months before study start (%)	76.2	100	0.0478
Concomitant diseases at study start (%)	85.7	100	0.2317
Concomitant medication at study start (%)	100	95.2	1.000
Oncological disease (%)	52.4	61.9	0.7557
Chemotherapy during last year (%)	14.3	23.8	0.6965
Radiation therapy during last year (%)	0	9.5	0.4878
Other tumor therapy during last year (%)	19.0	14.3	1.000
Weight loss during the last three months (%)	42.9	47.6	1.000
Nicotine consumption (%)	38.1	33.3	1.000
Alcohol abuse (%)	4.8	0	1.000
Drug abuse (%)	0	0	NA
On diet (not specified) before study start (%)	0	4.8	1.000

difference (mean difference ΔBMI(test group) – ΔBMI(control group) = 0.63 kg/m^2) revealed that the lower margin of the 97.5% CI ([– 0.07; ∞]) exceeded the pre-defined inferiority level of – 1.1 kg/m^2, indicating non-inferiority of the test lipid emulsion with respect to nutritional efficacy. BMI changes were neither correlated to the lipid emulsion assigned nor to the amount of lipid emulsion administered as revealed by covariance analyses.

BMI changes over the 8 weeks of HPN were based on a gain of body weight in both study groups (+ 3.7 ± 3.1 kg and + 2.0 ± 2.9 kg in test and control groups, respectively) which was also reflected by a comparable increase of body cell mass (BCM) in the test and control groups as determined via BIA ($\Delta BCM_{(test\ group)}$ = 3.4 ± 5.3%, $\Delta BCM_{(control\ group)}$ = 3.2 ± 7.7%). Covariance analyses revealed that weight gain was not correlated to the lipid emulsion assigned, the amount of lipid emulsion administered, weight loss within three month prior study start, or chemotherapy during the year before study start.

BMI increase and weight gain were more pronounced during the first 4 weeks of HPN: while body weight and BMI increased by 4.2 ± 3.9% and 2.6 ± 2.9% in test and control groups, respectively, during the first 4 weeks of HPN, BMI and body weight increased by 1.5 ± 3.0% and 0.6 ± 4.2% in test and control groups, respectively, during the subsequent 4 weeks of HPN (see also Table 3). Weight gain during the first 4 weeks of HPN was correlated to the conduct of chemotherapy during the year before study start.

Influence of nutritional regimen on fatty acid pattern

Lipid composition of erythrocytes, platelets and serum phospholipids was significantly altered after 8 weeks of administration of the test lipid emulsion. In the test group, the proportion of n-3 PUFAs (i. e. Eicosapentaenoic acid (EPA), Docosahexaenoic acid (DHA) and Docosapentaenoic acid (DPA)) increased while the proportion of n-6 PUFAs (i.e. Linoleic Acid (LA), Arachidonic Acid (AA), Dihomo-ɣ-linolenic acid (DGLA) and ɣ-Linolenic acid (GLA)) decreased in erythrocytes, platelets and serum phospholipids. In the control group, the proportion of n-3 PUFAs and n-6 PUFAs remained mostly stable (see Table 4). Significant treatment differences were detected for EPA, DHA and DPA in erythrocytes, platelets and serum phospholipids. Significant treatment differences for n-6 PUFAs were found in erythrocytes (AA, DGLA and GLA), platelets (LA, DGLA and GLA) and serum phospholipids (LA, AA).

Influence of nutritional regimen on inflammatory parameters

IL-10 and TNF-α values were within the reference range at baseline and stayed stable during nutritional treatment. IL-6 and CRP levels exceeded the reference range in both study groups at baseline, probably reflecting the high incidence of co-morbidities. Mean values of IL-6 and CRP increased in the test group during 8 weeks of HPN while they decreased in the control group. However, IL-6 and CRP values in the test group showed a broad distribution especially after 8 weeks of HPN (IL-6: min-value: 3.30 ng/l, max-value: 32.5 ng/l; CRP: min-value: 0.12 ng/l, max-value:

Table 3 Changes of parameters for nutritional efficacy during HPN

Efficacy parameter	Test group (MCT/LCT/FO-derived n-3 PUFAs) $N = 15$	Control group (MCT/LCT) $N = 18$
BMI (kg/m^2)		
Baseline	21.9 ± 2.4	20.7 ± 2.4
V1 (4 weeks HPN)	22.8 ± 2.2	21.2 ± 2.5
V2 (8 weeks HPN)	23.2 ± 2.6	21.3 ± 2.4
Mean treatment difference (V2-BL) = 0.63 kg/m^2, CI 95%: [– 0.07; 1.32], $p = 0.0768$, t-test		
Body weight (kg)		
Baseline	63.1 ± 13.0	62.9 ± 10.7
V1 (4 weeks HPN)	65.6 ± 12.9	64.4 ± 10.8
V2 (8 weeks HPN)	66.7 ± 13.9	64.8 ± 11.0
Mean treatment difference (V2-BL) = 1.70 kg, CI 95%: [– 0.44; 3.84], $p = 0.1153$, t-test		
Body cell mass (kg)*		
Baseline	24.5 ± 6.3	22.9 ± 4.5
V1 (4 weeks HPN)	25.0 ± 6.0	23.7 ± 4.7
V2 (8 weeks HPN)	25.4 ± 6.7	24.4 ± 5.4
Mean treatment difference (V2-BL) = – 0.01 kg, CI 95%: [– 1.33; 1.32], $p = 0.9939$, t-test		

*Missing values (test group): N_{miss}(Baseline, V1) = 1; N_{miss}(V2) = 3 Missing values (control group): N_{miss}(Baseline) = 2; N_{miss}(V1, V2) = 1

6.90 mg/dl) which is reflected by the high standard deviation for mean IL-6 and CRP-values in the test group (see Table 5). This indicates single outliers with a high impact on mean values due to the small number of patients included for this investigation ($N = 11$ in each group). No statistically significant differences could be detected between groups regarding the profile of inflammatory markers after 8 weeks of HPN Mean values of inflammatory parameters are displayed in Table 5.

Influence of nutritional regimen on quality of life

Evaluation of the EORTC-QLQ-C30 questionnaire revealed that scores for global health status increased equally during treatment with the test and the control lipid emulsion (test group: 46.21 ± 12.56 (BL) vs 52.08 ± 20.14; control group: 36.27 ± 22.62 (BL) vs. 44.44 ± 24.73 (V2); score range: 0–100). Statistical analysis of score changes between BL and V2 revealed no significant treatment dependent differences.

Safety of nutritional treatment

No differences could be detected between groups regarding the profile of laboratory parameters determined to monitor liver function, bone metabolism, renal function, metabolic activity, lipid metabolism, coagulation and haematology. All parameters stayed stable throughout the nutritional treatment (for mean values ± SD and reference ranges see Additional file 2). Only two individual clinically relevant abnormalities were reported (low platelet count, already present at baseline, and CRP elevation, reported as AE, both in the test group).

The number and intensity of reported adverse events (AEs) were comparable for test and control group. A total of 11 patients in the test group and 12 patients in the control group experienced at least one treatment emergent AE. In total, 76 AEs were reported (34 and 42 AEs in test and control groups, respectively).

No differences were detected regarding the AE pattern between study groups. Most AEs were classified as "Gastrointestinal disorders" (i.e. diarrhea, nausea and vomiting, constipation), "Musculoskeletal and connective tissue disorders" (mainly muscle spasm), "Nervous system disorders" (headache and somnolence), "General disorders and administration site conditions" (i.e. fatigue, chills and medical device complication), "Infections and infestations" (i.e. device related sepsis), and "Skin and subcutaneous tissue disorders". None of the AEs was considered to be related to the nutritional regimen.

A total of four patients in each treatment group experienced at least one AE that was rated as serious. In total, 10 serious treatment emergent AEs were recorded. Although none of these serious adverse events (SAEs) was related to the investigational products, the treatment was prematurely terminated due to inability to continue IP administration during hospitalisation in six patients ($n = 4$ and $n = 2$ in test and control groups, respectively). No unexpected SAEs occurred. The most frequent SAE (device related sepsis) was expected as it represents a common complication of PN therapy. No patient died during the study.

Table 4 Changes from Baseline of n-6 and n-3 PUFAs in Erythrocytes, Platelets and Serum Phospholipids upon 8 weeks of HPN

	Test group (MCT/LCT/FO-derived n-3 PUFAs) *N* = 11*	Control group (MCT/LCT) *N* = 9*
n-6 PUFAs		
Linoleic Acid (LA)		
Erythrocytes (%)		
Baseline	10.1 ± 1.0	10.2 ± 1.5
V2 (8 weeks HPN)	9.3 ± 0.9	10.6 ± 1.4
Mean treatment difference (V2-BL) = – 1.14%, CI 95 [– 2.0; – 0.3], *p* = 0.0107, t-test		
Platelets (%)		
Baseline	22.1 ± 3.1	16.9 ± 4.0
V2 (8 weeks HPN)	21.8 ± 2.9	20.9 ± 4.4
Mean treatment difference (V2-BL) = – 5.0%, CI 95 [– 7.3; – 2.7], *p* = 0.0002, t-test		
Serum Phospholipids (%)		
Baseline	20.0 ± 2.3	20.0 ± 3.1
V2 (8 weeks HPN)	18.1 ± 1.8	20.9 ± 2.6
Mean treatment difference (V2-BL) = – 3.3%, CI 95 [– 4.6; – 2.1, *p* < 0.0001, t-test		
Arachidonic Acid (AA)		
Erythrocytes (%)		
Baseline	16.8 ± 2.0	16.8 ± 1.3
V2 (8 weeks HPN)	13.2 ± 1.9	17.0 ± 2.4
Mean treatment difference (V2-BL) = – 3.8%, CI 95 [– 5.9; – 1.8], *p* = 0.0011, t-test		
Platelets (%)		
Baseline	10.9 ± 3.8	12.9 ± 4.0
V2 (8 weeks HPN)	8.4 ± 1.6	11.3 ± 4.2
Mean treatment difference (V2-BL) = – 1.3%, CI 95 [– 3.8; 1.2], *p* = 0.2883, t-test		
Serum Phospholipids (%)		
Baseline	10.6 ± 1.5	9.7 ± 2.2
V2 (8 weeks HPN)	8.2 ± 1.4	9.6 ± 1.9
Mean treatment difference (V2-BL) = – 2.7%, CI 95 [– 4.0; – 1.4], *p* = 0.0005, t-test		
Dihomo-γ-linolenic acid (DGLA)		
Erythrocytes (%)		
Baseline	2.2 ± 0.4	2.4 ± 0.5
V2 (8 weeks HPN)	1.7 ± 0.3	2.4 ± 0.5
Mean treatment difference (V2-BL) = – 0.4%, CI 95 [– 0.6; – 0.1], *p* = 0.0044, t-test		
Platelets (%)		
Baseline	1.7 ± 0.4	1.9 ± 0.4
V2 (8 weeks HPN)	1.1 ± 0.4	1.8 ± 0.4
Mean treatment difference (V2-BL) = – 0.4%, CI 95 [– 0.8; – 0.01], *p* = 0.0471, t-test		
Serum Phospholipids (%)		
Baseline	3.1 ± 1.0	4.2 ± 1.2
V2 (8 weeks HPN)	2.1 ± 0.9	3.8 ± 1.3
Mean treatment difference (V2-BL) = – 0.5%, CI 95 [– 1.2; 0.1], *p* = 0.1156, t-test		
γ-Linolenic acid (GLA)		
Erythrocytes (%)		
Baseline	0.08 ± 0.03	0.09 ± 0.4
V2 (8 weeks HPN)	0.05 ± 0.02	0.10 ± 0.05

Table 4 Changes from Baseline of n-6 and n-3 PUFAs in Erythrocytes, Platelets and Serum Phospholipids upon 8 weeks of HPN *(Continued)*

	Test group (MCT/LCT/FO-derived n-3 PUFAs) $N = 11$*	Control group (MCT/LCT) $N = 9$*
Mean treatment difference (V2-BL) = − 0.05%, CI 95 [− 0.09; − 0.01], $p = 0.0118$, t-test		
Platelets (%)		
Baseline	0.5 ± 0.3	0.4 ± 0.1
V2 (8 weeks HPN)	0.3 ± 0.1	0.5 ± 0.2
Mean treatment difference (V2-BL) = − 0.3%, CI 95 [− 0.5; − 0.1], $p = 0.0049$, t-test		
Serum Phospholipids (%)		
Baseline	0.14 ± 0.08	0.16 ± 0.07
V2 (8 weeks HPN)	0.07 ± 0.04	0.13 ± 0.04
Mean treatment difference (V2-BL) = − 0.03%, CI 95 [− 0.09; 0.04], $p = 0.3647$, t-test		
n-3 PUFAs		
Eicosapentaenoic acid (EPA)		
Erythrocytes (%)		
Baseline	0.7 ± 0.2	0.7 ± 0.2
V2 (8 weeks HPN)	2.8 ± 0.9	0.7 ± 0.1
Mean treatment difference (V2-BL) = 2.1%, CI 95 [1.4; 2.8], $p < 0.0001$, t-test		
Platelets (%)		
Baseline	0.7 ± 0.2	0.6 ± 0.2
V2 (8 weeks HPN)	4.3 ± 2.0	0.6 ± 0.2
Mean treatment difference (V2-BL) = 3.4%, CI 95 [2.1; 4.8], $p < 0.0001$, t-test		
Serum Phospholipids (%)		
Baseline	1.1 ± 0.3	1.1 ± 0.4
V2 (8 weeks HPN)	4.6 ± 1.5	1.0 ± 0.3
Mean treatment difference (V2-BL) = 3.5%, CI 95 [2.5; 4.5], $p < 0.0001$, t-test		
Docosahexaenoic acid (DHA)		
Erythrocytes (%)		
Baseline	4.5 ± 1.3	4.1 ± 1.1
V2 (8 weeks HPN)	6.5 ± 1.1	4.0 ± 0.5
Mean treatment difference (V2-BL) = 2.2%, CI 95 [1.0; 3.3], $p = 0.0008$, t-test		
Platelets (%)		
Baseline	1.8 ± 0.4	1.4 ± 0.5
V2 (8 weeks HPN)	3.6 ± 0.7	1.5 ± 0.4
Mean treatment difference (V2-BL) = 1.8%, CI 95 [1.3; 2.3], $p < 0.0001$, t-test		
Serum Phospholipids (%)		
Baseline	3.1 ± 0.7	2.7 ± 1.0
V2 (8 weeks HPN)	5.8 ± 1.6	2.7 ± 0.6
Mean treatment difference (V2-BL) = 2.6%, CI 95 [1.6; 3.6], $p < 0.0001$, t-test		
Docosapentaenoic acid (DPA)		
Erythrocytes (%)		
Baseline	2.9 ± 0.5	2.9 ± 0.5
V2 (8 weeks HPN)	4.0 ± 0.5	3.0 ± 0.7
Mean treatment difference (V2-BL) = 0.8%, CI 95 [0.3; 1.4], $p = 0.0058$, t-test		
Platelets (%)		
Baseline	0.9 ± 0.2	1.1 ± 0.3

Table 4 Changes from Baseline of n-6 and n-3 PUFAs in Erythrocytes, Platelets and Serum Phospholipids upon 8 weeks of HPN *(Continued)*

	Test group (MCT/LCT/FO-derived n-3 PUFAs) $N = 11$*	Control group (MCT/LCT) $N = 9$*
V2 (8 weeks HPN)	1.4 ± 0.2	1.0 ± 0.4
Mean treatment difference (V2-BL) = 0.5%, CI 95 [0.3; 0.7], $p = 0.0003$, t-test		
Serum Phospholipids (%)		
Baseline	1.0 ± 0.2	1.0 ± 0.3
V2 (8 weeks HPN)	1.6 ± 0.4	1.0 ± 0.3
Mean treatment difference (V2-BL) = 0.4%, CI 95 [0.2; 0.6], $p = 0.0009$, t-test		

* Number of baseline values (test group): $N = 14$; Number of baseline values (control group): $N = 13$

Discussion

HPN aims to prevent malnutrition in patients who cannot cover their nutritional requirements via the oral or enteral route for a prolonged period of time. This clinical trial was performed to compare the nutritional efficacy of two different lipid emulsions when administered as part of HPN for a duration of 8 weeks. Test and control lipid emulsions only differed in terms of lipid composition: the test lipid emulsion provided a mixture of MCT, LCT and FO-derived n-3 PUFAs (EPA and DHA) in a ratio of 5:4:1, while the control lipid emulsion provided a mixture of MCT and LCT in a 1:1 ratio.

Nutritional efficacy was assessed via changes of BMI during 8 weeks of HPN. BMI increased in both study groups during HPN treatment with a trend to higher BMI increases in the test group. Statistical analysis revealed non-inferiority of the test lipid emulsion to the reference lipid emulsion indicating that replacement of 10% LCT by FO-derived n-3 PUFAs does not affect nutritional efficacy and that PN regimes containing EPA and DHA are at least as efficient in maintaining as well as improving the nutritional status during HPN as PN regimens without those n-3 PUFAs.

It is well known that PUFAs are incorporated into cellular membranes [6]. In order to assess incorporation of PUFAs upon long-term HPN of 8 weeks, the FA pattern of cell-membrane phospholipids in erythrocytes and platelets as well as serum phospholipids was assessed in this clinical trial. FA analysis revealed significant treatment differences between test and control group. Upon

Table 5 Inflammatory parameters before and after 8 weeks of HPN

Inflammatory parameter	Test group (MCT/LCT/n-3 PUFA) $N = 11$	Control group (MCT/LCT) $N = 11$
IL-6 (ng/L)		
(reference range < 5 ng/L)		
Baseline	5.473 ± 2.501	7.050 ± 5.432
V2 (8 weeks HPN)	9.145 ± 8.614	4.364 ± 2.448
Mean treatment difference (V2-BL) = 4.8 ng/L, CI 95 [− 0.5; 10.1], $p = 0.0745$, t-test		
IL-10 (ng/L)		
(reference range < 5 ng/L)		
Baseline	5.000 ± 0.000	5.033 ± 0.115
V2 (8 weeks HPN)	5.000 ± 0.000	5.027 ± 0.090
Mean treatment difference (V2-BL) = − 0.03 ng/L, CI 95 [− 0.09; 0.03], $p = 0.3062$, t-test		
TNF-alpha (ng/L)		
(reference range < 15 ng/L)		
Baseline	11.918 ± 6.506	13.175 ± 6.996
V2 (8 weeks HPN)	10.673 ± 4.382	10.645 ± 4.457
Mean treatment difference (V2-BL) = 0.9 ng/L, CI 95 [− 2.5; 4.3], $p = 0.5801$, t-test		
CRP (mg/dL)*		
(reference range < 0.50 mg/dL)		
Baseline	0.691 ± 0.595	0.977 ± 1.370
V2 (8 weeks HPN)	1.453 ± 1.903	0.745 ± 0.541
Mean treatment difference (V2-BL) = 0.6 mg/L, CI 95 [− 0.4; 1.6], $p = 0.2231$, t-test		

*Number of values (test group): N(Baseline) = 14; N(V2) = 15 Number of values (control group): N(Baseline) = 18; N(V2) = 18

administration of n-3 PUFA for a period of 8 weeks, the proportion of n-3 PUFAs (i. e. EPA, DHA and DPA) was increased while the proportion of n-6 PUFAs (AA, DGLA and GLA) was decreased in cell-membrane phospholipids in erythrocytes and platelets as well as in serum phospholipids. The FA pattern in the control group remained mostly stable. The effect of n-3 PUFAs administration during 8 weeks is thus in line with several other studies that investigated on the incorporation of PUFAs into serum and cell-membrane phospholipids after administration of lipid emulsions (reviewed in [30]).

The n-3/n-6 ratio of phospholipids in cell-membranes is thought to play an important role in the modulation of inflammation [10]. In response to an inflammatory stimulus AA (n-6 PUFA) and EPA (n-3 PUFA) are both released from cell membranes and are metabolized by the same enzymes into eicosanoids that modulate the intensity and duration of inflammatory responses [8]. An elevation of the n-3/n-6 ratio is thus thought to result in less intense inflammatory reactions and also reduced amounts of inflammatory cytokines that in turn might prevent the development of life-threatening hyper-inflammatory states. This assumption is supported by findings in gastrointestinal surgical patients that show beneficial modulation of eicosanoids and cytokines and reduced length of hospital stay after administration of FO as a source of bioactive n-3 PUFAs (reviewed in [20]). Beneficial effects of n-3 PUFA administration (reduction of infection rate, reduced length of intensive care unit (ICU) and hospital stay, increased release of less potent inflammatory mediators and reduction of inflammatory cytokines) have also been reported in a meta-analysis of a pooled population of surgical and medical ICU patients [31]. Nevertheless, the state of evidence is less clear in critically ill medical patients [11]. Meta-analyses of studies in critically ill patients (excluding studies with surgical intensive care patients) indicated that FO administration may reduce mortality and duration of ventilation [32] or reduce the incidence of infectious complications and length of hospital [33]. However, other studies did not reveal any beneficial effects of n-3 PUFA administration on cytokine levels or primary outcome parameters in this patient population [34, 35].

Although this clinical trial was not powered to address the influence of FO-derived n-3 PUFA administration on inflammatory parameters, serum cytokine levels were analysed for explorative purposes. IL-10 and TNF-α values were within the reference range at baseline and were not altered during 8 weeks of HPN. Most patients had elevated IL-6 and CRP values already at study start, likely reflecting the high incidence of concomitant diseases – nearly all patients that participated in this study suffered from concomitant diseases – and indicating an elevated inflammatory state in both groups at study start. There was a trend towards higher IL-6 and CRP levels in the group receiving n-3 PUFAs paralleled by a trend towards lower IL-6 and CRP levels in the control group. However, no statistically significant group differences were detected and time profiles determined for IL-6 and CRP levels have to be interpreted very carefully due to broad data distribution, reflecting individual abnormally high values, and small sample size. Results of this clinical trial therefore do not allow to reveal whether administration of n-3 PUFAs influence serum cytokine levels in HPN patients, and adequately powered studies are required to address this aspect.

Maintenance and improvement of nutritional status are especially important during HPN as malnutrition has been shown to decrease quality of life in patients with both benign and malignant diseases of the digestive system [36, 37]. Assessment of quality of life in this clinical trial revealed that scores for global health status and functional scales were increased after 8 weeks of HPN in both groups. This indicates increased quality of life and a better functioning in daily life that was most probably due to an improved nutritional status achieved via HPN therapy. This is in line with other studies showing an increase in quality of life due to HPN [38–40].

Coagulation parameters assessed in this study were similar between treatment groups, remained stable throughout 8 weeks HPN and were within the reference range. In addition, there were no adverse events indicative for an increased risk of bleeding. In line with other publications, data derived from this study therefore does not indicate an increased risk of bleeding upon administration of n-3 PUFAs [22, 23].

In this study, administration of both lipid emulsions was safe for a period of eight weeks. No treatment related AE (i.e. no adverse drug reaction) was reported and there was no difference in the occurrence of AEs or SAEs between the test and control groups. All safety laboratory parameters determined to monitor hepatic metabolism, haematology/coagulation, lipid metabolism, and bone metabolism remained stable during 8 weeks of HPN in both treatment groups. These findings are in line with other studies assessing safety of long-term administration of different lipid emulsions that revealed good clinical tolerance and safety of all lipid emulsions tested (reviewed in [30]).

One limitation of this study is that several study participants were on HPN therapy already at the study start. It was intended to include only patients with a new indication for HPN in this study. However, recruitment of patients was very difficult, as patients had to be able and willing to mix the HPN regimen at home. The inclusion criteria therefore had to be amended in order to also allow study participation of patients already receiving HPN. BMI changes detected during this study therefore most probably underestimate the beneficial effects of

HPN on BMI. Furthermore, it cannot be excluded that differences between treatment groups (e.g. BMI increase, inflammatory parameters) would have been more pronounced if only patients with a new indication for HPN had been included. A further limitation is, that data regarding prior dietary intake was not collected. The correlation between prior HPN and treatment differences could therefore not be analysed. However, these limitations do not affect the assessment of efficacy and safety of the MCT/LCT/FO-derived n-3 PUFAs containing lipid emulsion.

Conclusions

This study revealed that the lipid emulsion containing MCT/LCT/FO-derived n-3 PUFAs is at least as efficient in maintaining or improving the nutritional status of patients requiring long-term HPN as the lipid emulsion containing MCT/LCT only. Administration of FO-derived n-3 PUFAs for a period of 8 weeks markedly altered the fatty acid profile of serum and cell-membrane phospholipids resulting in an increased proportion of n-3 PUFAs and a decreased proportion of n-6 PUFAs. In this study, both lipid emulsions were safe and well tolerated during 8 weeks of HPN.

Abbreviations

(S)AE: (Serious) Adverse Event; BCM: Body Cell Mass; BIA: Bio Impedance Analysis; BL: Baseline Visit; BMI: Body Mass Index; CI: Confidence Interval; EN: Enteral Nutrition; FAS: Full Analysis Set; FO: Fish Oil; HPN: Home Parenteral Nutrition; ICU: Intensive Care Unit; ITT: Intent-to-Treat; LCT: Long-chain triglycerides; MCT: Medium-chain triglycerides; PN: Parenteral Nutrition; PP: Per Protocol; PUFA: Polyunsaturated Fatty Acids; SD: Standard Deviation; V1: Visit, 4 weeks after study start; V2: Visit, 8 weeks after study start

Acknowledgements

Not applicable.

Funding

This study was funded by B. Braun Melsungen AG, Carl-Braun Str. 1, D-42327 Melsungen, Germany. Investigational test and reference products were produced and delivered by B. Braun Melsungen AG. B. Braun Melsungen AG was involved in protocol development, clinical trial application, monitoring, data management and statistics, writing of the study report, and provided writing assistance for this manuscript. The University of Southampton received funding for the fatty acid composition analysis.

Authors' contributions

HB and VM took part in the analysis and interpretation of the data and the writing of the manuscript. MM and JP revised the Manuscript. PT performed the data collection and the conception and design of the study. PCC supervised laboratory measurement of fatty acids and revised the draft manuscript. HB, MM, PCC, JP and VM read and approved the manuscript.

Authors' information

Not applicable

Competing interests

PCC has received speaking honoraria from B. Braun. For conflict of interest see "funding sources". Otherwise the authors have no conflict of interest to declare.

Author details

[1]Charité-Universitätsmedizin Berlin Department of Surgery, Campus Charité Mitte | Campus Virchow-Klinikum, Charitéplatz 1, 10117 Berlin, Germany. [2]Human Development and Health, Faculty of Medicine, University of Southampton, Southampton, UK. [3]NIHR Southampton Biomedical Research Centre, University Hospital Southampton NHS Foundation Trust and University of Southampton, Southampton, UK.

References

1. Staun M, Pironi L, Bozzetti F, Baxter J, Forbes A, Joly F, et al. ESPEN guidelines on parenteral nutrition: home parenteral nutrition (HPN) in adult patients. Clin Nutr. 2009;28:467–79. https://doi.org/10.1016/j.clnu.2009.04.001.
2. Pironi L, Goulet O, Buchman A, Messing B, Gabe S, Candusso M, et al. Outcome on home parenteral nutrition for benign intestinal failure: a review of the literature and benchmarking with the European prospective survey of ESPEN. Clin Nutr. 2012;31:831–45. https://doi.org/10.1016/j.clnu.2012.05.004.
3. McNamara MJ, Alexander HR, Norton JA. Cytokines and their role in the pathophysiology of cancer cachexia. JPEN J Parenter Enteral Nutr. 1992;16: 50S–5S. https://doi.org/10.1177/014860719201600603.
4. Bozzetti F, Gavazzi C, Ferrari P, Dworzak F. Effect of total parenteral nutrition on the protein kinetics of patients with cancer cachexia. Tumori. 2000;86:408–11.
5. Lawson RM, Doshi MK, Barton JR, Cobden I. The effect of unselected post-operative nutritional supplementation on nutritional status and clinical outcome of orthopaedic patients. Clin Nutr. 2003;22:39–46.
6. Wanten GJA, Calder PC. Immune modulation by parenteral lipid emulsions. Am J Clin Nutr. 2007;85:1171–84
7. Stapleton RD, Martin JM, Mayer K. Fish oil in critical illness: mechanisms and clinical applications. Crit Care Clin. 2010;26:501–14, ix. https://doi.org/10.1016/j.ccc.2010.04.009.
8. Calder PC. Marine omega-3 fatty acids and inflammatory processes: effects, mechanisms and clinical relevance. Biochim Biophys Acta. 2015;1851:469–84. https://doi.org/10.1016/j.bbalip.2014.08.010.
9. Waitzberg DL, Torrinhas RS, Jacintho TM. New parenteral lipid emulsions for clinical use. JPEN J Parenter Enteral Nutr. 2006;30:351–67. https://doi.org/10.1177/0148607106030004351.
10. Miles EA, Calder PC. Fatty acids, lipid emulsions and the immune and inflammatory systems. World Rev Nutr Diet. 2015;112:17–30. https://doi.org/10.1159/000365426.
11. Calder PC, Adolph M, Deutz NE, Grau T, Innes JK, Klek S, et al. Lipids in the intensive care unit: recommendations from the ESPEN expert group. Clin Nutr. 2017. https://doi.org/10.1016/j.clnu.2017.08.032.
12. Wachtler P, Konig W, Senkal M, Kemen M, Koller M. Influence of a total parenteral nutrition enriched with omega-3 fatty acids on leukotriene synthesis of peripheral leukocytes and systemic cytokine levels in patients with major surgery. J Trauma. 1997;42:191–8.
13. Grimm H, Mertes N, Goeters C, Schlotzer E, Mayer K, Grimminger F, Furst P. Improved fatty acid and leukotriene pattern with a novel lipid emulsion in surgical patients. Eur J Nutr. 2006;45:55–60. https://doi.org/10.1007/s00394-005-0573-8.
14. Morlion BJ, Torwesten E, Lessire H, Sturm G, Peskar BM, Furst P, Puchstein C. The effect of parenteral fish oil on leukocyte membrane fatty acid composition and leukotriene-synthesizing capacity in patients with postoperative trauma. Metabolism. 1996;45:1208–13.
15. Koller M, Senkal M, Kemen M, Konig W, Zumtobel V, Muhr G. Impact of omega-3 fatty acid enriched TPN on leukotriene synthesis by leukocytes after major surgery. Clin Nutr. 2003;22:59–64.
16. Wichmann MW, Thul P, Czarnetzki H-D, Morlion BJ, Kemen M, Jauch K-W. Evaluation of clinical safety and beneficial effects of a fish oil containing lipid emulsion (Lipoplus, MLF541): data from a prospective, randomized, multicenter trial. Crit Care Med. 2007;35:700–6. https://doi.org/10.1097/01.CCM.0000257465.60287.AC.
17. Liang B, Wang S, Ye Y-J, Yang X-D, Wang Y-L, Qu J, et al. Impact of postoperative omega-3 fatty acid-supplemented parenteral nutrition on clinical outcomes and immunomodulations in colorectal cancer patients. World J Gastroenterol. 2008;14:2434–9.

18. Weiss G, Meyer F, Matthies B, Pross M, Koenig W, Lippert H. Immunomodulation by perioperative administration of n-3 fatty acids. Br J Nutr. 2002;87(Suppl 1):S89–94.
19. Jiang ZM, Wilmore DW, Wang XR, Wei JM, Zhang ZT, Gu ZY, et al. Randomized clinical trial of intravenous soybean oil alone versus soybean oil plus fish oil emulsion after gastrointestinal cancer surgery. Br J Surg. 2010;97:804–9. https://doi.org/10.1002/bjs.6999.
20. Calder PC. Lipids for intravenous nutrition in hospitalised adult patients: a multiple choice of options. Proc Nutr Soc. 2013;72:263–76. https://doi.org/10.1017/S0029665113001250.
21. Dyerberg J, Bang HO. Haemostatic function and platelet polyunsaturated fatty acids in Eskimos. Lancet. 1979;2:433–5.
22. Wachira JK, Larson MK, Harris WS. N-3 fatty acids affect haemostasis but do not increase the risk of bleeding: clinical observations and mechanistic insights. Br J Nutr. 2014;111:1652–62. https://doi.org/10.1017/S000711451300425X.
23. Jeansen S, Witkamp RF, Garthoff JA, van Helvoort A, Calder PC. Fish oil LC-PUFAs do not affect blood coagulation parameters and bleeding manifestations: analysis of 8 clinical studies with selected patient groups on omega-3-enriched medical nutrition. Clin Nutr. 2018;37:948–57. https://doi.org/10.1016/j.clnu.2017.03.027.
24. Jones CJ, Calder PC. Influence of different intravenous lipid emulsions on fatty acid status and laboratory and clinical outcomes in adult patients receiving home parenteral nutrition: a systematic review. Clin Nutr. 2016. https://doi.org/10.1016/j.clnu.2016.12.026.
25. Klek S, Chambrier C, Singer P, Rubin M, Bowling T, Staun M, et al. Four-week parenteral nutrition using a third generation lipid emulsion (SMOFlipid)--a double-blind, randomised, multicentre study in adults. Clin Nutr. 2013;32: 224–31. https://doi.org/10.1016/j.clnu.2012.06.011.
26. Driscoll DF, Ling P-R, Bistrian BR. Pharmacopeial compliance of fish oil-containing parenteral lipid emulsion mixtures: globule size distribution (GSD) and fatty acid analyses. Int J Pharm. 2009;379:125–30. https://doi.org/10.1016/j.ijpharm.2009.06.021.
27. Versleijen MW, Roelofs HM, Rombouts C, Hermans PW, Noakes PS, Calder PC, Wanten GJ. Short-term infusion of a fish oil-based lipid emulsion modulates fatty acid status, but not immune function or (anti)oxidant balance: a randomized cross-over study. Eur J Clin Investig. 2012;42:290–302. https://doi.org/10.1111/j.1365-2362.2011.02582.x.
28. Barros KV, Cassulino AP, Schalch L, Della Valle Munhoz E, Manetta JA, Noakes PS, et al. Supplemental intravenous n-3 fatty acids and n-3 fatty acid status and outcome in critically ill elderly patients in the ICU receiving enteral nutrition. Clin Nutr. 2013;32:599–605. https://doi.org/10.1016/j.clnu.2012.10.016.
29. Friede T, Kieser M. Blinded sample size reassessment in non-inferiority and equivalence trials. Stat Med. 2003;22:995–1007. https://doi.org/10.1002/sim.1456.
30. Pironi L, Agostini F, Guidetti M. Intravenous lipids in home parenteral nutrition. World Rev Nutr Diet. 2015;112:141–9. https://doi.org/10.1159/000365608.
31. Pradelli L, Mayer K, Muscaritoli M, Heller AR. N-3 fatty acid-enriched parenteral nutrition regimens in elective surgical and ICU patients: a meta-analysis. Crit Care. 2012;16:R184. https://doi.org/10.1186/cc11668.
32. Manzanares W, Dhaliwal R, Jurewitsch B, Stapleton RD, Jeejeebhoy KN, Heyland DK. Parenteral fish oil lipid emulsions in the critically ill: a systematic review and meta-analysis. JPEN J Parenter Enteral Nutr. 2014;38: 20–8. https://doi.org/10.1177/0148607113486006.
33. Manzanares W, Langlois PL, Dhaliwal R, Lemieux M, Heyland DK. Intravenous fish oil lipid emulsions in critically ill patients: an updated systematic review and meta-analysis. Crit Care. 2015;19:167. https://doi.org/10.1186/s13054-015-0888-7.
34. Friesecke S, Lotze C, Köhler J, Heinrich A, Felix SB, Abel P. Fish oil supplementation in the parenteral nutrition of critically ill medical patients: a randomised controlled trial. Intensive Care Med. 2008;34: 1411–20. https://doi.org/10.1007/s00134-008-1072-1.
35. Palmer AJ, Ho CKM, Ajibola O, Avenell A. The role of ω-3 fatty acid supplemented parenteral nutrition in critical illness in adults: a systematic review and meta-analysis. Crit Care Med. 2013;41:307–16. https://doi.org/10.1097/CCM.0b013e3182657578.
36. Norman K, Kirchner H, Lochs H, Pirlich M. Malnutrition affects quality of life in gastroenterology patients. World J Gastroenterol. 2006;12:3380–5.
37. Gupta D, Lis CG, Granick J, Grutsch JF, Vashi PG, Lammersfeld CA. Malnutrition was associated with poor quality of life in colorectal cancer: a retrospective analysis. J Clin Epidemiol. 2006;59:704–9. https://doi.org/10.1016/j.jclinepi.2005.08.020.
38. Chambers A, Hennessy E, Powell-Tuck J. Longitudinal trends in quality of life after starting home parenteral nutrition: a randomised controlled study of telemedicine. Clin Nutr. 2006;25:505–14. https://doi.org/10.1016/j.clnu.2006.01.001.
39. Culine S, Chambrier C, Tadmouri A, Senesse P, Seys P, Radji A, et al. Home parenteral nutrition improves quality of life and nutritional status in patients with cancer: a French observational multicentre study. Support Care Cancer. 2014;22:1867–74. https://doi.org/10.1007/s00520-014-2164-9.
40. Vashi PG, Dahlk S, Popiel B, Lammersfeld CA, Ireton-Jones C, Gupta D. A longitudinal study investigating quality of life and nutritional outcomes in advanced cancer patients receiving home parenteral nutrition. BMC Cancer. 2014;14:593. https://doi.org/10.1186/1471-2407-14-593.

14

Maternal periconceptional consumption of sprouted potato and risks of neural tube defects and orofacial clefts

Wenli Ni[1,2], Tian Tian[1,2], Le Zhang[1,2], Zhiwen Li[1,2], Linlin Wang[1,2*] and Aiguo Ren[1,2]

Abstract

Background: The association between maternal consumption of sprouted potato during periconceptional period on the development of neural tube defects (NTDs) or orofacial clefts (OFCs) remains unclear. We aimed to examine the association between maternal consumption of sprouted potatoes during periconceptional period and risks of NTDs or OFCs.

Methods: Subjects included 622 NTD cases, 135 OFC cases and 858 nonmalformed controls, were recruited from a case-control study in Shanxi Province of northern China between 2002 and 2007. Information on demographics, maternal sprouted potato consumption, lifestyle behaviors and folic acid supplementation was collected.

Results: Consumption of sprouted potatoes was associated with elevated odds of total NTDs (OR = 2.20; 95% CI, 1.12–4.32) and anencephaly (OR = 2.48; 95% CI, 1.10–5.58); no association for spina bifida or encephalocele. Sprouted potato consumption increased the risk of total OFCs (OR = 3.49; 95% CI, 1.29–9.49) and cleft lip with or without cleft palate (CL ± P) (OR = 4.03; 95% CI, 1.44–11.28).

Conclusion: Maternal consumption of sprouted potatoes during periconceptional period may increase the risks of NTDs and OFCs. Given that potato is commonly consumed around the world, improper preservation and use should be a matter of concern in respect of the potential teratogenicity.

Keywords: Sprouted potato, Periconceptional period, Neural tube defects, Orofacial clefts

Background

Neural tube defects (NTDs) and orofacial clefts (OFCs) are relatively common congenital anomalies that have a significant impact on infant mortality, health, and quality of life [1–3]. NTDs result from failure of neural tube to close by the 28th day of postconception [4]. OFCs derive from an embryopathy with the tissues of the lip or palate not joining properly [5]. The etiologies of NTDs and OFCs are generally thought to be multifactorial, involving both genetic and environmental factors. Environmental factors such as maternal unhealthy diet, and exposure to smoking and alcohol consumption contribute to these congenital anomalies [6–10]. Nutrient deficiency as a part of harmful dietary factors, especially folic acid deficiency, has been shown to be associated with increased risks of NTDs and OFCs [11–13]. Toxins in food are another important part of harmful dietary factors, however, the role of toxins in the occurrence of these two birth defects remains largely unknown.

Toxins in staple food have a great influence on human health because of the large amount of consumption. Today potato, as the 4th major food crop after rice, wheat and maize, is cultivated worldwide under various climatic conditions, and is consumed commonly throughout the world [14, 15]. However, in the process of storage and transportation, potato is easy to become green and spout in inappropriate environment [16, 17]. Sprouted potato contains high concentration of solanine that is a toxic glycoalkaloid [18]. The reproductive toxicity of solanine has been assessed in vitro or in vivo animal studies [15, 19–23]. Steroidal glycoalkaloid from

* Correspondence: linlinwang@bjmu.edu.cn
[1]Peking University Institute of Reproductive and Child Health, National Health Commission Key Laboratory of Reproductive Health, Beijing 100191, China
[2]Department of Epidemiology and Biostatistics, School of Public Health, Peking University Health Science Center, Beijing 100191, China

potatoes could inhibit pre-implantation embryo development when exposing to oocytes and fertilized ova in vitro [15]. Additionally, solanine was found to have teratogenicity, such as inducing NTDs, OFCs, microcephaly, and severe muscular kinking in frog embryo, mice, or hamster [19–23]. However, only one study with a small sample size reported that sprouted potato consumption might be a risk factor for NTDs [24], while no study investigated the effect of maternal consumption of sprouted potato during periconceptional period on the development of OFCs in humans.

In the present study, we aimed to examine the association between maternal periconceptional consumption of sprouted potatoes and risks for NTDs and OFCs.

Methods

Study design

The data were from a case–control study of birth defects in four counties (Pingding, Xiyang, Taigu and Zezhou) of Shanxi province in northern China, which has been described elsewhere [25]. Concisely, a population-based surveillance system of birth defects was established in the study area in 2002. The surveillance system monitored major external structural birth defects through active case ascertainment. Cases with major external structural malformations were ascertained from live births, stillbirths, and elective terminations. County or township health workers verified the diagnoses by physical examination of the fetal body for all pregnancy outcomes and filled out a reporting form for each case. When a case infant was identified, a newborn control without any external structural birth defect was matched to the case infant by county, sex, maternal ethnic group, and date of the last menstrual period (±4 months). The study was approved by the Institutional Review Board of Peking University Health Science Centre. All participants provided written informed consent.

Data collection

Trained local health care workers conducted face-to-face interviews with mothers of cases and controls within 1 week of delivery or termination of pregnancies to collect the exposure information using a structured questionnaire. Data were collected on the mother's demographic characteristics, reproductive history, lifestyle, folic acid supplementation, smoking exposure (active or passive), and consumption of sprouted potato and other foods from 1 month before through 2 months after conception. Definition of maternal sprouted potato consumption is eating the sprouts of potato or any skin that started to turn green. Definition of passive smoking is staying in the tobacco smoking environmental for at least 30 min and at least 1 time per week. Definition of higher consumption of B vitamins is that maternal consumption of fresh vegetables and fresh fruit at ≥4 meals/week or maternal periconceptional use of folic acid, otherwise, it was lower consumption of B vitamins. Consumption of sprouted potato was classified as < 1 meal/week, 1–3 meals/week, 4–6 meals/week, or > 6 meals/week; we combined two frequency categories ("4–6 meals/week" and "> 6 meals/week") into a single group (referred to as "≥ 4 meals/week"), because subjects with the highest consumption of sprouted potato frequency of "> 6 meals/week" were few.

Study population

For this study, we used data collected from June 2002 through December 2007. The cases included newborns with NTDs or OFCs assigned an ICD-9 code of 740.0 (anencephaly), 741.0 (spina bifida), 742.0 (encephalocele), 749.0 (cleft palate), 749.1 (cleft lip), or 749.2 (cleft lip with cleft palate). A total of 1615 participants were available for analyses, including 622 NTD cases (281 with anencephaly, 293 with spina bifida, and 48 with encephalocele), 135 OFC cases (126 with cleft lip with or without cleft palate, 9 with cleft palate only), and 858 controls. Because OFCs and NTDs are rare diseases and few studies investigated the assocaition between sprouted potato consumption and birth defects, no information about the proportion of maternal sprouted potato exposure in control group or OR value can be referred for calculating sample size. In the present study, we used an empirical sample size. The statistical powers were 96.4% for NTDs and 99.7% for OFCs of this given the sample size (622 NTD cases, 135 OFC cases, and 858 controls) by PASS.11 software calculation, which were adequate to test the existence of significantly association between the sprouted potato consumption and NTDs and OFCs in this study.

Statistical analyses

The original study used a pair-matching design, but for some data about sprouted potato consumption were not available for evaluation, the matching was broken in this analysis. The differences in demographic and lifestyle characteristics between the case and control group were evaluated by Chi-square test or Fisher's exact test. Risk was estimated by the use of OR, and the precision of each OR was assessed by its 95% CI. We used the unconditional logistic regression and Chi-square trend test to evaluate the associations between sprouted potato consumption and risks of NTDs and OFCs, respectively. We calculated two adjusted OR (aOR) with different logistic models. The aOR_1 was adjusted only for demographic and obstetrics variables, including maternal age, BMI, education, occupation, parity, history of pregnancy affected by birth defects, infant sex, folic acid supplementation, season of conception, alcohol drinking, and maternal smoking exposure. Considering the other dietary characteristics which may generate confounding bias, we also estimated aOR_2 by additionally adjusting for consumption of meat or fish, consumption of egg or milk, consumption of fresh vegetable, consumption of fresh fruit, and consumption of legumes. Another, the associations between sprouted potato consumption and risks of NTDs and OFCs among mother with higher consumption of B vitamins consumption versus mother with lower consumption of B vitamins were conducted. We considered $p < 0.05$ statistically significant. All data were analyzed using SPSS 23.0 software (SPSS, Chicago, IL, USA).

Results

Characteristics of study population

The demographic and lifestyle characteristics of study participants are summarized in Table 1. More than 99% mothers were of Han ethnicity. Compared with control mothers, mothers of infants with NTDs were more likely to have a lower BMI and a lower education level, to be multiparous, to report a history of pregnancy affected by birth defects, to have alcohol drinking exposure, and to have smoking exposure; mothers of infants with OFCs were more likely to be not farmers, to have a lower education level, and to have a male infant.

Additional file 1: Table S1 shows the dietary characteristics of study participants. Compared to control mothers, mothers of infants with NTDs were more likely to have lower frequencies of meat or fish consumption, egg or milk consumption, fresh vegetables consumption, fresh fruit consumption, and beans or bean products consumption. There was no significant difference between OFC cases and controls with respect to dietary characteristics.

Table 2 shows the association between sprouted potato consumption and risks of total NTDs and subtypes of NTDs. When maternal consumption of sprouted potato at < 1 meal/week was used as the reference, increases in the risks for total NTDs of 2.20-fold (95% CI, 1.12–4.32) were observed for maternal consumption at ≥4 meals/week, respectively. The positive relationship was also present for anencephaly but not for spina bifida or encephalocele; the adjusted ORs for anencephaly in association with maternal consumption of sprouted potato at ≥4 meals/week were 2.48 (95% CI, 1.10–5.58). Trend analysis showed a clear positive dose-response relationship between risks for NTD or anencephaly and sprouted potato consumption (*P* for trend < 0.05).

Table 3 details the association between sprouted potato consumption and risks of total OFCs and CL ± P. When maternal consumption of sprouted potato at < 1 meal/week was used as the reference, increases in the risks for total OFCs and CL ± P of 3.49-fold (95% CI, 1.29–9.49) and 4.03-fold (95% CI, 1.44–11.28) were observed for maternal consumption at ≥4 meals/week, respectively.

We also assessed association between maternal sprouted potato consumption and risks of NTDs and OFCs in stratified by consumption of B vitamin (Additional file 1: Table S2 and S3).

Among mother with lower consumption of B vitamins, maternal consumption of sprouted potato at ≥4 meals/week, still were significantly associated with NTDs and OFCs, the aOR were 1.84 (1.02–7.86) for total NTD, 3.21(1.00–10.35) for anencephaly, 12.17(2.22–66.63) for total OFCs, and 15.65(2.68–91.40) for CL ± P. However, no significant associations were observed between maternal consumption of sprouted potato and NTDs and OFCs among mother with a higher consumption of B vitamins. Recall bias is the main concern in case-control studies. The women who have infant with birth defects might over-report unhealthy exposure. To assess whether such a recall bias existed in the present study, we further analyzed the distribution of consumption of sprouted potato during periconceptional period between women had infant with limb malformations (polydactylism, syndactylia, limb shortening, strephenopodia, or strephexopodia) without other malformations and controls (Additional file 1: Table S4). No difference was found in the distribution of sprouted potato consumption between cases and controls ($P = 0.066$).

Sensitivity analysis

To test the robustness of our results, we conducted a sensitivity analysis limited to the subjects without a history of pregnancy affected by birth defects. The results did not change after removing 65 subjects with a history of pregnancy affected by birth defects (Additional file 1: Tables S5 and S6).

Discussion

In this population-based case-control study, we examined potential association between maternal consumption of sprouted potatoes during periconceptional period and risks for NTDs and OFCs. Overall, we observed that maternal consumption of sprouted potatoes increased the risk for total NTDs, anencephaly, total OFCs, and CL ± P.

Few literatures reported the association between sprouted potato consumption and risk of NTDs in humans [24]. In our study, based on relatively large sample of NTD cases ($n = 622$) versus controls ($n = 858$), we found about 2.20-fold increased risks for NTDs among mothers who consumed sprouted potato at ≥4 meals/week and the risk increased with the rising consumption frequency of sprouted potato. One study reported that sprouted potato consumption was a risk factor affecting

Table 1 Characteristics of women who had pregnancies affected by NTDs or OFCs (cases) and women who delivered healthy infants (controls)

Characteristics	Controls ($n = 858$)	Cases			
		NTDs ($n = 622$)		OFCs ($n = 135$)	
	n(%)[a]	n(%)[a]	*p*-Value	n(%)[a]	*p*-Value
Maternal age (years)					
< 25	358(42.4)	249(40.8)	0.800	61(47.3)	0.140
25–29	268 (31.7)	196 (32.0)		45 (34.9)	
≥30	219 (25.9)	166 (27.2)		23 (17.8)	
BMI (kg/m^2)					
< 18.5	53 (6.3)	45 (7.5)	0.002	11 (8.5)	0.339
18.5–23.9	417 (49.8)	350 (58.0)		70 (53.8)	
≥ 24	368 (43.9)	208 (34.5)		49 (37.7)	
Ethnicity					
Han	853 (99.6)	620 (99.8)	1.000	135 (100)	1.000
Other	3 (0.4)	1 (0.2)		0 (0)	
Occupation					
Farmer	568 (66.9)	420 (69.2)	0.356	73 (54.1)	0.004
Other	281 (33.1)	187 (30.8)		62 (45.9)	
Education					
Primary or lower	51 (6.0)	101 (16.3)	< 0.001	18 (13.5)	0.002
Junior high	656 (76.9)	445 (71.8)		87 (65.4)	
High school or above	146 (17.1)	74 (11.9)		28 (21.1)	
Parity					
Primiparas	538 (62.8)	345 (56.4)	0.013	95 (70.9)	0.069
Multiparas	319 (37.2)	267 (43.6)		39 (29.1)	
History of pregnancy affected by birth defects					
Yes	18 (2.1)	42 (6.8)	< 0.001	5 (3.7)	0.360
No	838 (97.9)	573 (93.2)		130 (96.3)	
Infant sex					
Male	404 (47.6)	268 (43.9)	0.153	84 (62.2)	0.002
Female	444 (52.4)	343 (56.1)		51 (37.8)	
Folic acid supplementation					
Yes	113 (13.7)	65 (10.7)	0.090	20 (14.4)	0.690
No	709 (86.3)	540 (89.3)		113 (85.6)	
Maternal smoking exposure					
Yes	491 (57.6)	423 (68.6)	< 0.001	84 (62.2)	0.315
No	361 (42.4)	194 (31.4)		51 (37.8)	
Alcohol drinking					
Yes	5 (0.6)	9 (1.4)	0.107	4 (3.0)	0.024
No	848 (99.4)	613 (98.4)		131 (13.4)	
Season of conception					
Spring	202 (24.1)	156 (25.4)	0.657	36 (26.9)	0.857
Summer	206 (24.6)	142 (23.2)		29 (21.6)	
Autumn	207 (24.7)	164 (26.8)		33 (24.6)	
Winter	222 (26.5)	151 (24.6)		36 (26.9)	

[a]Values for some variables may not equal the total number of cases or controls because of missing data

Table 2 Sprouted potato consumption and risks of total NTDs and NTD subtypes

Sprouted potato consumption	Controls ($n = 858$)	Total NTDs ($n = 622$)		Anencephaly ($n = 281$)		Spina bifida ($n = 293$)		Encephalocele ($n = 48$)	
	n(%)	n(%)	OR (95% CI)	n(%)	OR (95% CI)	n(%)	OR (95% CI)	n(%)	OR (95% CI)
Crude OR									
< 1 meal/week	737 (85.9)	512 (82.1)	1.00	229 (81.5)	1.00	243 (83.0)	1.00	38 (79.2)	1.00
1–3 meals/week	99 (11.5)	79 (12.7)	1.15 (0.84–1.58)	34 (12.1)	1.11 (0.73–1.68)	37 (12.6)	1.13 (0.75–1.69)	8 (16.7)	1.57 (0.71–3.46)
≥ 4 meals/week	22 (2.6)	33 (5.3)	2.16 (1.24–3.75)	18 (6.4)	2.63 (1.39–5.00)	13 (4.4)	1.79 (0.89–3.60)	2 (4.2)	1.76 (0.75–1.69)
Adjusted OR_1[a]									
< 1 meal/week	737 (85.9)	512 (82.1)	1.00	229 (81.5)	1.00	243 (83.0)	1.00	38 (79.2)	1.00
1–3 meals/week	99 (11.5)	79 (12.7)	1.28 (0.88–1.87)	34 (12.1)	1.22 (0.74–2.02)	37 (12.6)	1.23 (0.77–1.97)	8 (16.7)	2.13 (0.86–5.27)
≥ 4 meals/week	22 (2.6)	33 (5.3)	2.22 (1.18–4.18)	18 (6.4)	2.42 (1.15–5.11)	13 (4.4)	2.03 (0.94–4.39)	2 (4.2)	2.22 (0.46–10.79)
Adjusted OR_2[b]									
< 1 meal/week	737 (85.9)	512 (82.1)	1.00	229 (81.5)	1.00	243 (83.0)	1.00	38 (79.2)	1.00
1–3 meals/week	99 (11.5)	79 (12.7)	1.11 (0.75–1.63)	34 (12.1)	1.06 (0.63–1.78)	37 (12.6)	1.23 (0.76–2.00)	8 (16.7)	1.82 (0.70–4.73)
≥ 4 meals/week	22 (2.6)	33 (5.3)	2.20 (1.12–4.32)	18 (6.4)	2.48 (1.10–5.58)	13 (4.4)	2.17 (0.97–4.85)	2 (4.2)	3.18 (0.61–16.65)
P for trend		0.009		0.011		0.117		0.203	

[a]Adjusted for maternal age, education, BMI, occupation, infant sex, parity, history of pregnancy affected by birth defects, folic acid supplementation, season of conception, alcohol drinking, and maternal smoking exposure

[b]Adjusted for maternal age, education, BMI, occupation, infant sex, parity, history of pregnancy affected by birth defects, folic acid supplementation, season of conception, alcohol drinking, maternal smoking exposure, consumption of meat or fish, consumption of egg or milk, consumption of fresh vegetable, consumption of fresh fruit, and consumption of legumes

the occurrence of NTDs in mothers with NTD fetuses ($n = 99$) and control mothers ($n = 99$) [24]. NTD subtype analysis was absent in the previous study due to the small sample size. To our knowledge, our study is the first to examine the association between maternal sprouted potato consumption during periconceptional period and risks for NTD subtypes. We found a 2.48-fold increased risk for anencephaly not for other NTD subtypes among mothers who consumed sprouted potato at ≥4 meals/week. Several previous animal studies support our findings. Water suspensions of sprouts from seven potato varieties, gavaged at concentration of 2.5–3.5 g/kg on days 8–15 of gestation, produced NTD abnormalities in one strain of hamsters [22]. Oral administration of solanines at 0.44 mmol/kg dose on days 8–15 of gestation could induce NTDs in Syrian hamsters [23]. Glycoalkaloids were also found to induce anencephaly, microcephaly, and severe muscular kinking at a dosage of 4–5 mg/L in frog embryo [19, 20].

No previous studies have examined the role of maternal consumption of sprouted potatoes during periconceptional period in OFCs in humans. In our study, we found a 3.49-fold elevated risk for OFCs among mothers who consumed sprouted potato at ≥4 meals/week. In animal experiment, potato sprouts has been shown to be teratogenic for OFCs. Hamsters gavaged sprouts of potato suspended in water at about 2.2 ± 0.3 g/kg dose on days 8–15 of gestation presented OFC phenotypes [21].

B vitamin consumption (folic acid supplementation) has been shown a beneficial factor against the occurrence of NTDs and OFCs [26, 27]. We, therefore, examined the association between maternal sprouted potato consumption and risks of NTDs and OFCs in stratified by consumption of B vitamin. Among mother with lower consumption of B vitamins, we still found maternal consumption of sprouted potatoes significantly associated with NTDs and OFCs, however, no significant associations were observed among mother with a higher consumption of B vitamins, which meaning that B vitamins maybe antagonize the toxicity of solanine. Previous study also showed that folic acid could decrease glycoalkaloids-induced polarization, and then decrease glycoalkaloid toxicity [19].

Potato is an important food crop and constitutes an integral part of diets in many countries around the world, including China [28]. During the storage process, potato is easy to sprout in inappropriate environment and produce a large amount of solanine, which can be increased to 500 mg/100 g and is far more than the safety standard (20 mg/100 g) [29]. Solanine is stable during cooking even in frying oil at 180 °C [19]. Home processing methods (boiling, cooking, frying, and microwaving) have small and variable effects on solanine [30, 31]. Therefore, most of solanines (potato glycoalkaloids) are taken into the bodies when pregnant women have sprouted or green potatoes. The mechanisms underlying the teratogenicity of solanines are little investigated. It has been suggested that potato glycoalkaloids interfere with transport across cell membranes of Ca^{2+} and Na^{+} ions [32–35]. The potential teratogenicity of sprouted

Table 3 Sprouted potato consumption and risks of total OFCs and OFC subtypes

Sprouted potato consumption	Controls (*n* = 858)	Total OFCs (*n* = 135)		CL ± P (*n* = 126)	
	n(%)	n(%)	OR(95% CI)	n(%)	OR(95% CI)
Crude OR					
< 1 meal/week	737 (85.9)	111 (82.2)	1.00	104 (82.5)	1.00
1–3 meals/week	99 (11.5)	16 (11.9)	1.07 (0.61–1.89)	14 (11.1)	1.00 (0.55–1.82)
≥ 4 meals/week	22 (2.6)	8 (5.9)	2.41 (1.05–5.56)	8 (6.3)	2.58 (1.12–5.94)
Adjusted OR_1[a]					
< 1 meal/week	737 (85.9)	111 (82.2)	1.00	104 (82.5)	1.00
1–3 meals/week	99 (11.5)	16 (11.9)	1.37 (0.70–2.69)	14 (11.1)	1.34 (0.67–2.68)
≥ 4 meals/week	22 (2.6)	8 (5.9)	2.99 (1.12–8.03)	8 (6.3)	3.17 (1.18–8.55)
Adjusted OR_2[b]					
< 1 meal/week	737 (85.9)	111 (82.2)	1.00	104 (82.5)	1.00
1–3 meals/week	99 (11.5)	16 (11.9)	1.10 (0.55–2.21)	14 (11.1)	1.20 (0.57–2.50)
≥ 4 meals/week	22 (2.6)	8 (5.9)	3.49 (1.29–9.49)	8 (6.3)	4.03 (1.44–11.28)
P for trend		0.094		0.099	

[a]Adjusted for maternal age, maternal education, BMI, occupation, infant sex, parity, history of pregnancy affected by birth defects, folic acid supplementation, season of conception, alcohol drinking, and maternal smoking exposure
[b]Adjusted for maternal age, maternal education, BMI, occupation, infant sex, parity, history of pregnancy affected by birth defects, folic acid supplementation, season of conception, alcohol drinking, maternal smoking exposure, consumption of meat or fish, consumption of egg or milk, consumption of fresh vegetable, consumption of fresh fruit, and consumption of legumes

potatoes may be involved in solanine direct or indirect adverse effects on transport across cell membranes [19].

There is strength in our study. It was a relatively large population-based study with collection of the information on sprouted potato consumption and other key confounding factors, which enables us to investigate the relationship between sprouted potato consumption and NTDs with adjustment of potential interference factors. However, our study has several limitations. An intrinsic limitation of the case-control study is recall bias. Case mothers may over-report factors they believe to be risk factors of birth defects in comparison with control mothers. For assessment of recall bias, we determined whether a difference existed in the distribution of maternal consumption of sprouted potatoes during periconceptional period between women have infant with and without limb malformations. The result showed that the distribution of sprouted potato consumption between limb malformation cases and controls is similar, suggesting that recall bias of over-report was small in this study. On the other hand, to further minimize the recall bias, participants were interviewed within the first week after delivery or pregnancy termination, and the researchers helped women to confirm the period of exposure according to the dates of their last menstrual period. Second, the sample size for some subgroups was small, which limited our ability to detect statistical differences. Third, the exposure information in this study was obtained from a questionnaire. We did not measure the solanine quantity in sprouted potato. So, we can not provide data on the amount of solanine contained in a sprouted potato and the amount of solanine consumed per meal. Finally, information about consumption of dietary we collected does not specify the frequency of certain food items consumption or the weight of food consumption, and just were roughly classified by consumption of meat or fish, egg or milk, fresh vegetable, fresh fruit, and legumes in present study. So we did not use a nutrient based adjustment procedures in this study.

Conclusions

In conclusion, maternal consumption of sprouted potatoes during periconceptional period may increase the risks for NTDs and OFCs. Our study is the first to examine the association between maternal periconceptional sprouted potato consumption and risks of NTD subtypes and OFCs in human. Our findings provide novel insight into the etiology of NTDs and OFCs and propose a new way to prevent from birth defects. Potato is a commonly consumed food items in the world, and improper preservation and use should be a matter of concern. The dietary guidance for pregnant women should be emphasized and the knowledge level of healthy fertility in reproductive woman should be improved. Maternal consumption of sprouted potato could be avoided through health education and pre-pregnancy care. Further studies aiming to replicate the findings in other racial groups and to construe the fundamental mechanism underlying the association of sprouted potato consumption and birth defects are needed.

Additional file

Additional file 1: Table S1. Dietary characteristics of women who had pregnancies affected by NTDs or OFCs (cases) and women who delivered healthy infants (controls). **Table S2.** Sprouted potato consumption and risks of total NTDs and NTD subtypes stratified by consumption of B vitamin. **Table S3.** Sprouted potato consumption and risks of total OFCs and OFC subtypes stratified by consumption of B vitamin. **Table S4.** The distribution of sprouted potato consumption between Limb malformation cases and controls. **Table S5.** Sensitivity analysis: Sprouted potato consumption and risks of total NTDs and NTD subtypes. **Table S6.** Sensitivity analysis: Sprouted potato consumption and risks of total OFCs and OFC subtypes.

Abbreviations

BMI: Body mass index; CI: Confidences interval; CL ± P: Cleft lip with or without cleft palate; NTDs: Neural tube defects; OFCs: Orofacial clefts; OR: Odds radio

Acknowledgments

We are grateful to the local healthcare workers in four counties (Pingding, Xiyang, Taigu and Zezhou) of Shanxi Province, China, for their assistance with data collection during the course of the study. We also thank the study participants for their contributions.

Funding

Supported by the National Natural Science Foundation of China (Grant No. 81472987 and 81773441); Beijing Natural Science Foundation (Grant No. 7162094); and the National Key Research and Development Program, Ministry of Science and Technology, P.R. China (Grant No. 2016YFC1000501).

Authors' contributions

LW conceived and designed the study; WN and LW posed the hypothesis, analyzed the data, and drafted the manuscript; AR and ZL established the population-based surveillance system; TT and LZ contributed to acquisition and cleaning of data; LW, ZL and AR contributed to reviewing the manuscript. All authors read and approved the final manuscript.

Competing interests

The authors declare that they have no competing interests.

References

1. Lockhart E. The mental health needs of children and adolescents with cleft lip and/or palate. Clin Child Psychol Psychiatry. 2003;8:7–16.
2. Hunt O, Burden D, Hepper P, Johnston C. The psychosocial effects of cleft lip and palate: a systematic review. Eur J Orthod. 2005;27:274.
3. Detrait ER, George TM, Etchevers HC, Gilbert JR, Vekemans M, Speer MC. Human neural tube defects: developmental biology, epidemiology, and genetics. Neurotoxicol Teratol. 2005;27:515–24.
4. Wilde JJ, Petersen JR, Niswander L. Genetic, epigenetic, and environmental contributions to neural tube closure. Annu Rev Genet. 2014;48:583–611.
5. Mossey PA, Little J, Munger RG, Dixon MJ, Shaw WC. Cleft lip and palate. Lancet. 2009;374:1773–85.
6. Shaw GM, Carmichael SL, Laurent C, Rasmussen SA. Maternal nutrient intakes and risk of orofacial clefts. Epidemiology. 2006;17:285–91.
7. Kirke PN, Daly LE, Elwood JH. A randomized trial of low-dose folic-acid to prevent neural-tube defects. Arch Dis Child. 1992;67:1442–6.
8. Grewal J, Carmichael SL, Ma C, Lammer EJ, Shaw GM. Maternal periconceptional smoking and alcohol consumption and risk for select congenital anomalies. Birth Defects Res A Clin Mol Teratol. 2008;82:519–26.
9. Krapels IP, van Rooij A, Ocke MC, West CE, van der Horst CM, Steegers-Theunissen RP. Maternal nutritional status and the risk for orofacial cleft offspring in humans. J Nutr. 2004;134:3106–13.
10. Sotresalvarez D, Siegariz AM, Herring AH, Carmichael SL, Feldkamp ML, Hobbs CA, Olshan AF. Maternal dietary patterns are associated with risk of neural tube and congenital heart defects. Am J Epidemiol. 2013;177:1279.
11. Berry RJ, Li Z, Erickson JD, Li S, Moore CA, Wang H, Mulinare J, Zhao P, Wong LYC, Gindler J. Correction: Prevention of neural-tube defects with folic acid in China. N Engl J Med. 1999;341:1864.
12. Figueiredo RF, Figueiredo N, Feguri A, Bieski I, Mello R, Espinosa M, Damazo AS. The role of the folic acid to the prevention of orofacial cleft: an epidemiological study. Oral Dis. 2015;21:240–7.
13. Johansen AM, Lie RT, Wilcox AJ, Andersen LF, Drevon CA. Maternal dietary intake of vitamin a and risk of orofacial clefts: a population-based case-control study in Norway. Am J Epidemiol. 2008;167:1164–70.
14. Paul V, Ezekiel R, Pandey R. Sprout suppression on potato: need to look beyond CIPC for more effective and safer alternatives. J Food Sci Technol. 2016;53:1–18.
15. Wang S, Panter KE, Gaffield W, Evans RC, Bunch TD. Effects of steroidal glycoalkaloids from potatoes (Solanum tuberosum) on in vitro bovine embryo development. Anim Reprod Sci. 2005;85:243–50.
16. Friedman M, Mcdonald GM. Glycoalkaloids in fresh and processed potatoes. Acs Symposium. 1996;631:189–205.
17. Hopkins J. The glycoalkaloids: naturally of interest (but a hot potato?). Food Chem Toxicol. 1995;33:323–8.
18. Barceloux D. Potatoes, tomatoes, and solanine toxicity (Solanum tuberosum L., Solanum lycopersicum L.). Dis Mon. 2009;55:391–402.
19. Friedman M. Potato glycoalkaloids and metabolites: roles in the plant and in the diet. J Agric Food Chem. 2006 54:8655–81.
20. Friedman M, Rayburn JR, Bantle JA. Structural relationships and development toxicity of Solanum alkaloids in the frog embryo teratogenesis assay-Xenopus. J Agric Food Chem. 1992;40:1617–24.
21. Keeler RF, Baker DC, Gaffield W. Spirosolane-containing Solanum species and induction of congenital craniofacial malformations. Toxicon Off J Int Soc Toxinol. 1990;28:873.
22. Keeler RF, Young S, Brown D, Stallknecht GF, Douglas D. Congenital deformities produced in hamsters by potato sprouts. Teratology. 1978;17:327.
23. Gaffield W, Keeler RF. Induction of terata in hamsters by solanidane alkaloids derived from Solanum tuberosum. Chem Res Toxicol. 1996;9:426.
24. F W, YF Y, PZ L. A case-control study on the risk factors of neural tube defects in Shanxi province. Chin J Epidemiol. 2008;29:771–4.
25. Li Z, Ren A, Liu J, Pei L, Zhang L, Guo Z Li Z. Maternal flu or fever, medication use, and neural tube defects: a population-based case-control study in northern China. Birth Defects Res A Clin Mol Teratol. 2007;79:295–300.
26. Millacura N, Pardo R, Cifuentes L, Suazo J. Effects of folic acid fortification on orofacial clefts prevalence: a meta-analysis. Public Health Nutr. 2017;20: 2260–8.
27. Berry RJ, Li Z, Erickson JD, Li S, Moore CA, Wang H, Mulinare J, Zhao P, Wong LY, Gindler J, et al. Prevention of neural-tube defects with folic acid in China. China-U.S. collaborative project for neural tube defect prevention. N Engl J Med. 1999;341:1485–90.
28. Hossain MB, Rawson A, Aguilo-Aguayo I, Brunton NP, Rai DK. Recovery of steroidal alkaloids from potato peels using pressurized liquid extraction. Molecules. 2015;20:8560–73.
29. Liu Chunhua LC, Guihao Y. Research Progress of Solanine in the potato and its product. J Anhui Agric Sci. 2010;38:3519–20.
30. Sizer CE, Maga JA, Craven CJ. Total glycoalkaloids in potatoes and potato chips. J Agric Food Chem. 1980;28:578–9.
31. Bushway RJ, Ponnampalam R. alpha.-Chaconine and .alpha.-solanine content of potato products and their stability during several modes of cooking. J Agric Food Chem. 1981;29:814–7.
32. Blankemeyer JT, Atherton R, Friedman M. Effect of Potato Glycoalkaloids .Alpha.-Chaconine and .Alpha.-Solanine on sodium active transport in frog skin. J Agric Food Chem. 1995;43:636–9.
33. Blankemeyer JT, Stringer BK, Rayburn JR, Bantle JA, Friedman M. Effect of potato glycoalkaloids, alpha-chaconine and alpha-solanine, on membrane potential of frog embryos. J Agric Food Chem. 1992;40:2022–5.
34. Michalska L, Nagel G, Swiniarski E, Zydowo MM. The effect of α-solanine on the active calcium transport in rat intestine. Gen Pharmacol. 1985;16:69–70.

15

Periconceptional folic acid supplementation and sex difference in prevention of neural tube defects and their subtypes in China: results from a large prospective cohort study

Jufen Liu[1,2], Zhiwen Li[1,2*], Rongwei Ye[1,2*], Jianmeng Liu[1,2] and Aiguo Ren[1,2]

Abstract

Background: Folic acid (FA) supplementation is known to prevent neural tube defects (NTDs). We examined whether this preventive effect differs by the sex of the infant.

Methods: Data were gathered from a large population-based cohort study in China that evaluated the effects of FA supplementation on NTDs. All births at 20 complete gestational weeks, including live births, stillbirths, and pregnancy terminations, and all NTDs, regardless of gestational age, were recorded. In a northern China province, a total of 30,801 singleton live births to women whose use of FA supplements during the first trimester was known at the time were included in the study. The birth prevalence of NTDs was classified by sex, subtype, and maternal FA supplementation. Male to female rate ratios [RR] and their 95% confidence intervals [CI] were calculated.

Results: A total of 106 NTDs cases were recorded. The overall prevalence of NTDs was 2.5‰ among males and 4.4‰ among females; NTDs were less prevalent among males than among females (RR, 0.58; 95% CI, 0.54–0.63). There was a higher prevalence of anencephaly (RR, 0.34; 95% CI, 0.27–0.43) and spina bifida (RR, 0.73; 95% CI, 0.63–0.84) among females. However, FA supplementation led to significantly greater decreases in the rates of anencephaly (4.8‰) and total NTDs (7.6‰) in females than in males (1.6‰ and 2.8‰, respectively).

Conclusions: FA supplementation successfully reduces the prevalence of NTDs in both male and female infants, although we found a significantly greater decrease in anencephaly and total NTDs in females than in males. How the protective effects of FA supplementation affect the sexes differently needs to be studied further.

Keywords: Periconceptional folic acid, Sex difference, Neural tube defects (NTDs), Difference in differences (DID) model

Key messages

- Periconceptional FA use reduces NTD risk, but whether the effect differs by infant sex is unknown.
- Daily FA use significantly decreased anencephaly and total NTDs among both males and females in the Chinese population studied.
- These decreases were significantly greater in females than in males.

Introduction

Many congenital malformations and birth defects, such as defects of the sex organs, urinary tract defects, gastrointestinal tract defects, are sex specific [1–3]. As early as the 1970s, scientists began to notice much higher rates of neural tube defects (NTDs) in females as in males, especially anencephaly [4, 5]. Almost a decade later, researchers suggested that certain environmental factors may contribute to higher rates of anencephalus in

* Correspondence: lizw@bjmu.edu.cn; yerw@bjmu.edu.cn
[1]Institute of Reproductive and Child Health / Key Laboratory of Reproductive Health, National Health Commission of the People's Republic of China, Peking University, Beijing 100191, People's Republic of China
Full list of author information is available at the end of the article

females, in particular [6, 7]. In a study that compared the effectiveness of periconceptional vitamin supplementation for the prevention of NTDs recurrence in England and Ireland, beneficial effects were apparent in both countries, and all but one recurrence occurred in male fetuses [8]. A subsequent population study revealed that females tend to have craniorachischisis, spina bifida involving the upper spine, anencephaly, and encephalocoeles more often than males, while males more often have spina bifida affecting the lower spine [9].

Although these findings support the supposition that the less commonly affected sex may be less responsive to environmental therapy, the different rates of NTDs according to sex are difficult to explain because neural tubes close before sex differentiation occurs [8]. While the sequence of maternal events that take place during the development of a fetus are slightly different depending on the sex of the fetus (at least early in pregnancy), the development of male fetuses may be better synchronized on average with these events than female fetuses, from the point of view of NTD [10]. The pattern of variation between the sexes seems to suggest that there are two causes of anencephaly; 1) an environmental cause that predominantly affects female embryos, or 2) an environmental or genetic cause that seems to affect the sexes in roughly equal numbers [6]. However, this difference could also be due to other reasons including sex differences in genetic risk, epigenetic factors, timing of neural tube formation, fetal loss rates, and susceptibility to environmental influences [11, 12].

Periconceptional supplementation with folic acid (FA) has been shown to dramatically reduce the risk for pregnancies complicated with NTDs in different countries including in northern China [13]. Indeed, a recent meta-analysis concluded that fortifying food with FA reduces the overall incidence of NTDs by about 37% globally [14]; however, how this effect may differ by sex is unclear. In addition, some previous studies on NTDs have lacked data on NTD type and/or the sex affected [15, 16]. Still, others did not find significant differences in the effects of FA according to NTD subtype [17] or tended to generalize the apparent protective effects of folate [18, 19]. Contrarily, a study in Mexico found that administration of 5 mg FA each week to be associated with a 50% reduction in the incidence of NTDs, the main effect was on spina bifida, with a higher reduction in female cases [12]. More recent studies in Chile and Argentina showed that folic acid fortification resulted in a greater reduction of anencephaly and cervico-thoracic spina bifida in females compared to males [20]. However, results are not widely generalizable due to the use of a cross-sectional study, as opposed to a population based study. An animal study demonstrated that high maternal FA levels alter gene expression in cerebral hemispheres in a sex-specific manner [21]. In some other studies, FA fortification decreased the rate of spina bifida in both sexes while anencephaly showed no decrease or the change was questionable [22, 23]. Hence, it remains unclear whether or not the effects of FA supplementation significantly differ by NTD subtype and/or the sex of the fetus.

Therefore, the potential sex differences in the preventive effects of FA supplementation on NTD prevalence were examined in northern China, based on a large cohort study in a public health campaign from 1993 to 1996.

Methods

Starting in 1993, the Chinese Ministry of Health conducted a public health campaign to evaluate the effects of FA on NTDs in 21 counties in southern (Zhejiang and Jiangsu) and northern (Hebei) China. The methods of the orginal study are well-described elsewhere [13, 24, 25]. There was no FA fortification, nor vitamin supplementation at the time the study conducted in China, because prenatal vitamin use was not considered part of routine antenatal care and women had little access to any vitamin supplements in the project areas at the time [24]. No folate related genotypes or family history of NTD were collected.

A well-organized pregnancy-monitoring system (PMS) was established to collect principal records of prenatal care and demographic information. All women who were preparing for marriage or who became pregnant in the project counties were registered. Women who registered with the PMS between October 1993 and September 1995, and who delivered by 31 December 1996, from five counties in northern China were included. There were 36,144 pregnancies among the enrolled subjects (37425), 97% of all pregnancies [13]. The enrolled women were advised to take a pill containing 400 μg FA every day, starting at the time of registration with the PMS and continuing until completion of the first trimester of pregnancy. If women consented to take FA, the pills were distributed at the time of registration. At the end of each month, health workers recorded the dates of all menstrual periods and how many pills remained in each bottle (if taking pills). A total of 31,960 women with detailed FA supplementation information were included in this analysis.

Ethics, consent and permissions

The project was approved by the institutional review boards of the US Centers for Disease Control and Prevention and Peking University Health Science Center. All women who took pills provided oral informed consent.

Definition of FA use

The classification and patterns of FA consumption were the same as previously reported [13]. Women who took FA pills at any time from the registration period until the end of the first trimester of pregnancy were classified as FA users. Women who did not agree to take FA or who were registered during the second trimester of pregnancy (i.e., did not have the opportunity to start taking FA by the end of the first trimester) were considered non-users. Three patterns of FA use were derived based on the start and stop date of supplement use. The groups included periconceptional use (Start: before LMP; Stop: at the end of the first trimester), preconceptional use (Start: before LMP; Stop: before LMP) and postconceptional use (Start: after LMP but within the first trimester; Stop: at the end of the first trimester). Compliance was computed as the percentage of folic acid pills that were taken as compared with the number that could have been taken; ≥80% was regarded as high compliance.

Identification of NTDs

NTDs were identified through a birth defects surveillance system [13]. This system, which was established in January 1993, collects detailed data on infants and fetuses with external structural birth defects. Live-born infants with birth defects are included in the surveillance system if they have a gestational age of at least 20 weeks and a birth defect diagnosed by 6 weeks of age. Photographs of every infant born with a suspected birth defect and all stillborn infants, whether or not a structural abnormality were collected for diagnosis. Information on all pregnancies, even those with gestations of less than 20 weeks that were electively terminated after the prenatal diagnosis of any birth defect, was also collected. Three pediatricians who were unaware of the women's pill-taking status independently reviewed the reports and photographs and assigned standard diagnostic codes; a clinical geneticist from USA validated the diagnoses. The NTDs included in our analyses were anencephaly (including iniencephaly, craniorachischisis,), spina bifida, and encephalocele. The prevalence of NTDs by infant sex was also analyzed by NTDs subtype. As anencephaly and spina bifida share causes [6], the prevalence of open NTDs was also determined.

Statistical analysis

Age, body mass index (BMI), ethnicity, education, occupation, and parity between the groups of women who had and had not taken FA, were compared. The treatment and control groups were compared to determine differences in mean body mass index (BMI), ethnicity, education, occupation, and parity using chi-square analysis and t-tests. We calculated the prevalence of NTDs and subtypes according to the patterns of FA intake. Male to female rate ratios [RR] and their 95% confidence intervals [CI] were calculated. Relative Rate of Prevalence decreased (%) = [(Prevalence of group without FA supplementation -Prevalence of group with FA supplementation)/ Prevalence of group without FA supplementation]*100%.

A difference in differences (DID) model was used to compare differences in the changes in prevalence of NTDs according to maternal FA use, and differences between FA and no-FA groups [26, 20]. All data were analyzed using the SPSS software (v. 20.0; SPSS, Chicago, IL, USA). A two-tailed $p \leq 0.05$ was considered statistically significant.

Results

Of the 31,960 women, we excluded 137 (0.4%) women with twins and multiple births, 958 (3.0%) women with unknown parity, and 81 (0.3%) infants with ambiguous or unknown sex. Hence, 30,801(96.4%) women were included in our analyses. Table 1 shows select characteristics of the participants according to periconceptional use of FA by sex of infant. A total of 18,201 (59.0%) women took FA during the periconceptional period and 12,664 (41.0%) had not taken FA at all. Women who took FA were on average 2.3–2.4 years younger and their BMIs were 0.3–0.4 kg/m^2 lower than those who did not take it. Women who took FA supplements were more likely to be primiparous, factory workers, and to have higher educational levels. There were no significant differences for ethnicity between mothers of male and female infants.

A total of 106 NTD cases were recorded: 45 anencephaly, 54 spina bifida, and 7 encephalocele. The overall prevalence of NTDs was 2.5‰ among males and 4.4‰ among females. Anencephaly had a higher prevalence among females (2.2‰) than males (0.7‰), regardless of FA supplementation. NTDs were significantly more prevalent in female infants of mothers who did not take FA supplement (8.8‰) than male infants (4.2‰) of such mothers. The rates were 1.4‰ for males and 1.3‰ for females in mothers who took FA supplement (Table 2).

The comparison of folic acid supplementation characteristics showed no significant difference in average months of folic acid supplementation, timing, and compliance between male and female infants, see Table 3. Most women took 5.5 months of folic acid tablets, 70% of them were periconceptional use, and 80% of them showed high compliance (≥80%).

Total NTDs were less prevalent among males than among females. For every 1 case of total NTDs among females, only 0.58 cases occurred among males (rate ratio [RR] 0.58; 95% confidence interval [CI], 0.54–0.63). For open NTDs, RR was 0.50 (95% CI, 0.5–0.6). There

Table 1 Characteristics of subjects by periconceptional folic acid use and sex of infant

Characteristics	Male infant					Female infant				
	Women with folic acid ($n = 9497$)		Women without folic acid ($n = 6644$)		*P* value	Women with folic acid ($n = 8652$)		Women without folic acid ($n = 6008$)		*P* value
	n(SD)	%	n(SD)	%		n(SD)	%	n(SD)	%	
Age at pregnancy, years	24.5(2.5)		26.8(3.9)		< 0.001	24.5(2.4)		26.9(4.0)		< 0.001
Body mass index, kg/m^2	21.2(2.0)		21.5(1.9)		< 0.001	21.2(2.0)		21.6(1.9)		< 0.001
Primiparous	9078	95.6	4211	63.4	< 0.001	8297	95.9	3758	62.5	< 0.001
Han ethnic group	9258	99.0	6544	99.2	0.123	8395	98.9	5914	99.2	0.092
Education										
High school or higher	869	9.3	505	7.7	0.001	773	9.1	442	7.4	0.001
Junior high school	7219	77.4	5212	79.0		6563	77.5	4704	79.0	
Primary school or lower, or unknown	1239	13.3	882	13.4		1127	13.3	811	13.6	
Occupation										
Farmer	8180	86.1	6058	91.2	0.000	7424	85.8	5494	91.4	< 0.001
Factory worker	944	9.9	443	6.7		836	9.7	380	6.3	
Other or unknown	373	3.9	143	2.2		392	4.5	134	2.2	

Values for some characteristics may not be equal to total numbers in each group because of missing values
SD standard deviation

was a higher prevalence of anencephaly (RR, 0.34; CI, 0.27–0.43) and spina bifida (RR, 0.73; CI, 0.63–0.84) among females, but this trend was only significant among infants born to mothers who did not take supplements (Table 4).

In our analyses, the decreases in the rates of anencephaly (4.8‰), open NTDs (7.5‰), and total NTDs (7.6‰) were significantly greater in females than in males (1.6‰, 2.6‰, and 2.8‰, respectively) (Table 5).

Discussion

NTDs are serious birth defects that occur during early pregnancy and affect the spine (e.g., spina bifida) and the brain (e.g., anencephaly). A large number of studies have found that 50–70% of these defects can be prevented by women consuming sufficient FA daily before conception and throughout the first trimester of pregnancy [13, 27, 28]. In our study, 41% of women didn't take folic acid supplementation, among those who took folic acid, the compliance≥80% was 81%, which indicated half of mothers in our study achieved sufficient FA daily intake. Based on a large prospective cohort study, we found that FA supplementation had beneficial effects for the prevention NTDs in both males and females. However, our most important finding is that the effect was much stronger among females, both for open NTDs (including anencephaly and spina bifida) and total NTDs. The prevalence of NTDs in females was 7.6‰ lower compared to a 2.8‰ reduction in males among infants born to mothers who took FA versus mothers who did not. Similarly, the prevalence of anencephaly in females was 4.8‰ lower compared to 1.6‰ reduction in males among infants born to mothers who took FA versus mothers who did not.

Since many countries have adopted mandatory fortification of cereal grain products or dietary supplements containing FA, the prevalence of spina bifida and anencephaly has declined significantly [22]. Based on eight population-based surveillance systems that included prenatal ascertainment of these types of birth defects in the United States (USA), the number of NTD-affected pregnancies in the United States declined from 4000 in 1995–1996 (before the FA mandate) to 3000 in 1999–2000 (after the FA mandate). This decline highlights the partial success of the USA FA fortification program as a public health strategy [29]. However, few studies have investigated sex differences in the NTD-prevention effects of adequate maternal FA intake.

Table 2 Prevalence of NTDs by sex and folic acid supplementation in northern China, 1993–1995 (per 1000 births)

Folic acid	N	Open NTDs			Anencephaly			Spina Bifida			Encephalocele			Total NTDs		
		Male	Female	Total	Male	Female	Total	Male	Female	Total	Male	Female	Total	Male	Female	Total
Yes*	18,201	1.2	1.2	1.2	0.1	0.2	0.2	1.1	0.9	1.0	0.2	0.1	0.2	1.4	1.3	1.3
No	12,664	3.8	8.7	6.1	1.7	5.0	3.2	2.1	3.7	2.8	0.5	0.2	0.3	4.2	8.8	6.4
Total	30,801	2.2	4.2	3.2	0.7	2.2	1.4	1.5	2.0	1.8	0.3	0.1	0.2	2.5	4.4	3.4

NTD neural tube defect
*Compared to group without folic acid supplementation, $P < 0.001$

Table 3 Characteristics of folic acid supplementation by sex of infant in northern China

Characteristics	N	Women with male infants	Women with female infants	*P*-value
Folic acid supplementation (Months)	18,201	5.5(2.4)	5.5(2.4)	0.180
Timing				0.369
Periconception	12,779	70.5	70.4	
Preconception	3623	20.1	19.8	
Postconception	1714	9.7	9.4	
Compliance				0.190
< 80%	3310	17.9	18.6	
≥80%	14,839	82.1	81.4	

In China, since a massive nationwide FA supplementation program was started in 2009, an increasing number of women have begun to consume adequate amounts of FA. The program provides FA supplements, free of charge, to all women who have a rural registration (as opposed to urban registration) and who plan to become pregnant [30]. Hence, it is more important than ever to further elucidate the effects of FA supplementation on infants in China, in particular, how these effects may differ by sex.

One previous case-control study, conducted in China in 2006, reported a female predominance among anencephaly cases (RR, 0.49; 95% CI, 0.30–0.79) but not among spina bifida (RR, 0.90; 95% CI, 0.55–1.45) or encephalocele (RR, 1.03; 95% CI, 0.40–2.69) cases [31]. In our study, we found that females had a higher prevalence of anencephaly and spina bifida, particularly among infants whose mothers did not take FA supplements (anencephaly: RR, 0.34; CI, 0.27–0.43; spina bifida: RR, 0.73; CI, 0.63–0.84). In addition, the male–female ratio was higher for anencephaly and spina bifida in the group associated with FA supplements than in the non-FA group. The fact that FA prevented more female anencephaly cases may indicate heterogeneity in the causes of NTDs. One animal study revealed that female embryos tend to have more NTDs than males [32]. This could be an epigenetic phenomenon considering females methylate most of the DNA in the large inactive X chromosome after each cell division. Consequently, methylation needs for other cells may not be met [33]. Genetic and environmental factors contribute to increase sex ratios in exencephaly (an early stage of anencephaly) and spina bifida, due to preferential lethality of females [34]. Burren et al. [35], however, reported that folate deficiency resulted in an increased frequency of cranial NTDs in embryos carrying the Sp^{2H}, which carries an intragenic deletion in the Pax3 gene. Remarkable differences between sexes were observed in response to FA supplementation, with no treatment effect observed among females. In contrast, our findings suggest that open NTDs (including anencephaly) in female human embryos are responsive to FA. Other possible explanations include folic acids exertion of a protective effects through varying mechanisms that more strongly impact females. For example, epigenetic X-inactivation, among other mechanisms, may proceed through different pathways in males and females [20].

The present study had several strengths. First, it was based on a well-organized population-based monitoring system, that used quality control to ensure data quality [13], including village health workers distributed, counted and recorded the dates of menstrual periods for women enrolled and the pills to reflect FA supplementation, the independent, blind and standard diagnosis and final validation of NTDs diagnosis. The use of a population-based surveillance system that covered all live births, all stillbirths at 20 or more gestational weeks, and pregnancy terminations after the prenatal diagnosis of any birth defect at any gestational age was a second strength of the study. This could lay the groundwork for more precise estimations of NTDs than hospital-based surveillance systems [36], especially considering that the

Table 4 Male:female rate ratio of NTDs by folic acid supplementation in northern China, 1993–1995

Folic acid	N	Open NTDs		Anencephaly		Spina bifida		Encephalocele		Total NTDs	
		RR	95% CI	RR	95% CI	RR	95% CI	RR	95% CI	RR	95% CI
Yes	18,201	1.00	0.69–1.46	0.46	0.02–8.62	1.14	0.73–1.77	1.82	0.10–34.48	1.08	0.77–1.50
No	12,664	0.43	0.39–0.49	0.33	0.26–0.42	0.58	0.46–0.72	2.71	0.20–37.04	0.48	0.43–0.53
Total	30,801	0.53	0.48–0.57	0.34	0.27–0.43	0.73	0.63–0.84	2.27	0.58–8.59	0.58	0.54–0.63

NTD neural tube defect, *RR* rate ratio, 95%CI, 95% confidence interval

Table 5 Change in prevalence rates of NTDs due to FA supplementation by NTD type and sex in northern China, 1993–1995 (per 1000 births)

Change	Male rate	Female rate	Female–Male DID Value	*P* value
Open NTDs	2.6	7.5	4.9	0.000
Anencephaly	1.6	4.8	3.2	0.000
Spina bifida	1.1	2.7	1.6	0.083
Encephalocele	0.2	0.1	−0.1	0.587
Total NTDs	2.8	7.6	4.8	0.000

Rate of prevalence decrease = Prevalence of group without FA supplementation − Prevalence of group with FA supplementation
NTD neural tube defect, *FA* folic acid

majority of fetuses with NTDs are terminated following prenatal diagnosis before 28 gestational weeks in China [37]. Third, we obtained data for NTDs before the national FA supplementation program, which could best reflect the natural status of the population. Fourth, we compared the folic acid supplementation characteristics between mothers of male infants and female infants, which showed no significant difference. Our study revealed the sex-specific effects of folic acid supplementation in a large prospective study.

However, a couple limitations should also be noted. One limitation was that we did not include the detailed subtype of spina bifida (e.g., severe vs. mild), which may be heterogeneous in cause. A further study may be useful to address this. In addition, we did not collect information on the diets of women, which could have influenced the results. However, the study area was in northern China, and the majority of participants were of Han ethnicity, thus there may be a traditional northern diet pattern in play and would likely not affect the overall trends observed in the study. The third limitation was no folate related genotypes or family history of NTD was collected.

Conclusions

Overall, FA supplementation successfully reduces the prevalence of NTDs in both male and female infants, although there is a significantly greater decrease in anencephaly and total NTDs in females than in males. How the protective effects of FA supplementation affect the sexes differently needs to be studied further. In addition to genetic and environmental factors in determining sex ratios, future studies are needed to investigate the importance of epigenetic factors, imprinting effects, methylation status, and the folate supplementation effect pathway in altering NTDs risk.

Abbreviations

BMI: Body mass index; DID: Difference in differences; FA: Folic acid; NTD: Neural tube defects; PMS: Pregnancy-monitoring system

Acknowledgements

We are grateful to the thousands of health workers, village doctors from the study counties, and the staffs of Institute of reproductive and child health, who participated the project.

Funding

This work was supported in part by the National Key Research and Development Program, Ministry of Science and Technology, P.R. China (grant No. 2016YFC1000500), National Natural Science Foundation of China (No. 81373014 and No. 81202265). The original project was supported by a cooperative agreement between the US Centers for Disease Control and Prevention and Peking University (grant No. U01 DD000293). There is no role of the funding body in the design of the study and collection, analysis, and interpretation of data and in writing the manuscript.

Authors' contributions

JFL analyzed the data and wrote the first draft of the manuscript, ZWL designed the research and analyzed the data, RY collected the data and interpreted the data, AR interpreted the data and revised the draft, JML revised the draft and provided critical suggestions on the study. All authors read, reviewed and approved the final manuscript.

Competing interests

The authors declare that they have no competing interests.

Author details

[1]Institute of Reproductive and Child Health / Key Laboratory of Reproductive Health, National Health Commission of the People's Republic of China, Peking University, Beijing 100191, People's Republic of China. [2]Department of Epidemiology and Biostatistics, School of Public Health, Peking University, Beijing 100191, People's Republic of China.

References

1. Hay S. Sex differences in the incidence of certain congenital malformations: a review of the literature and some new data. Teratology. 1971;4:277–86.
2. Fernando J, Arena P, Smith DW. Sex liability to single structural defects. Am J Dis Child. 1978;132:970–2.
3. Lary JM, Paulozzi LJ. Sex differences in the prevalence of human birth defects: a population-based study. Teratology. 2001;64:237–51.
4. Timson J. The sex ratio in anencephaly. Genetica. 1970;41:457–65.
5. Mayo O. Sex ratio in spina bifida and anencephaly. Genetica. 1971; 42:437–44.
6. James WH. The sex ratio in anencephaly. J Med Genet. 1979;16:129–33.
7. Machin GA. Etiology of neural tube defect in man--do teratogens play any part? Evidence from sex ratios. Med Hypotheses. 1979;5:277–88.
8. Seller MJ, Nevin NC. Periconceptional vitamin supplementation and the prevention of neural tube defects in south-East England and Northern Ireland. J Med Genet. 1984;21:325–30.
9. Seller MJ. Sex, neural tube defects, and multisite closure of the human neural tube. Am J Med Genet. 1995;58:332–6.
10. James WH. A possible mechanism underlying the sex selectivity of neural tube defect. J Med Genet. 1985;22:319.
11. Brown AS, Susser ES. Sex differences in prevalence of congenital neural defects after periconceptional famine exposure. Epidemiology. 1997;8:55–8.
12. Martinez de Villarreal LE, Arredondo P, Hernandez R, Villarreal JZ. Weekly administration of folic acid and epidemiology of neural tube defects. Matern Child Health J. 2006;10:397–401.
13. Berry RJ, Li Z, Erickson JD, Li S, Moore CA, Wang H, Mulinare J, Zhao P, Wong LY, Gindler J, Hong SX, Correa A. Prevention of neural-tube defects with folic acid in China. China-U.S. collaborative project for neural tube defect prevention. N Engl J Med. 1999;341:1485–90.
14. Brinkhof M, Meier S, Chamberlain J, Mader L. The impact of folic acid food fortification on global incidence of neural tube defects: systematic

review, meta-analysis and estimate of preventable cases. Int J Epidemiol. 2015;44:143.
15. Kirke PN, Daly LE, Elwood JH. A randomised trial of low dose folic acid to prevent neural tube defects. The Irish vitamin study group. Arch Dis Child. 1992;67:1442–6.
16. Smithells RW, Sheppard S, Schorah CJ, Seller MJ, Nevin NC, Harris R, Read AP, Fielding DW. Apparent prevention of neural tube defects by periconceptional vitamin supplementation. 1981. Int J Epidemiol. 2011;40: 1146–54.
17. MRC Vitamin Study Research Group. Prevention of neural tube defects: results of the Medical Research Council vitamin study. Lancet. 1991;338:131–7.
18. Shaw GM, Todoroff K, Lammer EJ. NTD phenotypes in infants and fetuses whose mothers used multivitamins containing folic acid in early pregnancy compared to those who did not. Am J Med Genet. 1997;70:330–1.
19. Seller MJ. Multi-site neural tube closure in humans and maternal folate supplementation. Am J Med Genet. 1995;58:222–4.
20. Poletta FA, Rittler M, Saleme C, Campana H, Gili JA, Pawluk MS, Gimenez LG, Cosentino VR, Castilla EE, Lopez-Camelo JS. Neural tube defects: sex ratio changes after fortification with folic acid. PLoS One. 2018;13:e0193127.
21. Barua S, Kuizon S, Brown WT, Junaid MA. High gestational folic acid supplementation alters expression of imprinted and candidate autism susceptibility genes in a sex-specific manner in mouse offspring. J Mol Neurosci. 2016;58:277–86.
22. Honein MA, Paulozzi LJ, Mathews TJ, Erickson JD, Wong LY. Impact of folic acid fortification of the US food supply on the occurrence of neural tube defects. JAMA. 2001;285:2981–6.
23. Williams LJ, Mai CT, Edmonds LD, Shaw GM, Kirby RS, Hobbs CA, Sever LE, Miller LA, Meaney FJ, Levitt M. Prevalence of spina bifida and anencephaly during the transition to mandatory folic acid fortification in the United States. Teratology. 2002;66:33–9.
24. Li Z, Ye R, Zhang L, Li H, Liu J, Ren A. Periconceptional folic acid supplementation and the risk of preterm births in China: a large prospective cohort study. Int J Epidemiol. 2014;43:1132–9.
25. Li N, Li Z, Ye R, Liu J, Ren A. Impact of Periconceptional folic acid supplementation on low birth weight and small-for-gestational-age infants in China: a large prospective cohort study. J Pediatr. 2017;187:105–10.
26. Ashenfelter O, Card D. Using the longitudinal structure of earnings to estimate the effect of training-programs. Rev Econ Stat. 1985;67:648–60.
27. Oakley GP Jr, Erickson JD, James LM, Mulinare J, Cordero JF. Prevention of folic acid-preventable spina bifida and anencephaly. CIBA Found Symp. 1994;181:212–23 discussion 23-31.
28. Czeizel AE, Dudas I. Prevention of the first occurrence of neural-tube defects by periconceptional vitamin supplementation. N Engl J Med. 1992;327: 1832–5.
29. Mersereau P, Kilker K, Carter H, Fassett E, Williams J, Flores A, Prue C, Williams L, Mai C, Mulinare J. Spina bifida and anencephaly before and after folic acid mandate - United States, 1995-1996 and 1999-2000 (Reprinted from MMWR, vol 53, pg 362, 2004). JAMA. 2004;292:325–6.
30. Ren AG. Prevention of neural tube defects with folic acid: the Chinese experience. World J Clin Pediatr. 2015;4:41–4.
31. Li Z, Ren A, Zhang L, Ye R, Li S, Zheng J, Hong S, Wang T, Li Z. Extremely high prevalence of neural tube defects in a 4-county area in Shanxi Province, China. Birth Defects Res A Clin Mol Teratol. 2006;76:237–40.
32. Chen X, Watkins R, Delot E, Reliene R, Schiestl RH, Burgoyne PS, Arnold AP. Sex difference in neural tube defects in p53-null mice is caused by differences in the complement of X not Y genes. Dev Neurobiol. 2008;68: 265–73.
33. Juriloff DM, Harris MJ. Hypothesis: the female excess in cranial neural tube defects reflects an epigenetic drag of the inactivating X chromosome on the molecular mechanisms of neural fold elevation. Birth Defects Res A Clin Mol Teratol. 2012;94:849–55.
34. Martin LJ, Machado AF, Loza MA, Mao GE, Lee GS, Hovland DN Jr, Cantor RM, Collins MD. Effect of arsenite, maternal age, and embryonic sex on spina bifida, exencephaly, and resorption rates in the splotch mouse. Birth Defects Res A Clin Mol Teratol. 2003;67:231–9.
35. Burren KA, Savery D, Massa V, Kok RM, Scott JM, Blom HJ, Copp AJ, Greene ND. Gene-environment interactions in the causation of neural tube defects: folate deficiency increases susceptibility conferred by loss of Pax3 function. Hum Mol Genet. 2008;17:3675–85.
36. Ministry of Health C. China Birth Defects Prevention report (2012). 2012.
37. Li K, He XB, Zhang L, Li ZW, Ye RW, Liu JM, Zhai RQ, Duan XJ, Ren AG. Impact of pregnancy terminations before 28 weeks of gestation on the overall prevalence of neural tube defects in two counties of Shanxi province. Zhonghua Liu Xing Bing Xue Za Zhi. 2012;33:509–12.

16

The relationship between the leptin/ghrelin ratio and meals with various macronutrient contents in men with different nutritional status

Edyta Adamska-Patruno[1*], Lucyna Ostrowska[2], Joanna Goscik[1], Barbara Pietraszewska[2], Adam Kretowski[1,3] and Maria Gorska[3]

Abstract

Background: Hormones, which influence satiety and hunger, play a significant role in body energy balance regulation. Ghrelin is a peptide that plays an important role in short-term appetite regulation, whereas leptin is a factor that controls long-term energy balance and is considered as a satiety hormone. The aim of this study was to evaluate the leptin/ghrelin ratio in a fasting state and after the intake of meals with varying macronutrient contents and to assess the possible differences between normal body weight and overweight/obese men.

Methods: We examined 46 healthy adult men (23 with normal body weight and 23 overweight/obese) aged 21–58, who were divided into two groups. In the crossover study, participants received isocaloric (450 kcal) meals with different macronutrient contents: men from the first group received high-carbohydrate (HC) and normo-carbohydrate (NC) meals, and in the second group, participants received high-carbohydrate and high-fat (HF) meals. The ratio of leptin/ghrelin levels was calculated from leptin and total ghrelin serum concentrations in a fasting state and 30, 60, 120, 180 and 240 min after meal intake. One-way ANOVA and Wilcoxon signed-rank tests were carried out. The normality of the variable distribution was checked with the Shapiro–Wilk test, the homogeneity of variances was verified with the Levene test, and the false discovery rate *p*-value adjustment method was used.

Results: The leptin/ghrelin ratio was significantly higher in overweight/obese men than individuals with normal body weight in a fasting state, as well as postprandially. We observed trends towards a higher leptin/ghrelin ratio values from the 60 min after HC-meal intake compared to the NC- and HF-meals in normal body weight participants, while in overweight/obese men, we did not note any significant differences dependent on the meal type.

Conclusions: We have observed a significantly different postprandial leptin/ghrelin ratio in normal body weight and overweight/obese men, and our results suggest that in men with normal body weight, a greater feeling of satiety may occur after high-carbohydrate meal intake, which was not noted in the overweight/obese individuals.

Keywords: Leptin/ghrelin ratio, Postprandial state, High-carbohydrate meal, High-fat meal, Normo-carbohydrate meal, Normal body weight men, Overweight/obesity

* Correspondence: edyta.adamska@umb.edu.pl
[1]Clinical Research Centre, Medical University of Bialystok, Sklodowskiej 24A, 15-276, Bialystok, MC, Poland
Full list of author information is available at the end of the article

Background

Obesity is a chronic disease caused mostly by an excessive supply of energy delivered with food in relation to energy expenditure, which leads to fat accumulation in adipose tissue [1]. Although the basic function of adipose tissue is energy storage, it is also an organ of endocrine secretion, which produces hormones, adipokines and cytokines [2], such as leptin, adiponectin, which are involved in body energy homeostasis and many other pathways [3]. In the central regulation of energy balance, other peripherally produced signals also participate in this process, such as fatty acids, insulin, glucagon-like peptide-1 (GLP-1), ghrelin, cholecystokinin (CCK), peptide YY (PYY) [4, 5], as well as several other molecules recently linked to energy homeostasis regulation, such as chemerin, total bile acids, fibroblast growth factor 21 (FGF-21), secreted frizzled-related protein-4 (SFRP4), irisin, and heme oxygenase-1(HO-1) [6], which can be regulated by the macronutrient composition of the diet [4–6]. As listed above, many factors are involved in energy balance control, but one of the key roles in hormonal regulation of food intake is played by ghrelin and leptin, and their interactions, since these hormones affect the energy balance antagonistically [7–9].

Ghrelin is an orexigenic hormone secreted primarily by P/D1 cells, located in the mucosa of the stomach fundus, pancreatic epsilon cells, kidneys, gonads and adipose tissue [7]. Ghrelin plays an important role in short-term appetite regulation and is characterized by increased concentrations before meal intake, and decreased levels after meal ingestion [10]. The orexigenic action of ghrelin is based on increasing gastrointestinal peristalsis and reducing insulin secretion, and despite its appetite stimulation effects, it was found that obesity, type 2 diabetes mellitus and metabolic syndrome are associated with lower serum ghrelin concentrations [7, 8, 11].

Leptin is another important signal that influences energy balance, suggested to reduce food intake and increases energy expenditure. Leptin is a hormone synthesized mainly by adipocytes but also by the stomach [12], and it inhibits appetite by counteracting the action of neuropeptide Y (NPY) and anandamines, as well as by stimulating α-Melanocyte-stimulating hormone (α-MSH) synthesis [7]. Leptin secretion is proportional to the total amount of adipose tissue, and its serum concentration increases significantly in obesity [9]. A few years ago, it was thought that leptin played a significant role only in long-term energy balance; however, the data suggest that leptin is also involved in short-term food intake and body weight regulation [10, 12]. Therefore, in the analysis of hormonal response after meal intake, it is reasonable to combine these two hormones together, and due to their interaction, the ratio of their concentrations (leptin/ghrelin ratio) is defined as a hunger signal, called the "ghrelin-leptin tango" [13]. It has been found that leptin and ghrelin concentrations depend on body weight and postprandially, on meal composition, but studies on their ratio are very limited with varying results [11, 14, 15].

Because obesity has become a global problem, the mechanisms of its development, and the identification of effective prevention and treatment strategies are of high priority. The aim of our study was to investigate the leptin/ghrelin ratio in response to meal intake with various macronutrient contents in a crossover designed study, as well as to assess the fasting and postprandial differences between normal body weight and overweight/obese men.

Methods

The study protocol was approved by the local Ethics Committee (R-I-002/35/2009 approval of Bioethical Committee of Medical University of Bialystok, Poland). Participants were informed about the purpose and study signed informed consent consciously and voluntarily.

Study design and population. The study groups, study procedures and statistical analysis were previously described in detail [16, 17], and the presented results are part of a bigger project [18–20]. Briefly, the study was conducted among 46 non-diabetic men. Anthropometric measurements (body weight, height, and calculated BMI), and percentage of adipose tissue (bioimpedance method, InBody, InBody 220, Biospace, Korea) were performed. The participants were randomly divided into two groups. Each group included men with normal body weight (BMI $< 25\ kg/m^2$) and overweight/obesity (BMI $> 25\ kg/m^2$) (Table 1). The study was carried out by the crossover method. The subjects received standardized isocaloric (450 kcal) meals with different contents of basic nutrients during two subsequent visits (Fig. 1). Group I: 11 men with normal body weight (N1) and 12 subjects with overweight/obesity (O/O1) received a high-carbohydrate/fat-free meal (HC-meal, *Nutridrink Fat Free, Nutricia, Poland*) and a normo-carbohydrate/high-protein meal (NC-meal, *Cubitan, Nutricia, Poland*); and Group II: 12 men with normal body weight (N2), and 11 subjects with overweight/obesity(O/O2) received the high-carbohydrate/fat-free meal (HC-meal, *Nutridrink Fat Free, Nutricia, Poland*) and a high-fat/low-carbohydrate meal (HF-meal, *Calogen, Nutricia, Poland*). The energy and macronutrient contents for all meals are presented in Table 2. The study duration was approximately 3 weeks and included a screening visit and two meal challenge test visits, during which participants received the test meals, with 1–2 week intervals between tests. Subjects were asked to maintain their usual diet and lifestyle throughout the study. After at least 12-h fasting, at approximately 08.00–08.30 AM, all anthropometric measurements were performed, and a cannula was inserted into the vein. To determine leptin and

Table 1 Study population characteristics

		Normal body weight men	Overweight/obese men	*p*-value
Group I	n	11	12	
	Age (years)	33 ± 2	40 ± 2	0.01
	BMI (kg/m^2)	23.8 ± 0.5	31.4 ± 1.5	0.0002
	Body fat content (%)	17.9 ± 1.0	28.6 ± 1.7	0.00003
Group II	n	12	11	
	Age (years)	33 ± 3	36 ± 3	0.24
	BMI (kg/m^2)	23.9 ± 0.2	33.7 ± 2.2	0.000001
	Body fat content (%)	18.6 ± 1.5	31.9 ± 2.7	0.0002

The results are presented as mean values ± SE

ghrelin concentrations, which were used for leptin/ghrelin ratio calculations, venous blood was collected immediately prior to meal intake (0 min), and at 30, 60, 120, 180 and 240 min after meal intake.

Biochemical analysis. Blood was drawn, centrifuged, stored at − 80 °C, and prepared for testing as previously described, in accordance with the recommendations and procedures provided by the laboratory kit producers. Leptin concentration was measured using an enzyme immunoassay (Human Leptin ELISA, BioVendor, Czech Republic). Total ghrelin concentration was measured using a radioimmunoassay (Ghrelin (total) RIA, Millipore, USA).

Statistical analysis. The statistical analysis has been described in detail previously [17]. The mean value and its standard error were calculated, and two hypotheses were stated: (1) the type of meal does not influence the postprandial leptin/ghrelin ratio (the normal body weight and overweight/obese men were analysed separately), and (2) there is no statistically significant difference in postprandial leptin/ghrelin ratio between normal body weight and overweight/obese individuals (the types of meals were analysed separately).

Since participants in every group received two different meals, the lack of independence was taken into consideration. One-way ANOVA (analysis of variance), or the Wilcoxon signed-rank test, both for paired samples, were carried out, dependent on fulfilment of the normality of variable distribution, which was checked by the Shapiro–Wilk test.

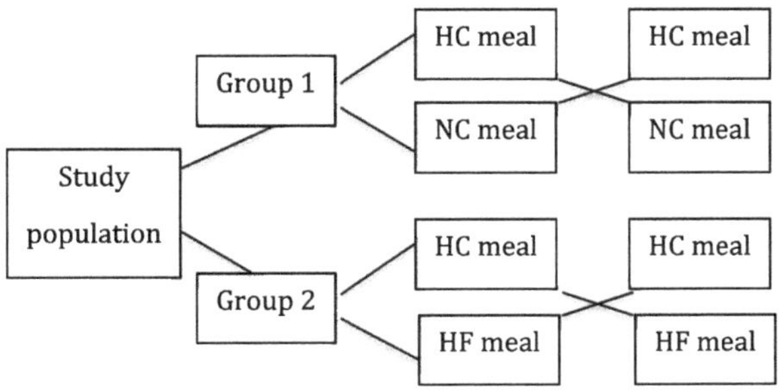

Fig. 1 Study design. HC-meal (high-carbohydrate meal); NC-meal (normo-carbohydrate meal); HF-meal (high-fat meal)

The goal of the second hypothesis was to investigate whether there are any significant differences in the postprandial leptin/ghrelin ratio between normal body weight and overweight/obese men. We used one-way ANOVA or the Wilcoxon rank-sum test, depending on the normality of variable distribution, and the homogeneity of variances (verified with the Levene test). The false discovery rate *p*-value adjustment method was used to address the issue of multiple hypothesis testing. For all analyses, the alpha level was set at 0.05.

Results

In Group I, the leptin/ghrelin ratio after the HC-meal intake vs. the leptin/ghrelin ratio after the NC-meal intake was analysed. In N1 subjects we observed a trend towards higher leptin/ghrelin ratio values from 60 min after the HC-meal compared to the NC-meal (Table 3). In O/O1 men we did not notice any significant differences in the leptin/ghrelin ratio between both meals.

In Group II, the leptin/ghrelin ratio after the HC-meal intake vs. the leptin/ghrelin ratio after the HF-meal intake was analysed. In N2 subjects we noted a trend towards higher leptin/ghrelin ratio values at 60 min of testing after the HC-meal intake when compared to the HF-meal, and at 120 min the difference almost reached statistical significance ($p = 0.06$), which was not observed in the O/O2 subjects (Table 4).

Subsequently, the leptin/ghrelin ratio was compared between normal body weight and overweight/obese individuals after meal intake in Group I (Fig. 2) and Group II (Fig. 3). We noticed that the leptin/ghrelin ratio was significantly higher in overweight/obese men, compared to normal body weight participants in a fasting state, as well as postprandially in both groups and after all the three meals. A more favourable leptin/ghrelin ratio in normal body weight men was observed after the HC-meal intake compared to the NC- and HF-meals, while in overweight/obese individuals, we did not note any significant differences dependent on the meal type.

Table 2 The energy and macronutrient composition of tested meals

	High-carbohydrate meal	Normo-carbohydrate meal	High-fat meal
Energy (kcal)	450	450	450
Carbohydrate (g)	100.5	51.1	4.0
Carbohydrate (% of total energy)	89.3	45.1	4.0
Fat (g)	0	12.6	47.5
Fat (% of total energy)	0	25.2	96
Protein (g)	12	36	0
Protein (% of total energy)	10.7	29.7	0
Fibre (g)	0	0.1	0

Discussion

Energy balance is regulated by central and peripheral signals, but the final clinical effect is not a consequence of the individual action of only one hormone, but depends on their interactions [9]. Therefore in our study we analysed the ratio of two crucial hormones that impact hunger and satiety feelings- the leptin to total ghrelin concentrations. The main finding of our study is that in normal body weight men, a more beneficial leptin/ghrelin ratio was noted after the HC-meal intake, compared to the NC- and HF-meals. The other observation is that overweight/obese men presented with a significantly higher leptin/ghrelin ratio in a fasting state, as well as after intake of each of the three meals, compared to normal body weight participants.

Our results seem to confirm the observations of Sanchez J et al. [21], who noted higher inhibition of stomach ghrelin production after a high-carbohydrate diet compared to a high-fat diet in Wistar rats. Moreover, the authors also noticed that carbohydrate intake (but not fat intake) stimulated gastric leptin expression, though the gastric leptin levels decreased after food intake without any differences between carbohydrate or fat intake. Other authors [22] noted that a higher leptin to ghrelin ratio was significantly correlated with a lower resting metabolic rate. These results are consistent with the findings of our studies, since in the overweight/obese group, in which we observed a higher leptin/ghrelin ratio in the current study, we also noted in a previously published analysis a lower energy expenditure in a fasting state, as well as postprandially [17]. It has been shown that leptin increases energy expenditure in particular through its effects on the cardiovascular system, as well as on brown adipose tissue thermogenesis via the hypothalamus [23], while ghrelin was found to decrease energy expenditure, mainly through stimulating the activity of neuropeptide Y/agouti-related protein (NPY/AgRP) and hypocretin/orexin cells, and decreasing the activity of proopiomelanocortin (POMC) and corticotropin releasing hormone (CRH) cells [24].

A significantly higher leptin/ghrelin ratio was observed in overweight/obese subjects in a fasting state, as well as after intake of each of the tested meals, which undoubtedly is a result of its higher fasting level in overweight/obese men. However, we have noted that in normal body weight men, there is strong tendency for an increased leptin/ghrelin ratio after the HC-meal than after the NC-meal intake, especially after 120–180 min. The opposite trends were noted in the overweight/obese group, where the increase of the leptin/ghrelin ratio was more

Table 3 Comparison of the leptin/ghrelin ratio after the HC- and NC-meal intake, in the population of study Group I

G1	Time (min)	0	30	60	120	180	240
High-carbohydrate (HC) meal vs normo-carbohydrate (NC) meal	N1-HC	5.01 ±1.75	4.71 ±1.55	5.28 ±2.00	6.74 ±2.39	5.59 ±1.79	4.92 ±1.47
	N1-NC	3.50 ±1.21	4.25 ±1.63	3.11 ±0.80	3.04 ±0.96	3.32 ±0.91	2.92 ±0.67
	†p=	0.59	0.57	0.17	0.06	0.07	0.14
	O/O1-HC	21.00 ±5.25	17.44 ±4.91	17.84 ±3.74	18.40 ±3.72	20.05 ±4.41	17.63 ±4.36
	O/O1-NC	19.25 ±7.10	16.49 ±4.05	19.87 ±4.33	24.15 ±8.84	20.85 ±5.28	19.15 ±4.40
	‡p=	0.26	0.57	0.67	1.0	0.34	0.68

The results are presented as mean values ± SE. † comparison between the high-carbohydrate (HC) and normo-carbohydrate (NC) meals in the normal body weight (N1) group; ‡ comparison between the high-carbohydrate (HC) and normo-carbohydrate (NC) meals in the overweight/obesity (O/O1) group

Table 4 Comparison of the leptin/ghrelin ratio after the HC- and HF-meal intake, in the population of study Group II

G2	Time (min)	0	30	60	120	180	240
High-carbohydrate (HC) meal vs high-fat (HF) meal	N2-HC	7.02 ±1.49	7.43 ±1.41	8.70 ±1.73	8.83 ±2.10	8.18 ±1.68	7.31 ±1.25
	N2-HF	7.01 ±1.66	6.19 ±1.45	6.97 ±1.77	6.91 ±1.54	7.55 ±2.06	6.84 ±1.51
	†p=	0.99	0.22	0.10	0.06	0.63	0.67
	O/O2-HC	38.21 ±14.50	31.55 ±12.12	30.58 ±10.20	32.45 ±10.82	37.57 ±14.44	28.04 ±10.01
	O/O2-HF	27.50 ±10.84	29.77 ±10.11	29.76 ±9.51	33.56 ±11.89	25.63 ±7.84	28.37 ±8.38
	‡p=	0.27	0.88	0.59	0.45	0.22	0.50

The results are presented as mean values ± SE. † comparison between the high-carbohydrate (HC) and high-fat (HF) meals in the normal body weight (N2) group; ‡ comparison between the high-carbohydrate (HC) and high-fat (HF) meals in the overweight/obesity (O/O2) group

marked after the NC-meal intake, while after the HC-meal, the mean values decreased postprandially. However, the differences were not significant, most likely due to the high standard error. We observed similar results in the G2 group. The tendency of an increase the leptin/ghrelin ratio was noted in normal body weight men after the HC- compared to the HF-meal, especially 120 min after meal intake, while in the overweight/obese group, the mean values decreased postprandially, and increased after the HF-meal intake, but the differences were not significant, maybe due to too high standard error, or too small a study sample.

To our knowledge, there are not any data that we can compare our leptin/ghrelin ratio results to, but different ghrelin and leptin concentrations have been demonstrated to be dependent on nutritional status [11], as well as on meal composition [25]. We decided to analyse leptin and ghrelin together, as the leptin/ghrelin ratio, since these are two of the main hormones that influence the metabolic status of the body, appetite and hunger sensations, etc., which are an effect of the hormone interactions, rather than an effect of only one individual hormone's action. Therefore, with a higher leptin/ghrelin ratio, we can expect more beneficial effects in suppressing the feeling of hunger. However neither the relationship between leptin/ghrelin ratio to hunger and satiety regulation, nor the metabolic states and consequences, have been published so far. Previous studies have found that increased ghrelin to leptin ratio correlated with increased hunger and appetite [26, 27]; therefore, we can suppose that with a higher leptin to ghrelin ratio, hunger and appetite should decrease. The only three studies that analysed the leptin/ghrelin ratio were focused on the relationship with child obesity [28] and resting metabolic rate, and this ratio was considered as a possible biomarker for predicting metabolic adaptations to energy restriction treatment [22], and as a non-invasive tool

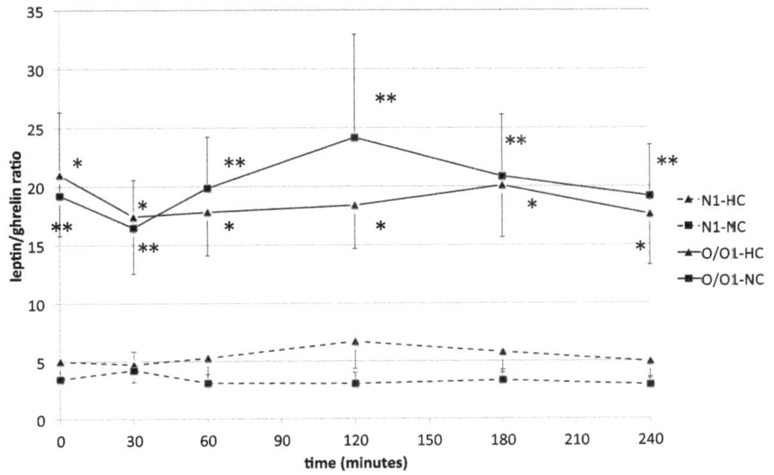

Fig. 2 Comparison of the leptin/ghrelin ratio between normal body weight and overweight/obese men. The results are presented as mean values ± SE. N1, broken line- men with normal body weight; O/O1, solid line- overweight/obese subjects; HC- high-carbohydrate meal; NC- normo-carbohydrate meal. The comparison between the N1 and O/O1 study groups after HC-meal intake *$p < 0.05$, and after NC-meal intake **$p < 0.05$

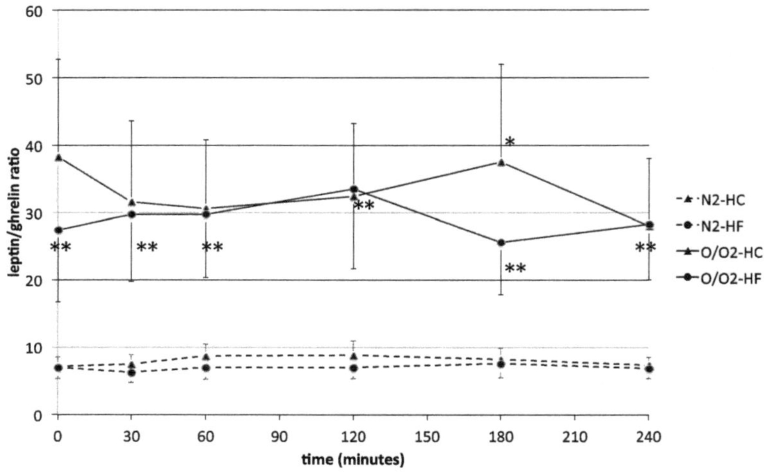

Fig. 3 Comparison of the leptin/ghrelin ratio between normal body weight and overweight/obese men. The results are presented as mean values ± SE. N2, broken line- men with normal body weight; O/O2, solid line- overweight/obese subjects; HC- high-carbohydrate meal; HF- high-fat meal. The comparison between the N2 and O/O2 study groups after HC-meal intake $*p < 0.05$, and after HF-meal intake $**p < 0.05$

for the discrimination of patients with obesity who are more likely to regain weight after therapy for obesity [29].

Our experiment also has some limitations. The presented study is a part of our larger project, with very long and labourious protocol procedures, and it was difficult to find volunteers who agreed to participate in the three meal challenge tests, with all of the tested meals. Therefore, if we wanted to follow a crossover study design, it was needed to divide participants into two groups (Group I and Group II) to compare the effects of different meals intake in the same individuals. The other major limitation is that normal body weight men in Group 1 were a little bit younger than the overweight/obese individuals, what could affect the results when comparing the differences after the HC- and NC-meal intake dependently on the body weight in this group, but it did not affect the results from comparing the HC- with NC-meal. The other limitations include the small sample size, enrolling only the male participants, and the liquid form of meals. Some of them were intentional, to reduce the impact of possible confounding factors, such as the influences of sex hormones and sex differences; or to decrease the time of meal digestion and absorption, to not discourage the volunteers with a long time spent at each visit etc. However, the mentioned factors could affect our results, and therefore, our observations and the relationship between leptin/ghrelin ratio and metabolic changes need further investigation.

Conclusions

In conclusion, the trends observed in our study show that in men with normal body weight, we can expect a more beneficial leptin/ghrelin ratio after HC-meal intake, whereas in overweight/obese individuals, we can expect this after meals with limited carbohydrate content. Therefore, the recommendation for overweight/obese men to choose meals with lower carbohydrate content, could be a practical implication of this study.

Abbreviations

AgRP: Agouti-related protein; ANOVA: One-way analysis of variance; BMI: Body mass index; CCK: Cholecystokinin; CRH: Corticotropin releasing hormone; ELISA: Enzyme-linked immunosorbent assay; FGF-21: Fibroblast growth factor 21; GLP-1: Glucagon-like peptide-1; HC: High-carbohydrate; HF: High-fat; HO-1: Heme oxygenase-1; NC: Normo-carbohydrate; NPY: Neuropeptide Y; NPY: Neuropeptide Y; POMC: Proopiomelanocortin; PYY: Peptide YY; RIA: Radioimmunoassay; SFRP4: Secreted frizzle-related protein-4; α-MSH: Stimulating the α-Melanocyte-stimulating hormone; α-MSH: α-Melanocyte-stimulating hormone

Acknowledgements

The authors would like to thank the Study Team of the Clinical Research Centre and Department of Endocrinology, Diabetology and Internal Medicine of Medical University of Bialystok for technical support.

Funding

The present study was supported by grants from the Medical University of Bialystok, Poland.

Authors' contributions

EAP, LO, AK and MG conceived and designed the study, analysed and interpreted the data and drafted the manuscript; JG analysed the data; JG and BP helped draft the manuscript. All authors performed critical revision for important intellectual content and approved the final version of the manuscript.

Competing interests
The authors declare that they have no competing interests.

Author details
[1]Clinical Research Centre, Medical University of Bialystok, Sklodowskiej 24A, 15-276, Bialystok, MC, Poland. [2]Department of Dietetics and Clinical Nutrition, Medical University of Bialystok, Mieszka I-go 4B, 15-054, Bialystok, Poland. [3]Department of Endocrinology, Diabetology and Internal Medicine, Medical University of Bialystok, Sklodowskiej 24A, 15-276, Bialystok, MC, Poland.

References
1. Ng M, Fleming T, Robinson M, Thomson B, Graetz N, Margono C, Mullany EC, Biryukov S, Abbafati C, Abera SF, et al. Global, regional, and national prevalence of overweight and obesity in children and adults during 1980-2013: a systematic analysis for the global burden of disease study 2013. Lancet. 2014;384:766–81.
2. Khan M, Joseph F. Adipose tissue and adipokines: the association with and application of adipokines in obesity. Scientifica (Cairo). 2014;2014:328592.
3. Guerre-Millo M. Adipose tissue and adipokines: for better or worse. Diabetes Metab. 2004;30:13–9.
4. Little TJ, Feltrin KL, Horowitz M, Meyer JH, Wishart J, Chapman IM, Feinle-Bisset C. A high-fat diet raises fasting plasma CCK but does not affect upper gut motility, PYY, and ghrelin, or energy intake during CCK-8 infusion in lean men. Am J Physiol Regul Integr Comp Physiol. 2008;294:R45–51.
5. Bodnaruc AM, Prud'homme D, Blanchet R, Giroux I. Nutritional modulation of endogenous glucagon-like peptide-1 secretion: a review. Nutr Metab (Lond). 2016;13:92.
6. Gavrieli A, Mantzoros CS. Novel molecules regulating energy homeostasis: physiology and regulation by macronutrient intake and weight loss. Endocrinol Metab (Seoul). 2016;31:361–72.
7. Verdeş G, DuŢă CC, Popescu R, MituleŢu M, Ursoniu S, Lazăr OF. Correlation between leptin and ghrelin expression in adipose visceral tissue and clinical-biological features in malignant obesity. Romanian J Morphol Embryol. 2017;58:923–9.
8. Rodríguez A. Novel molecular aspects of ghrelin and leptin in the control of adipobiology and the cardiovascular system. Obes Facts. 2014;7:82–95.
9. Shah, NN, MU D, TJ V: The role of neurohormonal Imbalances in Obesity. . vol. 7. pp. 182–183: Advances in Obesity, Weight Management & Control; 2017:182–183.
10. Klok MD, Jakobsdottir S, Drent ML. The role of leptin and ghrelin in the regulation of food intake and body weight in humans: a review. Obes Rev. 2007;8:21–34.
11. Korek E, Krauss H, Gibas-Dorna M, Kupsz J, Piątek M, Piątek J. Fasting and postprandial levels of ghrelin, leptin and insulin in lean, obese and anorexic subjects. Prz Gastroenterol. 2013;8:383–9.
12. Picó C, Oliver P, Sánchez J, Palou A. Gastric leptin: a putative role in the short-term regulation of food intake. Br J Nutr. 2003;90:735–41.
13. Konturek PC, Konturek JW, Cześnikiewicz-Guzik M, Brzozowski T, Sito E, Konturek SJ. Neuro-hormonal control of food intake: basic mechanisms and clinical implications. J Physiol Pharmacol. 2005;56(Suppl 6):5–25.
14. Poppitt SD, Leahy FE, Keogh GF, Wang Y, Mulvey TB, Stojkovic M, Chan YK, Choong YS, McArdle BH, Cooper GJ. Effect of high-fat meals and fatty acid saturation on postprandial levels of the hormones ghrelin and leptin in healthy men. Eur J Clin Nutr. 2006;60:77–84.
15. Briggs DI, Andrews ZB. Metabolic status regulates ghrelin function on energy homeostasis. Neuroendocrinology. 2011;93:48–57.
16. Adamska E, Ostrowska L, Gościk J, Waszczeniuk M, Krętowski A, Górska M. Intake of meals containing high levels of carbohydrates or high levels of unsaturated fatty acids induces postprandial Dysmetabolism in young overweight/obese men. Biomed Res Int. 2015;2015:147196.
17. Adamska-Patruno E, Ostrowska L, Golonko A, Pietraszewska B, Goscik J, Kretowski A, Gorska M. Evaluation of energy expenditure and oxidation of energy substrates in adult males after intake of meals with varying fat and carbohydrate content. Nutrients. 2018;10.
18. Adamska E, Kretowski A, Goscik J, Citko A, Bauer W, Waszczeniuk M, Maliszewska K, Paczkowska-Abdulsalam M, Niemira M, Szczerbinski L, et al. The type 2 diabetes susceptibility TCF7L2 gene variants affect postprandial glucose and fat utilization in non-diabetic subjects. Diabetes Metab. 2017.
19. Kretowski A, Adamska E, Maliszewska K, Wawrusiewicz-Kurylonek N, Citko A, Goscik J, Bauer W, Wilk J, Golonko A, Waszczeniuk M, et al. The rs340874 PROX1 type 2 diabetes mellitus risk variant is associated with visceral fat accumulation and alterations in postprandial glucose and lipid metabolism. Genes Nutr. 2015;10:454.
20. Adamska E, Waszczeniuk M, Gościk J, Golonko A, Wilk J, Pliszka J, Maliszewska K, Lipińska D, Milewski R, Wasilewska A, et al. The usefulness of glycated hemoglobin A1c (HbA1c) for identifying dysglycemic states in individuals without previously diagnosed diabetes. Adv Med Sci. 2012;57:296–301.
21. Sánchez J, Oliver P, Palou A, Picó C. The inhibition of gastric ghrelin production by food intake in rats is dependent on the type of macronutrient. Endocrinology. 2004;145:5049–55.
22. Labayen I, Ortega FB, Ruiz JR, Lasa A, Simón E, Margareto J. Role of baseline leptin and ghrelin levels on body weight and fat mass changes after an energy-restricted diet intervention in obese women: effects on energy metabolism. J Clin Endocrinol Metab. 2011;96:E996–1000.
23. Pandit R, Beerens S, Adan RAH. Role of leptin in energy expenditure: the hypothalamic perspective. Am J Physiol Regul Integr Comp Physiol. 2017;312:R938–47.
24. Abizaid A, Horvath TL. Ghrelin and the central regulation of feeding and energy balance. Indian J Endocrinol Metab. 2012;16:S617–26.
25. Romon M, Lebel P, Fruchart JC, Dallongeville J. Postprandial leptin response to carbohydrate and fat meals in obese women. J Am Coll Nutr. 2003;22: 247–51.
26. Spiegel K, Tasali E, Penev P, Van Cauter E. Brief communication: sleep curtailment in healthy young men is associated with decreased leptin levels, elevated ghrelin levels, and increased hunger and appetite. Ann Intern Med. 2004;141:846–50.
27. Hanlon EC, Van Cauter E. Quantification of sleep behavior and of its impact on the cross-talk between the brain and peripheral metabolism. Proc Natl Acad Sci U S A. 2011;108(Suppl 3):15609–16.
28. Miljković M, Šaranac L, Bašić J, Ilić M, Djindjić B, Stojiljković M, Kocić G, Cvetanović G, Dimitrijević Nb: Evaluation of ghrelin and leptin levels in obese, lean and undernourished children., vol. 74. pp. 963–969. VOJNOSANITETSKI PREGLED2017:963–969.
29. Crujeiras AB, Díaz-Lagares A, Abete I, Goyenechea E, Amil M, Martínez JA, Casanueva FF. Pre-treatment circulating leptin/ghrelin ratio as a non-invasive marker to identify patients likely to regain the lost weight after an energy restriction treatment. J Endocrinol Investig. 2014;37:119–26.

17

Impact of three different plate colours on short-term satiety and energy intake

Asli Akyol*†, Aylin Ayaz†, Elif Inan-Eroglu, Cansu Cetin and Gulhan Samur

Abstract

Background: Plate colour was previously shown to alter the amount of food consumption due to its environmental effect on food intake. However, different studies have indicated that the effect of plate colour cannot be generalized. In light of this finding, the main objective of this study was to determine whether food consumption during an open buffet meal was different when using same-sized white, red or black plates.

Methods: This study was a crossover study conducted with 54 female participants aged 18–30 years with normal BMIs. On experimental days, participants ate a standard breakfast and were then randomly assigned to eat ad libitum lunch (pasta with tomato sauce and soft drinks) using white, red or black plates. Visual analogue scale (VAS) scores on satiety outcomes were measured for all meals. Energy and macronutrient intake during lunch was recorded.

Results: The results showed that plate colour exerted a significant effect on food intake during the test days ($p = 0.021$). The average total energy intake with red (1102.16 ± 47.12 kcal, $p = 0.05$) and black plates (1113.19 ± 47.12 kcal, $p = 0.034$) was significantly increased when compared to that with white plates (945.72 ± 47.12 kcal). There were no differences between red and black plates ($p = 0.985$). Overall, mean VAS scores did not indicate a significant difference between the groups.

Conclusions: Plate colour may be a crucial determinant of energy intake.

Keywords: Colour, Plate, Food, Energy intake, Satiety response

Background

There is strong interest in identifying environmental factors linked with overeating because improvement of those factors might prevent or reverse obesity [1]. Over the last 30 years, eating patterns have changed, and the number of meals eaten outside the home, commercial portion sizes, and dishware sizes have increased both at home and outside the home [2, 3]. These alarming trends in the food environment may have contributed to difficulty in restraining food intake and thus increased prevalence of overweight and obesity as a result of increased energy consumption. The need for efficient strategies in restraining food intake is evident as self-regulation of appetite and appetitive behaviour, which depend on several factors, becomes difficult in modern societies [4].

Several studies reported that modifications in food environments may alter eating patterns [5, 6]. For instance, environmental factors, such as the presence of other people [7], location [8], portion size [9] and time of consumption [10], appear to affect food intake and food choice. More specifically, the colour of the plate ware, of the packaging, and of the surrounding environment has been shown to influence food consumption [11]. In light of these outcomes, assessing the environmental and situational colour-related cues that induce inhibitory reactions towards food intake can be beneficial to improve and regulate healthy eating habits.

Recent studies showed that red can be a cognitive and behavioural stimulus in humans due to its high visibility

* Correspondence: asli.akyol@hacettepe.edu.tr
†Equal contributors
Department of Nutrition and Dietetics, Hacettepe University, Sihhiye, 06100 Ankara, Turkey

and its perception as a signal of danger [12, 13]. The observations originating from these studies introduced the hypothesis that using red plates may elicit similar avoidance behaviour towards food intake. Genschow et al. [14] reported that individuals drank and ate less from red labelled cups and red plates than from blue labelled cups and blue and white plates. Similarly, another study demonstrated reduced consumption of popcorn and chocolate chips when the foods were served on red plates [15]. However, other studies reported that red plate was not always a valid predictor of food intake [16]. Instead, the reaction towards the intake of food from different coloured plates developed through several adaptations. One of these adaptations depended on the perceived healthiness of the food, as Reutner et al., [17] indicated that the impact of red colour decreased when food options became healthier. Second, the contrast between the plate colour and the food colour appeared to be an important factor [16]. van Ittersum and Wansink [16] reported that contrast, instead of the specific colour of the plate, was the main factor in restricting food intake. Since the effect of plate colour on food intake remains unresolved in these studies, there is a need for further studies with different types of foods and contrasts [14, 15].

In the present study, the main aim was to examine energy intake in the context of three different plate colours (white, red and black) during an open buffet meal. The open buffet meal consisted of pasta and non-carbonated soft drinks, which were consumed during a regular meal time since most of the studies conducted to assess the effect of plate colour on food intake were conducted with snack foods [14, 15, 18]. In addition, the current study included three different plate colours with measured colorimetric coordinates. White plates were used as the control group, and black plates were used to test the contrast difference with respect to red plates. As subjective satiety outcomes are influenced by external factors and are related to subsequent food intake, the second aim of the study was to measure participant's satiety outcomes using the visual analogue scale (VAS) [19].

Methods

Subjects

Fifty-four female subjects were recruited from Hacettepe University and the surrounding community through poster advertisements and announcements. A questionnaire examining general health and nutritional habits was used for screening all volunteers. Inclusion criteria included women in good health between the ages of 18–30 years who were non-smokers, not dieting and not diagnosed with any metabolic disease. They could not be colour blind, be professional athletes, possess food allergies or extreme dislikes for specific foods or be pregnant or lactating. None of the participants were taking medications known to affect appetite or weight regulation. Regular breakfast, snack, and lunch consumption was an additional inclusion criterion for participants. Each subject signed an informed consent document before the study. Subjects having extreme dislikes for specific foods were also excluded. Subjects were excluded if they scored > 9 on a Beck depression scale due to predisposition to depression and had a measured body mass index (BMI) < 18 or > 25 kg/m^2. Participants' body weight, height, and body compositions in terms of lean body mass (kg) and fat percentage (%) were measured with a Jawon XScan Plus (Jawon Medical, Gyeongsang, Korea). Since the menstrual cycle may affect appetite ratings, experiment days were arranged one week before menstruation for all participants. The Non-Interventional Clinical Studies Ethics Board of Hacettepe University (GO16/751–16) provided ethical approval on the 6th of December 2016.

Study design and experimental protocol

This study was a crossover study conducted at the Nutrition Laboratory in the Department of Nutrition and Dietetics, Hacettepe University, Ankara, Turkey. The experimental protocol of this study used the European consensus on postprandial studies evaluating appetite measures and eating behaviours [20]. The study was carried out on three separate days, with one to two weeks washout period between each study day. On each test day, participants were randomly assigned to eat lunch using a plastic white, red or black plate. A randomization scheme was generated using the website "randomization.com" to allocate participants to the different plate colours [21]. Each plate colour was named W, R and B in the randomization system, and then, plates were served to the corresponding subject according to the randomization letters by an investigator who was not involved in the trials. Participants were informed that the topic of the research was to examine their energy intake on different test days.

On experimental days, participants arrived at 08.00 h after fasting for 12 h and left at 14.00 h. On the previous evening, participants were guided to have dinner, namely, a bowl of tomato soup (200 mL), grilled meat (60 g), salad (200 g), white bread (50 g) (total, 602 kcal) and adequate water, and on the following morning, they were served breakfast, namely, two thin slices of white bread (50 g), a slice of cheese (30 g), and a cup of tea at 08.30 h (total, 250 kcal). Participants were asked to consume the full breakfast within 15 min. Additional food or beverage intake was not allowed until the open buffet lunch. At 12.00 h, an ad libitum buffet-style lunch was served. Lunch consisted of pasta and soft drinks. The recipe for the pasta was as follows: 500 g pasta was boiled in hot water with 50 g sunflower oil. Then, pasta was added to 300 g ready-to-eat Napolitana sauce and mixed until homogenously distributed. The nutritional value of 100 g of this recipe was 287 kcal, 44.8 g carbohydrates, 8.0 g protein and 8.2 g fat. The soft drinks were served in their original containers in order to simulate a typical situation and assess the effect of plate colour alone. The nutritional value of 100 mL of fruit juices (orange, peach and mixed) was between 63 and 90 kcal, with 12.7–20. 0 g carbohydrates.

The serving table was a separate dining table at a moderately close distance where the subjects sat. On each test day, the same amounts and types of foods were served, and the buffet items were identical. The same portion sizes, serving cutlery, and serving bowls were used on the test days. The subjects were instructed to have lunch until comfortably satisfied and allowed to re-fill their plate whenever they wanted.

Throughout the study, participants were in the same room and were allowed to read or use laptops throughout the experiment. Physical activity and social interaction were limited. Subjects were not allowed to see how much other subjects consumed. Energy and macronutrient intakes of subjects were measured by weighing the amounts of food and drink consumed and converting these values into energy (kcal) and macronutrients based on the manufacturer's labelling.

VAS

The VAS was used to assess hunger, satiety, prospective food consumption, amount of food they could consume, and desire for sugary foods throughout the study period [22]. Appetite ratings were recorded on a 100 mm visual analogue scale (VAS) with words anchored at each end describing the extremes of a unipolar question (for hunger: "I am not hungry at all"/"I have never been more hungry"; for satiety: "I am not sated at all"/"I have never been more sated"; for prospective food consumption: "I cannot consume any food at all"/"I have never wanted to consume food that much"; for desire for a sugary snack: "I do not want to consume a sugary snack at all"/"I have never wanted to consume a sugary snack that much"; for amount of food: "I can only have a small amount of food"/"I can eat a large amount of food"). The baseline VAS scores were measured before breakfast at 08.00 am. Then, participants were asked to consume breakfast until 08.30. After breakfast, participants filled in VAS questionnaires every 15 min until lunch and afterwards for a total of 23 times. Before the study period, subjects were informed as to how to fill out VAS forms.

Photometric measurements

The colorimetric coordinates of the plates used in the study are shown in Table 1. The measurements were performed with a Datacolor Mercury ™ 2000 Color Measurement System under a Xenon pulsed lamp with a spectral gap of 400–700 nm, a measuring range of 0–200% reflection and a bandwidth efficiency/resolution of 100 nm/2 nm. The colour difference equation was used according to CIE2000.

Table 1 Colorimetric coordinates of the white, red and black plates used in the study

	L	a	b	c	H
White	88.88	−1.37	−2.44	2.79	240.73
Red	47.76	0.28	−1.46	1.49	280.99
Black	30.50	45.94	25.83	52.7	29.35

L: The L dimension of the space is roughly proportional to log-luminance and captures perceived changes along the black–white achromatic colour continuum. a, b: The a and b dimensions define a chromatic plane with axes corresponding to the red–green and blue–yellow opponent continua. c: Chroma is the perceived strength of a surface colour and the degree of visual difference from a neutral grey of the same lightness. H: Hue is the attribute of appearance that is often colloquially called colour

Statistical analysis

Data were analysed using the Statistical Package for the Social Sciences (SPSS) version 22 (SPSS Inc., Chicago, IL, USA). The primary outcome of this trial was the effect of different coloured plates on energy intakes during an ad libitum lunch. For the primary outcome, data were analysed using a general linear model and ANOVA. The secondary outcome variables were subjects' VAS scores. For the secondary outcome, data were analysed using a repeated-measures ANCOVA with baseline measurement as the covariate. Subjects and test day were included in the procedure, in addition to the plate colours/time interaction. Bonferroni post hoc analysis was used for comparisons between black and red plates. Data for the area under the curve (AUC) for VAS scores were obtained using GraphPad Prism version 6 (GraphPad Software Inc., La Jolla, CA, USA). Baseline values were added as covariates in AUC data. Data are given as the mean ± standard error of mean unless otherwise stated. $P < 0.05$ was considered statistically significant. Power analysis indicated that at least 24 subjects per condition were required in order to estimate a minimum effect size of 18.35% (for energy intake differences) for comparisons between treatment arms (yielding a power of 0.80 and alpha of 0.05) [23].

Results

All of the participants completed the study successfully. All subject data were analysed for each test meal. Participants were 22.22 ± 0.14 years of age, with an average BMI of 21.29 ± 0.12 kg/m^2, and had a waist circumference of 70.09 ± 0.48 cm. Body composition data for the participants were 44.19 ± 0.31 kg lean body mass and 23.91 ± 0.33% fat.

Figure 1 shows the mean VAS-rated hunger, satiety, prospective food consumption, amount of food that could be consumed, and desire for sugary foods for the

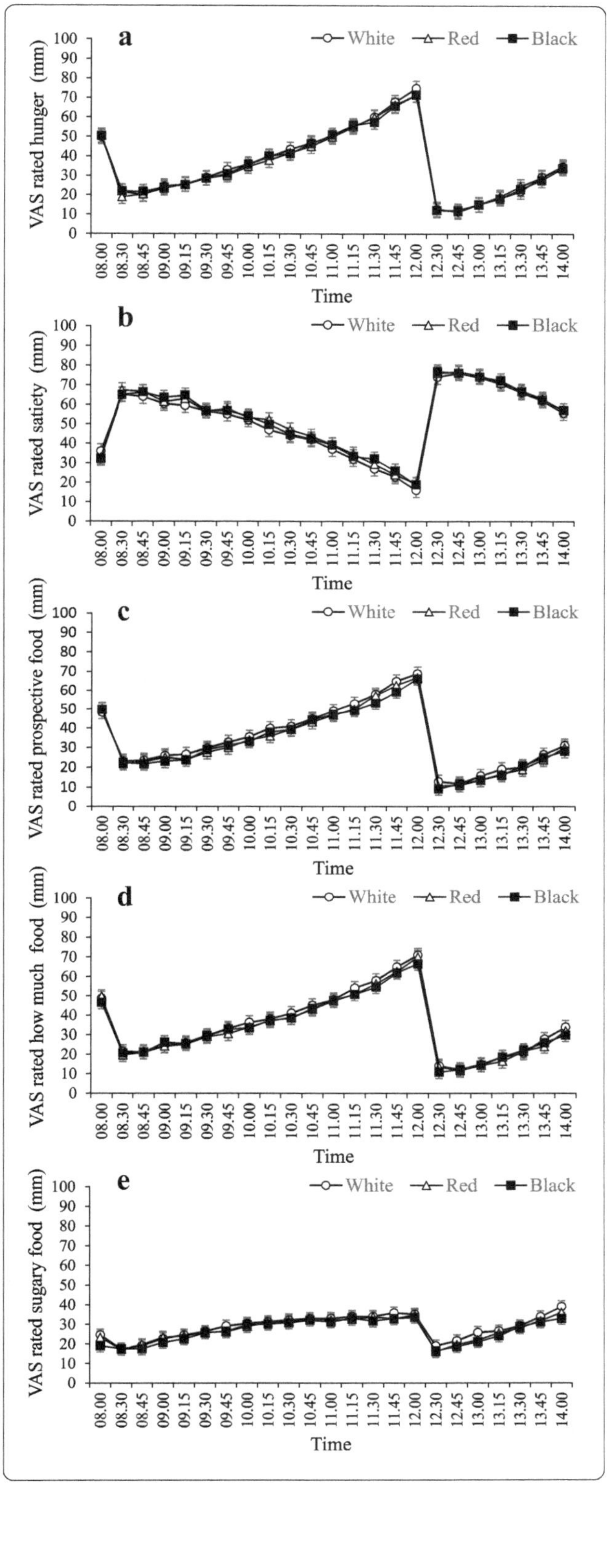

Fig. 1 Mean VAS scores (± SEM) during the three test days, $n = 54$. (**a**) VAS-rated hunger, (**b**) VAS-rated satiety, (**c**) VAS-rated prospective food consumption, (**d**) VAS-rated amount of food that could be consumed, (**e**) VAS-rated desire for a sugary snack. A light breakfast was served at 08.00 h, immediately after recording baseline VAS scores. Lunch was served at 12.00 h. Repeated measures indicated that there were no statistically significant differences between white, red and black plates ($P > 0.05$)

total study period. Baseline values did not differ between test days ($P > 0.05$). VAS scores indicated that both breakfast and lunch significantly influenced VAS scores ($P < 0.001$). However, plate colour did not affect VAS scores during the test days ($P > 0.05$). No interaction was detected between plate colour and time. In addition, AUC data of VAS scores did not show a significant difference between the groups (Table 2) ($P > 0.05$).

Energy intakes from pasta and drink during the open buffet lunch are shown in Table 3. Participants were allowed to refill their plates by visiting the serving table as much as they wanted in the present study. To distinguish exact calories between multiple visits to the buffet, the energy intake of each participants was separately recorded for refilled plates (2nd visit). At the first visit, participants' energy intake from pasta was significantly increased with red and black plates when compared to that with white plates ($P = 0.025$). The energy intake from soft drinks was similar for all plate colours ($P > 0.05$). Overall, the data indicated that the total energy intake (pasta and drink) of participants at the first visit to the buffet was significantly higher with red and black plates than with white plates ($P = 0.03$) (Table 3). Thirteen participants with white plates, sixteen participants with red plates and fifteen participants with black plates visited the buffet a second time, and participants did not have additional drinks. At this stage of the study, plate colours did not exert a significant effect on energy intake ($P > 0.05$) (Table 3). None of the participants visited the buffet a third time. When the total energy intake was evaluated, using red and black plates resulted in higher energy intake than using white plates ($P = 0.021$) (Table 3). Energy intake from red and black plates was similar.

Discussion

The present study examined whether or not three different colours (white, red or black) of plates would exert a significant effect on short-term satiety and food intake. Interestingly, for the first time, the results of this study demonstrated that energy intake from red and black plates was significantly increased when compared to white plates in women of a normal weight who were allowed to eat freely during lunch. With respect to VAS scores, subjective reporting of satiety-related parameters was similar between the three plate colours. Although

Table 2 Area under curve (AUC) data for VAS scores

VAS questions	Plate colours		
	White	Red	Black
Hunger	217.4 ± 25.3	212.4 ± 25.1	214.0 ± 24.6
Satiety	303.7 ± 28.7	320.80 ± 29.3	320.2 ± 29.7
Prospective consumption	215.5 ± 21.2	201.9 ± 20.6	200.0 ± 20.4
Amount of food that could be consumed	215.7 ± 24.8	203.1 ± 23.6	203.8 ± 23.7
Desire for sugary snack	174.3 ± 19.1	164.7 ± 17.4	159.2 ± 16.5

Mean VAS scores (± SEM) during the three test days ($n = 54$). There were no statistically significant differences between treatments ($P > 0.05$)

red was considered to evoke danger- and stop-related signals towards food intake in different studies [14, 15], our results suggested the possible role of additional factors that could be related to colour cues and food consumption.

Most of the studies that evaluated the effect of plate colour on food intake used rather snacks due to their independent effect on total energy intake [15, 18]. Since the composition and quantity of the main meals constitute a crucial part of daily energy intake [24, 25], the current study was particularly interested in the effect of plate colour on regular meals that occur on a daily basis. Therefore, the open buffet meal in the present study consisted of pasta with tomato sauce as a healthy and commonly consumed food. Our results showed that red plate colour did not reduce food intake compared to white plate. In addition to this effect, the presence of healthy food resulted in the consumption of larger amounts of food without any inhibitory effect. Notably, this impact was observed during only the first visit to the serving table. The initial food consumption might have compromised the further influence of having more food during a regular meal time, or simply, this effect might have been lessened over consumption time of the meal. As discussed by Genschow et al. [14], the link between the red plate and amount of energy intake from healthy or unhealthy foods was an open question, and in line with their speculation, this link appeared to be dependent on the type of food. Hence, in light of our results, it can be suggested that using red plates to control food intake might be an ineffective strategy in individuals who are healthy and consuming healthy foods.

The consumption of larger amounts of food from red or black plates can be explained by the contrast hypothesis rather than the specific effect of the plate colour [15]. In a related study, van Ittersum and Wansink [16] reported that participants consumed significantly more pasta when the colour contrast was lower between the pasta and the plate. For instance, participants had larger amounts of pasta when offered red sauce on red plates or white sauce on white plates. This finding seems to be consistent with our data, although van Ittersum and Wansink reported the serving size instead of the actual energy intake [16]. Since the present study recorded food intake and consumed amounts at every visit to the buffet, it can be concluded that contrast could be an important factor for the determination of the effect of plate colour on energy intake. Although the colour coordinates of the pasta with tomato sauce were not measured in the current study due to the heterogeneous texture of the food, it was observed that the colour of the served pasta was closer to red when compared to white because of the colour of the sauce. However, given that the black plate was also associated with the consumption of higher amounts of pasta, the simpler explanation of the similarity between the red sauce and red plate may not be accurate, as the colour coordinates of red and black plates that were used in the present study were distinct. Were et al. [15] reported that the defined direction of the contrast did not exert a significant effect, as they observed similar influence of red plates on popcorn and chocolate chip consumption. Similarly, the second study of Genschow et al. [14] showed the reduced food intake in red plates, as in their study, participants consumed significantly fewer pretzels with blue or white plates. Therefore, further examinations including different types of foods and plate colours are needed to elucidate the contrast issue.

Taste expectations were shown to be mediated according to different colour plates [26]. Piqueras-Fiszman et al. [18] demonstrated that participants rated the intensity of the flavour more when the mousse sample was served on white plates in comparison to black plates. In this context, the specific effect of the colour black on food consumption is unknown. Data generated from these studies introduced interesting questions of whether the resulting perception of consumers according to different plate colours will influence the consumption of these foods. As black plates induced a higher energy intake in the present study, a possible explanation may be that black plates can make food more appealing than white plates. Genschow et al. [12] addressed this issue in a further analysis. Despite finding that red plates were liked more and were rated more attractive compared to white plates, food intake from red

Table 3 Energy intake during the open buffet lunch meal

	Plate colours								
Energy intake (kcal)	White (Pasta energy)	White (Drink energy)	White (Total energy)	Red (Pasta energy)	Red (Drink energy)	Red (Total energy)	Black (Pasta energy)	Black (Drink energy)	Black (Total energy)
1st visit	740.67 ± 28.84	100.02 ± 15.28	850.70 ± 33.81	842.79 ± 28.84§	90.35 ± 15.32	957.89 ± 33.81*	837.29 ± 28.84§	96.33 ± 15.65	964.97 ± 33.81*
2nd visit	337.89 ± 69.26	–	337.89 ± 69.26	402.38 ± 62.43	–	402.38 ± 62.43	514.93 ± 64.48	–	514.93 ± 64.48
Total	902.65 ± 30.24	100.02 ± 15.28	947.72 ± 47.12	1084.45 ± 32.85‡	90.35 ± 15.32	1102.16 ± 47.12†	1095 ± 36.20‡	96.33 ± 15.65	1113.19 ± 47.12†

Mean energy intake scores (± SEM) during the three test days ($n = 54$). All participants visited the serving table for the 1st round with white, red or black plates (n = 54). Data on the 2nd visits to the serving table consisted of $n = 13$ participants for white plates, $n = 16$ participants for red plates, and $n = 15$ participants for black plates. § indicates the significant effect of plate colour on energy intake from pasta at the first visit to the serving Table ($P = 0.025$). * indicates the significant effect of plate colour on energy intake from pasta and drink at the first visit to the serving Table ($P = 0.03$). ‡ indicates the significant effect of plate colour on energy intake from pasta in total ($P = 0.028$). † indicates the significant effect of plate colour on energy intake from pasta and drink in total ($P = 0.021$). Post hoc tests did not show a significant difference between red and black plates ($P > 0.05$)

plates was still reduced. The present study did not examine the perception of flavour, quality, aesthetics of plates or liking for open buffet lunch. However, the VAS scores examined related parameters, such as the desire for sugary snacks or prospective food consumption, and all of these parameters were similar between the three plate colours. This result may suggest a possible direct effect of plate colours instead of an interaction with perceptive parameters. At present, how subjective perception, plate colour and food intake interact with each other is an open question. Future research may aim to investigate these connections on different occasions.

The current study has several limitations that should be addressed. First, this experiment was conducted in a laboratory where healthy participant's usual eating habits might be affected due to the different environment. Regarding the effects of plate colour on perception in an ecologically natural setting, one study confirmed that using white or black plates resulted in significantly different perception of the food in a restaurant [27]. In addition, the health status of the participants in such studies can also determine the observed effects, as one study showed that a high contrast intervention (red) versus baseline (white) resulted in significantly higher food and drink intake in patients with severe Alzheimer's disease [28]. Therefore, future studies may continue to perform similar research under natural settings and with different clinical groups. Second, the open buffet lunch consisted of pasta and soft drinks in the current study. It is well known that multi-item buffet meals can encourage overeating and increase food intake [29]. When the possible influence of food colour and interactions between other environmental colours and food colour is considered [30, 31], testing related hypotheses with a multi-item buffet meal can help us understand the current issues better. Third, eating behaviours are known to be influenced by sex differences [32]. Conducting similar experiments with male subjects can extend the current findings in future studies.

Conclusions

In conclusion, the present study demonstrated that red and black plates did not induce avoidance behaviour in healthy women during lunch. The results of this study suggest that the influence of plate colour on food intake may depend on other factors, such as the type of the food and contrast interaction between the colours of the plate and the served food. As the need for efficient strategies in restricting food intake is crucial to combating overeating and increased energy intake, research assessing the impact of colour on eating behaviour should be continued in future studies.

Acknowledgements

The authors are grateful to the study participants for their cooperation.

Funding

This research received no specific grant from any funding agency in the commercial or not-for-profit sectors.

Authors' contributions

AAk, AAy and GS designed and conducted the study. EIE and CC collected data. AAk performed statistical analyses and wrote the manuscript. AAy and GS helped draft the manuscript and interpret the data. All authors read and approved the final manuscript.

Competing interests

The authors declare that they have no competing interests.

References

1. Sofer S, Stark AH, Madar Z. Nutrition targeting by food timing: time-related dietary approaches to combat obesity and metabolic syndrome. Adv Nutr. 2015;6:214–23.
2. Nielsen SJ, Popkin BM. Patterns and trends in food portion sizes, 1977-1998. JAMA. 2003;289:450–3.
3. Piernas C, Popkin BM. Food portion patterns and trends among U.S. children and the relationship to total eating occasion size, 1977-2006. J Nutr. 2011;141:1159–64.
4. Young-Hyman D. Introduction to special issue: self-regulation of appetite-it's complicated. Obesity (Silver Spring). 2017;25(Suppl 1):S5–7.
5. Emilien C, Hollis JH. A brief review of salient factors influencing adult eating behaviour. Nutr Res Rev. 2017;19:1–14.
6. Wansink B. From mindless eating to mindlessly eating better. Physiol Behav. 2010;100:454–63.
7. Hetherington MM, Anderson AS, Norton GN, et al. Situational effects on meal intake: a comparison of eating alone and eating with others. Physiol Behav. 2006;88:498–505.
8. Markovski K, Nenov A, Ottaway A, et al. Does eating environment have an impact on the protein and energy intake in the hospitalised elderly? Nutr Diet. 2017;74:224–8.
9. Zuraikat FM, Roe LS, Privitera GJ, et al. Increasing the size of portion options affects intake but not portion selection at a meal. Appetite. 2016;98:95–100.
10. Roe LS, Meengs JS, Rolls BJ. Salad and satiety. The effect of timing of salad consumption on meal energy intake. Appetite. 2012;58:242–8.
11. Piqueras-Fiszman B, Spence C. Colour, pleasantness, and consumption behaviour within a meal. Appetite. 2014;75:165–72.
12. Elliot AJ, Maier MA, Moller AC, et al. Color and psychological functioning: the effect of red on performance attainment. J Exp Psychol Gen. 2007;136: 154–68.
13. Young SG, Elliot AJ, Feltman R, et al. Red enhances the processing of facial expressions of anger. Emotion. 2013;13:380–4.
14. Genschow O, Reutner L, Wänke M. The color red reduces snack food and soft drink intake. Appetite. 2012;58:699–702.
15. Bruno N, Martani M, Corsini C, et al. The effect of the color red on consuming food does not depend on achromatic (Michelson) contrast and extends to rubbing cream on the skin. Appetite. 2013;71:307–13.
16. van Ittersum K, Wansink B. Plate size and color suggestibility: the Delboeuf Illusion's Bias on serving and eating behavior. JCR. 2011;39:215–28.
17. Reutner L, Genschow O, Wänke M. The adaptive eater: perceived healthiness moderates the effect of the color red on consumption. Food Qual and Prefer. 2015;44:172–8.
18. Piqueras-Fiszman B, Alcaide J, Roura E, et al. Is it the plate or is it the food? Assessing the influence of the color (black or white) and shape of the plate on the perception of the food placed on it. Food Qual and Prefer. 2012;24: 205–8.
19. Herman CP, Polivy J. External cues in the control of food intake in humans: the sensory-normative distinction. Physiol Behav. 2008;94:722–8.
20. Blundell J, de Graaf C, Hulshof T, et al. Appetite control: methodological aspects of the evaluation of foods. Obes Rev. 2010;11:251–70.

21. Randomization Plans. http://www.randomization.com/. Accessed on 25 October 2017.
22. Flint A, Raben A, Blundell JE, et al. Reproducibility, power and validity of visual analogue scales in assessment of appetite sensations in single test meal studies. Int J Obes Relat Metab Disord. 2000;24:38–48.
23. Tabachnick BG, Fidell LS. Using multivariate statistics. 3rd ed. New York (NY): HarperCollins College Publishers; 1996.
24. Ovaskainen ML, Reinivuo H, Tapanainen H, et al. Snacks as an element of energy intake and food consumption. Eur J Clin Nutr. 2006;60:494–501.
25. Kim SY, Kim SM. Energy intake and snack choice by the meal patterns of employed people. Nutr Res Pract. 2010;4:43–50.
26. Tu Y, Yang Z, Ma C. The taste of plate: how the spiciness of food is affected by the color of the plate used to serve it. J Sens Stud. 2016;3:50–60.
27. Piqueras-Fiszman B, Giboreau A, Spence C. Assessing the influence of the color of the plate on the perception of a complex food in a restaurant setting. Flavour. 2013;2:24.
28. Dunne TE, Neargarder SA, Cipolloni PB, Cronin-Golomb A. Visual contrast enhances food and liquid intake in advanced Alzheimer's disease. Clin Nutr. 2004;23:533–8.
29. Brondel L, Romer M, Van Wymelbeke V, et al. Variety enhances food intake in humans: role of sensory-specific satiety. Physiol Behav. 2009;97:44–51.
30. Zampini M, Sanabria D, Phillips N, et al. The multisensory perception of flavor: assessing the influence of color cues on flavor discrimination responses. Food Qual Prefer. 2007;18:975–84.
31. Shankar MU, Levitan CA, Prescott J, et al. The influence of color and label information on flavor perception. Chemosens Percept. 2009;2:53–8.
32. Asarian L, Geary N. Sex differences in the physiology of eating. Am J Physiol Regul Integr Comp Physiol. 2013;305:R1215–67.

18

The effect of a portion size intervention on French fries consumption, plate waste, satiety and compensatory caloric intake: an on-campus restaurant experiment

Marie Vermote[1*], Vickà Versele[1], Marijn Stok[2,3], Patrick Mullie[1,4], Eva D'Hondt[1], Benedicte Deforche[1,5], Peter Clarys[1] and Tom Deliens[1]

Abstract

Background: One of the driving factors of dietary overconsumption throughout the last decennia is the increase of food portion sizes. Larger portions induce higher daily energy intake, so reducing portion size may reduce intake of excess calories. However, real-life studies about the effects of portion size reduction are lacking. Therefore, this study examined the effect of a French fries portion size reduction on French fries consumption, French fries plate waste, satiety and caloric intake during the subsequent afternoon among university students and employees in a Belgian on-campus restaurant setting. Moreover, this study evaluated consumers' perception about the portion size reduction.

Methods: The study took place over a two-time (i.e. baseline and intervention week) 4-day period (Tuesday–Friday) in the on-campus restaurant where ±1200 meals are served every day. French fries' portions were reduced by 20% by replacing the usual porcelain bowl served during the baseline week (±200 g) with smaller volume paper bags during the intervention week (±159 g) in a pre-post real-life experiment. French fries consumption and plate waste were measured in 2056 consumers at baseline and 2175 consumers at intervention. Additionally, interviews were conducted directly after lunch and again between 4 and 6 p.m. on the same day to assess satiety and caloric intake at pre and post in a small subsample of both French fries consumers ($n = 19$) and non-French fries consumers ($n = 14$). Post-intervention, the same subsample was interviewed about their perception of the portion size reduction ($n = 28$).

Results: Total French fries intake decreased by 9.1%, and total plate waste decreased by 66.4%. No differences were found in satiety or caloric intake between baseline and intervention week among the French fries' consumers. The majority ($n = 24$, 86%) of French fries consumers noticed the reduction in portion size during the intervention. Although most participants ($n = 19$, 68%) perceived the reduced portion size as sufficient, only a minority of participants ($n = 9$, 32%) indicated post-intervention that they would agree with a permanent implementation.

Conclusions: Reducing portion size may lead to reduced caloric intake, without changing perceived levels of satiety.

Keywords: Portion size, Consumption, Plate waste, Satiety, Caloric intake, University, Nudging, Choice architecture

* Correspondence: marie.vermote@vub.be
[1]Department of Movement and Sport Sciences, Vrije Universiteit Brussel, Pleinlaan 2, 1050 Brussels, Belgium
Full list of author information is available at the end of the article

Background

Colleges and universities have the ability, like most educational institutions [1–5], to set up public health initiatives for their students via education, physical activity, but also via food environments [6–8]. In this perspective, they provide the ideal setting to promote healthy eating [6–8]. It has been demonstrated that, on average, college and university students gain a substantial amount of weight during their years at college or university [9, 10]. Research also shows that this weight gain coheres with poor diets, including low intakes of fruits and vegetables, insufficient variety in food consumption, and consumption of large portions [11, 12]. Moreover, it was found that students were more likely to gain weight when eating more frequently at the university restaurant [13]. A similar relation was found for those students frequently eating French fries [13]. Obviously, colleges and universities provide also services and employment for a large number of employees. Since the low intakes of fruits and vegetables and high fat intake is not only manifested in students, but also in the adult population in general [14], strategies that produce opportunities for healthy choices are also needed for employees [14]. Because adults spend most of their waking hours at work, the workplace can be a good setting for health related interventions [15]. When installing an intervention in a worksite cafeteria or restaurant a large number of people with varying age and socioeconomic status can be reached [16]. From this perspective dietary interventions conducted in a workplace setting are plentiful but not recent and little innovative, as most of workplace interventions used a labelling system or provided product information [14, 17–22]. However, few dietary interventions approached both students and employees simultaneously.

With regard to intervention development, manipulating the physical environment, may be recommended because one can easily and instantly reach larger groups of people [15]. According to Roy et al. [7] and Thorndike et al. [23], simple environmental interventions in food settings can lead to healthier food choices among (young) adults. Recently, environmental interventions in food settings are becoming very popular in the form of nudge and choice architecture studies [5, 24–27]. However, in order to have a chance of success, behavioural approaches must generally be 'easy' by reducing the effort to participate to a minimum [28].

A relatively easy environmental intervention, which has the potential to control people's energy intake is portion size modification [29, 30]. Rolls et al. [31], for example, showed that portion size is positively related to daily energy intake. Beside the fact that (in general) people are consuming more kilocalories than they are expending [30], today's portions of high-caloric foods contain larger quantities than recommended by dietary guidelines, even in Europe [32]. These findings raise the argument to decrease portion sizes in the battle against overweight and obesity.

Rolls et al. [31] proved that a reduction in portion size of 25% of all foods on two consecutive days led to a reduced food intake of approximately 10%. In their study, however, participants (i.e. randomly recruited young women) were invited in a laboratory setting, where the portion sizes and energy density of the foods of daily menus were changed. From a scalability and public health point of view, it is clear that confirmation by real-life setting trials is needed. To our knowledge, only one US study reduced the portion size of a calorie-dense food product (i.e. French fries) served in an on-campus university restaurant, presented in plain paper bags [33]. This experiment showed that reducing the portion size of French fries by 50% resulted in a 30% decrease in French fries consumption per consumer as well as 31% reduction in plate waste per consumer [33]. In an intercept survey, 70% of the 322 questioned French fries consumers indicated they did not notice the change in portion size [33]. In the latter study, consumers consisted primarily of US freshmen while dietary intake, and thus also dietary compensational effects during the rest of the day were not assessed. So, from this study we cannot conclude that portion size reduction will lead to reduced food intake, as the 50% reduction in French fries consumption may have been compensated for later on the day. In the laboratory experiment by Rolls et al. [34], ratings of hunger decreased as the size of the package containing potato chips increased, but this did not lead to a reduced energy intake at the subsequent dinner later that day. Such possible adjustments were also checked in a study by Jeffery et al. [35], where unannounced 24-h dietary recalls were conducted by phone after a 50% reduction of pre-packaged lunches in a naturalistic setting. Results showed that mean 24-h energy intake decreased with 278 kcal/day when a small lunch was served in comparison with a large one [35]. A British study investigating the effects of reducing breakfast both on hunger feelings and subsequent energy intake, showed no influence on subsequent energy intake but did show a significance difference in hunger feeling after reducing the portion with 40%. However, this study was conducted in an overweight population in a laboratory setting [36].

In summary, no real-life experimental studies including portion size modification assessed level of satiety and dietary compensational behaviour during the hours immediately after consumption. Since European research about portion size reduction is limited and US results cannot be extrapolated due to the different eating habits between both continents [37–39], more European studies are desirable. Therefore, the primary aim of the present study was to investigate the effect of a French fries portion size reduction on French fries consumption and plate waste among university students and employees in a Belgian on-campus university restaurant setting. Secondly, we aimed to investigate the effect of the intervention on level of satiety and caloric intake during the afternoon. Thirdly, we aimed to evaluate consumers' perceptions about the portion size reduction.

Methods

Participants and design

The study was conducted in the on-campus restaurant of the Vrije Universiteit Brussel (Brussels, Belgium). The restaurant operates by a free-flow system which gives consumers the ability to choose daily between six different types of menus (i.e. menu 1 (generally meat dish), menu 2 (generally meat dish), fish-menu, vegetarian/vegan-menu, pasta menu, wok menu) or the salad bar. Consumers are free to choose a starchy side dish (French fries, mashed potatoes, boiled potatoes, or rice) when choosing one of the first four menus. Next to the main dish, a typical menu consists of soup of the day and a dessert (i.e. choice between fruit, yoghurt, pudding, cookies, or ice cream) and costs €5 for students and employees of the university, visitors pay a non-sponsored price (€10). French fries were chosen as the food of interest for the current study because it is high in calories, frequently chosen by students and employees, and relatively easy to manipulate in terms of portion sizes. Participants were university students and employees consuming one of the above mentioned menus as lunch at the on-campus restaurant during the experimental period. The on-campus restaurant is open on weekdays (Monday–Friday) from 11:30 a.m. till 1:45 p.m. and only serves lunch meals. Approximately 1200 to 1300 meals are served every day in the on-campus restaurant and all students and employees visiting the free-flow system of the on-campus restaurant were exposed to the experiment.

The study consisted of a real-life experiment during which French fries consumption and French fries plate waste were measured in 2056 consumers during baseline week and 2175 consumers during intervention week. In addition, a convenient subsample of as much students and employees as possible (n = 296) was recruited on the spot to voluntarily participate in face-to-face and telephone interviews assessing level of satiety and dietary intake during lunch and later in the afternoon. Dietary intake was measured by means of a 4-h dietary recall. Dietary recall has been validated against a 4-day food record and provides a good overall ranking of intake [40]. These assessments were performed during both the pre-intervention and intervention week. Post intervention, students and employees who consumed French fries during the intervention week were asked about their perception of the portion size reduction in a post-intervention week. Figure 1 represents how the experiment was conducted. This study was approved by the medical ethics committee of the university hospital (Vrije Universiteit Brussel, Brussels, Belgium, B.U.N. 143201732012).

Procedure

The experimental study took place over a two times (i.e. baseline and intervention week) 4-day period (Tuesday–Friday) during the opening hours of the on-campus restaurant (11:30 a.m. to 1:45 p.m.).

The course of the intervention was visually presented by Fig. 1. During the first (i.e. baseline) week, baseline data were collected of French fries consumption by registering the amount of portions of French fries (served in the usual porcelain bowls) purchased, the amount of French fries produced, and by weighing the wasted amount of French fries. Further, level of satiety shortly after completing lunch and caloric intake of the lunch were assessed using face-to-face interviews in a conveniently chosen group of students and employees immediately after having completed their lunch meal. Four hours after finishing these face-to-face interviews (between 4 and 6 p.m.), level of satiety of that exact moment and caloric intake and physical activity (as control for compensational behaviour for the larger/smaller portion) during the afternoon were assessed during telephone interviews within the same subgroup of students and employees who participated earlier that noon.

The second and third week were used as intermediate weeks during which no manipulations or assessments were carried out. This was due to the Easter holiday, during which the on-campus restaurant was less visited by students and employees.

During the fourth (i.e. intervention) week, French fries portion sizes were reduced by replacing the usual porcelain bowl containing approximately 200 g of French fries by smaller volume paper bags containing approximately 160 g French fries (Fig. 2), which corresponds to a reduction of 20%. Similar to the baseline week, French fries consumption, the amount of French fries produced and French fries plate waste were measured. Using telephone interviews, level of satiety and caloric intake were again assessed twice (right after lunch, and 4 h later) in the same subgroup of students and employees as in the baseline week. Because not everyone ate in the on-campus restaurant again, a part of this subgroup dropped out. At the end of the intervention week, two groups (French fries consumers and non-French fries consumers) were formed based on the side dish choice of the consumers. To avoid meal bias (i.e. some main

Dependent variable(s)	Week 1	Week 2 & 3	Week 4	Week 5
	PRE-INTERVENTION WEEK (BASELINE)	*INTERMEDIATE WEEKS*	*INTERVENTION WEEK*	*POST-INTERVENTION WEEK*
Consumption and plate waste	**No French fries portion size reduction** Measurements: French fries production French fries purchase French fries plate waste	No manipulation/ no measurements	**20% French fries portion size reduction** Measurements: French fries production French fries purchase French fries plate waste	No manipulation/ no measurements
Level of satiety and caloric intake	**Interviews with French fries and non-French fries eaters:** - Immediately after lunch: Face-to-face interview: satiety and caloric intake - Between 4 - 6 p.m.: Telephone interview: satiety and caloric intake		**Interviews with French fries and non-French fries eaters of the pre-intervention week:** - Immediately after lunch Telephone interview: satiety and caloric intake - Between 4 - 6 p.m.: Telephone interview satiety and caloric intake	
Perception of portion size reduction	No measurement(s)		No measurement(s)	**Interviews with French fries eaters of the intervention week** - Assessment of perception of portion size reduction - Estimation of the change in portion size - Sufficiency of the portion - Agreement with permanent implementation

Fig. 1 Flow diagram of the portion size experiment

dishes are more likely to go with French fries on the side than others), the same menus were provided during both baseline and intervention week.

In a fifth and last week (post intervention) all interviewed French fries consumers during the intervention week were asked about their perception of the portion size reduction.

Measurements

Consumption and plate waste

Consumers needed to identify themselves at the cash registers by their student/employee card. Four to six observers registered whether or not French fries were chosen and if the menu was purchased by a student or employee. Two student assistants in the tray return area separated all un-eaten French fries from the total plate waste by throwing these into a separate bin. French fries waste was then determined by weighing the un-eaten French fries after restaurant closing-time.

Satiety and caloric intake

In the face-to-face interviews level of satiety was assessed shortly after completing their meal in the on-campus restaurant by means of the Satiety Labelled Intensity Magnitude (SLIM) scale. This scale consists of a vertical line scale including 11 labels describing different levels of hunger and fullness ranging from 'greatest imaginable fullness' to 'greatest imaginable hunger'. Intermediate verbal labels

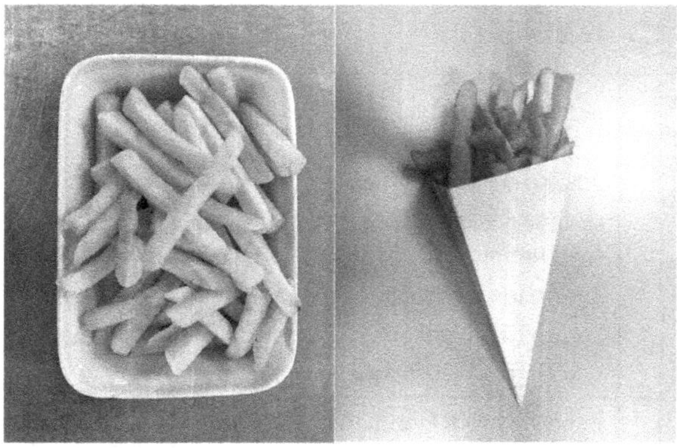

Fig. 2 Comparison of the French fries served in the porcelain bowls and in the paper bags

were placed at the appropriate distance along the top and bottom of the scale in accordance with their transformed magnitude estimates [41]. In this way, every label gets a score from + 100 (greatest imaginable fullness) to – 100 (greatest imaginable hunger) [41]. During the interviews, consumers indicated which label of the SLIM scale best suited to their level of satiety. The labels were then converted to their respective scores as described by Cardello et al. [41].

Furthermore, consumers were asked about which meal and starchy side dish they had chosen, which dessert, whether or not they had chosen for soup and their choice of beverage. All food items consumed next to the lunch were reported as well. Leftovers were estimated in quantities in proportion to the normal portion served per container (e.g., bowls, cups, and glasses). Additionally, socioeconomic status (assessed for employees only), sex, age and cell phone number (to be able to re-contact the consumers later in the afternoon) were assessed.

Between 4 and 6 p.m. on the same day the interviewees were re-contacted by telephone and asked again to indicate their level of satiety by discussing the SLIM scale orally. Food and beverages intake during this interval were questioned (~ dietary recall), as control for compensational behaviour for the larger/smaller portion. This was done by questioning what and how much specifically they had eaten or drunk. Nubel (Nutrition analysis software program) was used to calculate the caloric value of the consumed food and beverages, by multiplying the estimated amount consumed (of a certain food/beverage product, in grams/ml) with the caloric values per gram/ml. Additionally, physical activity was questioned. This was done by asking the consumers to report the type and duration of any physical activity done between lunch and the moment of the phone call and whether or not they had sweated during this activity. Height and weight of interviewee were additionally questioned to calculate participants' body mass index (BMI) and to be able to calculate the energy-expenditure of the physical activities by using 'Appendix B: Energy expenditure in household, occupational, recreational, and sports activities' of Katch, Katch, & McArdle William D [42].

Every consumer was phoned a maximum of three times on different times during this 2-h period before they were deemed to have dropped out. During the intervention week the same measurements were conducted in the same subgroup of students and employees, only if they again consumed a meal at the restaurant. A difference with the baseline week was that both interviews (i.e. directly after lunch and during the late afternoon) were conducted by telephone to be sure to include the same consumers as during baseline week. The time of ending the meal of the pre-intervention week was taken into account for the interviews directly after lunch in the intervention week. Again, everyone was phoned a maximum of three times on different times.

Only students and employees visiting the on-campus restaurant during both the baseline and intervention week were eligible to be allocated to the experimental or control group. The experimental group was formed by students and employees choosing French fries along with the same main dish on the same day of both weeks. In contrast, the control group consisted of students and employees choosing the same side dish different from French fries along with the same main dish on the same day of both weeks. Students and employees who chose a different main or side dish during the intervention week compared to the control week were excluded.

Perception of portion size reduction

During the fifth (i.e. post-intervention) week, all consumers of the experimental group were re-contacted by telephone. Consumers were asked whether or not they had noticed the reduced French fries portion size during the intervention week. If so, they were also asked to estimate the extent of alteration in portion size. Finally, participants were asked if the smaller portion was sufficient and whether or not a portion size reduction could be permanently implemented in the on-campus restaurant.

Data analysis

During the preparation phase of the experiment the difference between fried and deep-frozen French fries was measured in order to be able to calculate how many kilograms of fried French fries came out of the deep-frozen French fries. The weight of fried French fries was equal to approximately 73% of the weight of deep-frozen French fries. French fries were fried for 3 min in vegetable oil (Vandemoortele® Risso Chef), consisting of palm oil, rapeseed oil, sunflower oil, and corn oil, at a temperature of 175 °C. Total French fries consumption (in kg) was calculated by subtracting the total plate waste (in kg) from the total amount produced (i.e. kg of deep-fried French fries used multiplied by 73%). Consumption per consumer was calculated by dividing the total French fries consumption by the number of French fries consumers. A similar calculation was done to determine portion waste. By dividing total French fries consumed per portion by the amount produced per portion, the ratio of consumed French fries per portion was calculated. A similar calculation was done to determine the ratio of waste per portion.

R version 3.4.0 and IBM SPSS Statistics 24 were used for data analyses. Since the proportions of French fries and plate waste were used as the outcome measures, a binomial test for one proportion (performed in R) was used to analyse differences in French fries consumption and plate waste between the baseline and intervention week. The same test was used to analyse whether or not the amount of consumers differed between the baseline and intervention week.

Drop-out analyses for the subgroup interviews were conducted using independent samples t-tests for baseline age and BMI and chi2 for sex. Repeated measures ANOVA mixed design was used to analyze differences in satiety and caloric intake between the baseline and intervention week in both the French fries consumers (i.e. experimental group) and the non-French fries consumers (i.e. control group). Furthermore, partial eta squared (partial η^2) was calculated and reported as an estimate of effect size. Observed power (1-ß) was calculated as well. The statistical significance level was set at $\alpha = 0.05$.

Descriptive statistics on portion size perception, satisfaction about the portion size, and feasibility of long-term implementation were calculated (in %). Finally, data (i.e. quotes) representing reasons why they would or would not agree with a permanent smaller portion were examined for recurrent instances and grouped together into similar categories.

Results

A total of 4511 consumers were registered during the baseline week and 4868 during the intervention week. Of these consumers, 2056 (i.e. 45.6%) chose French fries during the baseline week, while 2175 (i.e. 44.7%) did during the intervention week. There was no significant difference in the relative number of consumers choosing French fries between the baseline or intervention week ($p = 0.200$).

Consumption and plate waste

Figure 3 shows the respective differences in French fries consumption and French fries plate waste between the baseline and intervention week. An overview of the effect of the portion size reduction on total French fries produced, consumed and wasted and the values for the individual portions can be found in Table 1. During the baseline week, consumers ate on average 88.1% (i.e. 177 g) of the available portion, whereas during the intervention week, consumers ate 95.2% (i.e. 152 g) of the available portion. Thus, although the absolute amount of French fries eaten was smaller in the intervention week, the proportion of the available portion eaten was greater.

Subgroup interviews

Table 2 gives an overview of the demographics and characteristics of the 296 consumers which were interviewed face-to-face during the baseline week immediately after

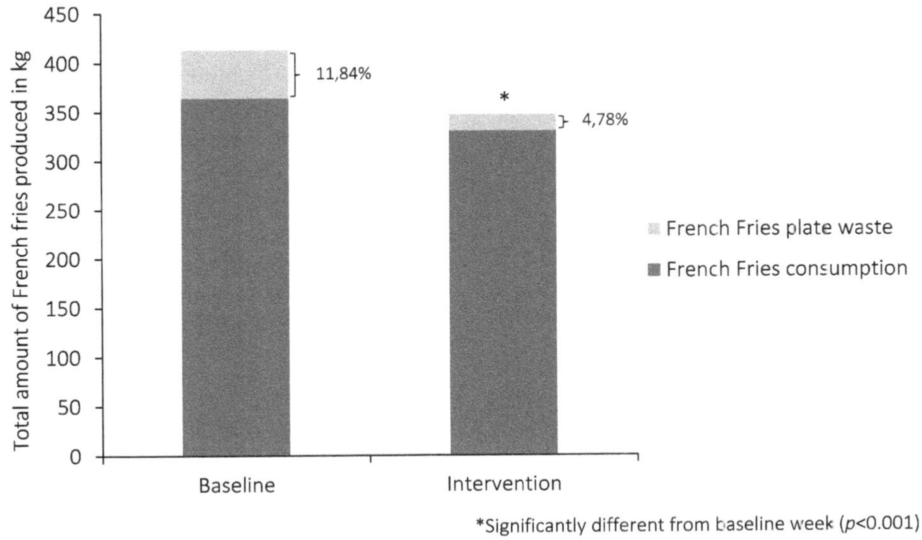

Fig. 3 Changes in French fries consumption and plate waste between baseline and intervention week

Table 1 Effect of French fries portion size reduction on consumption and plate waste

	Average portion size (g)	Total consumers of the on-campus restaurant	French fries consumers	Total French fries produced (kg)	Total French fries wasted (kg)	Total French fries consumed (kg)	French fries consumption per portion (g)	French fries plate waste per portion (g)
Baseline week	201.0	4511	2056	413.3	49.1	364.2	177.1	23.9
Intervention week	159.8	4868	2175	347.5	16.5	331.0	152.2	7.6
Difference	*20.9%*			*16.0%**	*66.4%*	*9.1%**	*14.1%*	*68.3%*

*Significant differences between baseline and intervention week ($p < 0.001$)

completing their lunch at the on-campus restaurant. Figure 4 shows a flow chart of these subgroup interviews, together with drop-out reasons and shows that the final sample consisted of 66 participants (68.2% males).

There were significant baseline differences in sex ($chi^2 = 8.519$, $p = 0.004$) and age ($t = 2.256$, $p = 0.025$) between the retention ($n = 66$; 68.2% males; age = 30.9 ± 13.5 years) and the drop-out group ($n = 230$; 47.8% males; age = 27.1 ± 11.6 years), whereas no significant difference in BMI ($t = 0.940$, $p = 0.348$) was found between both groups (BMI retention = 23.6 ± 3.8 kg/m2, BMI drop-out = 23.1 ± 3.5 kg/m2).

Of the 66 people who remained to be interviewed in the late afternoon of the intervention week, only those who consumed the same menu with the same side dish during the baseline and intervention week were used for analysis ($n_{experimental\ group} = 19$; $n_{control\ group} = 14$). Consequently, 33 consumers were excluded for further analyses.

Satiety and caloric intake

Table 3 shows the effect of the reduced French fries portion size on satiety and caloric intake during the afternoon. There was no significant interaction effect between the two groups (control and experimental) and the 2 weeks (baseline and intervention) for satiety ($F = 0.034$, $p = 0.855$, partial $\eta^2 = 0.001$, 1-ß = 0.054) and caloric-intake ($F = 3.176$, $p = 0.085$, partial $\eta^2 = 0.093$, 1-ß = 0.408). There were no significant differences between the experimental and control group concerning satiety ($F = 1.578$, $p = 0.218$, partial $\eta^2 = 0.048$, 1-ß = 0.230) and caloric intake ($F = 1.036$, $p = 0.317$, partial $\eta^2 = 0.032$, 1-ß = 0.167) and there were no significant differences between the baseline and intervention week in level of satiety ($F = 0.025$, $p = 0.875$, partial $\eta^2 = 0.001$, 1-ß = 0.053) and caloric intake ($F = 0.045$, $p = 0.834$, partial $\eta^2 = 0.001$, 1-ß = 0.055).

Table 2 Demographics and experiment related characteristics of interviewees during baseline and intervention weeks (Mean ± SD,%)

	Baseline ($n = 296$)	Intervention ($n = 66$)
Sex (% males)	52.4	68.2
Age (years)	27.9 ± 12.1	30.9 ± 13.5
Occupation (% students)	60.8	43.9
BMI (kg/m^2)	23.2 ± 3.6	23.6 ± 3.8
Underweight (%)	4.4	3.1
Normal weight (%)	72.3	69.2
Overweight or obese (%)	23.3	27.7
Food choice (%)		
French fries	48.3	50.0
Other	51.7	50.0

Perception of portion size reduction

During the fifth and final week of the experiment, all French fries consumers interviewed during the intervention week ($n = 31$) were re-contacted. Because three participants could not be reached, 28 French fries consumers were interviewed about their perception of the portion size reduction. Of these 28 people, 86% noticed the smaller portion and, on average, estimated a reduction of 29.5 ± 10.6%. Respectively 14 and 54% of the participants reported that the reduced French fries portion size was more than enough or sufficient, while respectively 25 and 7% found the French fries portion size insufficient or largely insufficient. When the interviewer suggested a permanent implementation of smaller French fries portions, 18% completely disagreed, 29% disagreed, 21% were neutral, 25% agreed and 7% completely agreed. Commonly mentioned reasons for disagreeing were the absence of price adjustments (i.e. smaller portions should equalize lower prices) ($n = 2$), the reduced portion being too small ($n = 7$), the fact that people like to eat a lot of French fries ($n = 1$) and other reasons ($n = 3$). Commonly mentioned reasons for agreeing were that the smaller portion was enough ($n = 4$), the reduction of plate waste ($n = 2$), and the fact that a smaller portion is better for one's health ($n = 3$).

Discussion

This study aimed to investigate the effect of a French fries portion size reduction on French fries consumption and French fries plate waste among university students and employees in a Belgian on-campus restaurant setting. Secondly, this study aimed to investigate the effect of the intervention on satiety and caloric intake during

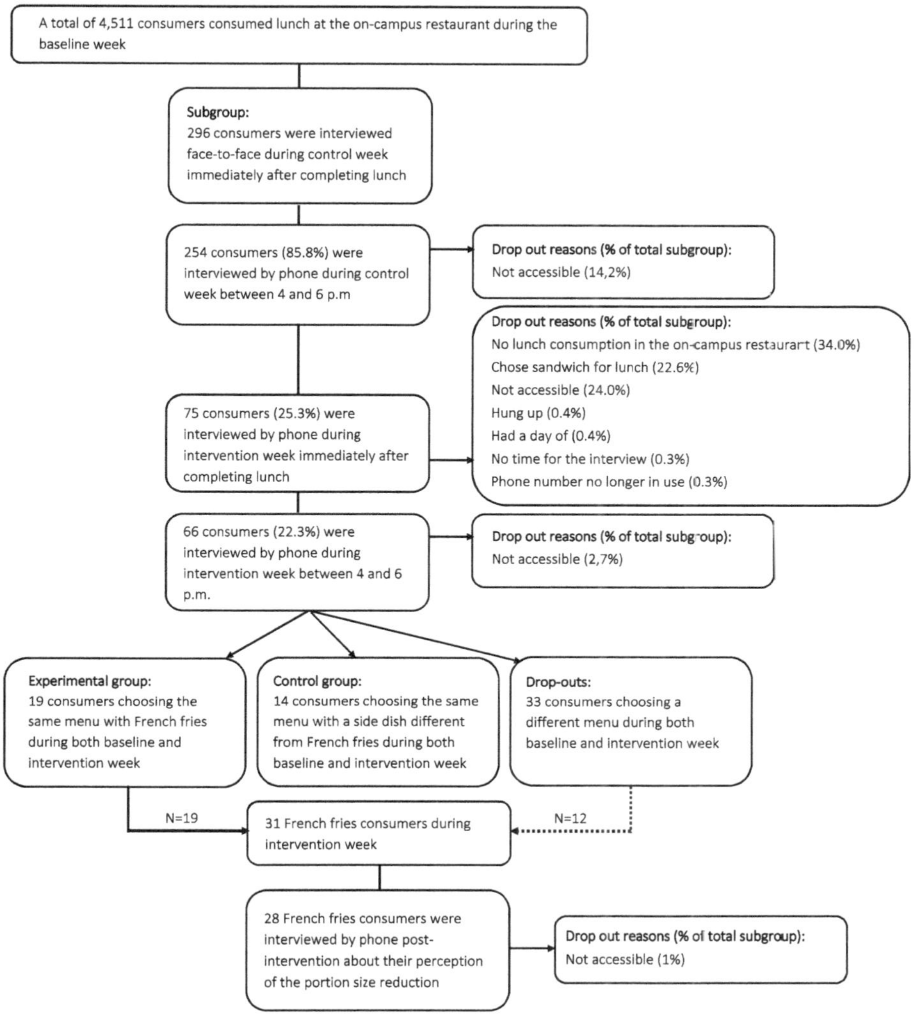

Fig. 4 Flow chart of subgroup interviews

the subsequent afternoon. Thirdly, we aimed to evaluate consumers' perception about the portion size reduction.

Results showed that decreasing portion size was effective in reducing French fries consumption and French fries plate waste. A decrease of 20.9% in portion size resulted in a total French fries intake reduction of 9.1% and a relative decrease of 66.4% in French fries plate waste. Furthermore, level of satiety did not change when a smaller portion was served and consumers did not calorically compensate during the subsequent afternoon.

Table 3 Satiety and caloric intake during afternoon after portion size reduction (Mean ± SD, *F*-values, *p*-values)

	Baseline week	Intervention week	$F_{\text{time x group}}$	$p_{\text{time x group}}$	F_{time}	p_{time}
Satiety[a]			0.034	0.855		
Experimental group (*n* = 19)	23.1 ± 36.9	25.6 ± 36.8			0.071	0.793
Control group (*n* = 14)	10.9 ± 31.8	10.8 ± 40.7			0.000	0.987
Caloric intake[b]			3.176	0.085		
Experimental group (*n* = 19)	182.4 ± 319.0	84.5 ± 96.2			1.539	0.231
Control group (*n* = 14)	45.3 ± 69.2	122.4 ± 159.0			3.871	0.071

Experimental group *n* = 19; Control group *n* = 14. [a]SLIM scale was divided as follows: greatest imaginable fullness = 100.0; extremely full = 79.4; very full = 74.3; moderately full = 46.7; slightly full = 31.9; neither hungry nor full = 0.0; slightly hungry = −18.6; moderately hungry = − 38.2; very hungry = −56.2; extremely hungry = −67.4; greatest imaginable hunger = −100.0. [b]All the food and beverages consumed by the interviewee between their lunch and the time of the call between 4 and 6 p.m. in kcal

Our results are in line with other studies showing that portion size reduction can positively affect food intake. Although, compared to the study of Freedman et al. [33] in which a French fries portion size reduction by 50% resulted in a significant decrease by ±30% in French fries consumption and plate waste, our study showed that a smaller portion size reduction (i.e. 20.9%) results in a greater decrease in total plate waste (66.4%). However, it is important to mention that even a 9.1% reduction in French fries consumption can be useful to match the recommended dietary guidelines for total energy intake. On the other hand, reduction in French fries plate waste can be positive for the sustainability of the planet, since reducing food waste also reduces emissions of greenhouse gases [25]. Yet, it has to be mentioned that the use of paper bags in this intervention was not environmental friendly. When installing a permanent reduced portion, one should look for more sustainable alternatives.

The fact that the level of satiety of the French fries consumers in our study did not differ between the baseline and intervention week is in accordance with the study by Rolls et al. [31], in which consumers rated the portions as 'smaller' during the experimental week compared to the usual portion sizes, while ratings of fullness and hunger during both conditions did not differ. Also the absence of compensation at subsequent consumption after a portion size reduction is in line with previous research. Lewis et al. [36] found no differences in energy intake during lunch and the rest of the day after reducing the portion size of breakfast by 20 and 40% respectively. It should be mentioned, however, that the study of Lewis et al. [36] was conducted in an overweight population and in a laboratory setting. Further, Jeffery et al. [35] reported no compensation effects when consuming a lunch containing 1528 kcal compared to one of 767 kcal. It should be mentioned, however, that it is very important to interpret our findings with caution since the low statistical power observed. The results of the assessment of satiety and dietary intake can be false-negatives, since the great chance of type II errors. However, the observed effect sizes were very low too.

The results of the perception interviews, where 86% of the consumers noticed the smaller portion size, are not in line with those found by Freedman et al. [33], in which only 30% noticed the smaller portion. This difference could be due to the change of container between baseline and intervention week in our study, or due to the fact that the interviews made the consumers more aware of the portion size intervention.

A permanent implementation of a smaller portion may be recommended to health promoters, university policy makers and restaurant operators, since 68% of the French fries consumers in the present study had sufficient or more than enough with the smaller portions.

A strength of the present study is that we used a real-life setting which maximises the external validity of the intervention. Secondly, we anticipated that consumers would feel that certain main dishes matched better with French fries than with rice or (mashed) potatoes. Therefore, we excluded meal bias by providing the same menus during the baseline and intervention week. Furthermore, to counter testing bias, we did not communicate about the content and the duration of the portion size experiment. However, the majority of consumers did notice the smaller portion and the unusual paper bags, which could have influenced consumers' food choice anyway. But our results showed that there was no difference in the amount of French fries portions sold per capita between the baseline and the intervention week. Finally, we checked for compensation effects during the subsequent afternoon. Although some studies already showed that there were no compensational effects seen after a portion size increase [35] or decrease [36], our study was, to our knowledge, the first real-life experimental study taking caloric intake throughout the subsequent afternoon into account when reducing portion size.

The first and possibly most important limitation of this study was the focus on consumption and plate waste of French fries and not on other food groups. Measuring plate waste of the whole lunch could have given us insights in the compensational behaviour of consumers during lunch, i.e. it may be that participants consumed more of the other food items of the chosen lunch when reducing French fries portion. Rolls et al. [31], for example, showed that focusing on several foods may be effective in monitoring consumption and energy intake. Unfortunately, it was practically impossible to measure plate waste of the whole lunch because of the difficulty of separating the wastes of every food product for French fries vs. non-French fries consumers. Secondly, although the present study found no compensational effects during the afternoon, participants may have compensated for the reduction in portion size by eating more during dinner. Therefore, it may be interesting to include this in future studies. However, several studies showed no compensational behaviour in subsequent meals after portion size modifications [31, 35, 36]. A third limitation of the present study is that we did not include a control setting. Because there are no similar on-campus restaurants available with comparable food availability, this was not possible. Also, for the measurement of French fries consumption and French fries plate waste in this study, it was not feasible to include a control group of students and employees because it was practically impossible to offer one part of the consumers less French fries (in the paper bags) while another part would still receive the usual portion (in the porcelain bowls). Lack of control may have jeopardized the internal validity of our study. Fourthly, our intervention was of short duration (i.e. only 1 week) and no follow-up measurements were conducted. Therefore, it is not clear whether this intervention effect would sustain in the long run. One study showed that the opposite, i.e. increasing the portion size of lunch with 50% over a longer period of time (4 weeks), resulted in a higher energy intake during the day, without compensation over time [35]. It should be noted, however, that 4 weeks can hardly be classified as "long-term". It is clear that more studies investigating the long-term effectiveness of portion size reductions are needed. Fifthly, it must be mentioned that for the subgroup interviews drop-out was large, causing a small sample size for the comparisons of satiety and dietary (caloric) compensation effects. This may have caused selection bias. For example, it may be that only those with a particular interest in health remained in the study. In contrast to sex and age, however, there was no difference in BMI between the retention and drop-out group. The above limitation shows the difficulty and complexity of such real-life trials and should be taken into account when conducting future research. It can be said that future studies with larger sample sizes are needed to confirm our results. Furthermore, it must be repeated that the interpretation of the results of the assessment of satiety and dietary intake should be taken with caution, since the small subsample may be the reason for the low statistical power. Future research should take this in mind and should try to work with sufficiently large samples, to obtain more statistical power. Sixthly, concerning consumption and plate waste, it was not feasible to investigate differences between students and employees, because it was practically impossible to weigh every paper bag sold to students versus employees. Also, separating students' plate waste from that of employees was not feasible. Seventh, the price of the reduced portion of French fries was not adjusted, which may have been of influence on the choice of the consumer to choose French fries or not. Especially, students, who are more sensitive to price changes than employees, could have opted a side dish different from French fries during the intervention week. However, since there was no significant difference in the number of consumers choosing French fries (and the proportion of students within these French fries consumers) between the baseline or intervention week, a lack of price adjustment was probably not crucial for the consumers' choice. However, the lack of price adjustment came up for discussion in the perception interview, when asking why people would or would not agree with a permanent implementation. The share of consumers indicating this as stumbling block was minimal, as only two out of 28 interviewees addressed this reason to disagree with a permanent implementation. Attractiveness of the French fries served in paper bags could have influenced the consumers' choice. Introducing paper bags before the baseline week could have ruled out a possible attractiveness effect ensuring a 'true' effect of the reduced portion was observed. However, no significant difference in the number of consumers choosing French fries between the baseline and intervention week was found. Misinterpretation of the terms satiety and fullness could also have influenced our results. Since satiety was questioned as a rating of fullness in the face-to-face interview, consumers could have reported a full feeling after consuming a 50 cl bottle of diet soda or water, which would not have corresponded with the calculated caloric intake. However, the study of Tremblay et al. [43] concludes that the use of VAS (visual analogue scale) scores, using ratings of hunger or fullness, has high relevance and is a simple and valid tool to predict variations in energy intake. Finally, this study only focused on one single energy dense food product and did not investigate possible effects on other foods. Also, focusing on different food products could have given us insight into which kind of portion size reduction consumers are most susceptible for. Therefore, future studies should examine whether portion size reduction of other foods will have similar effects and whether or not decreasing portion size of one food has an effect on the intake of other foods.

Conclusion

Reducing the portion size of French fries was effective in reducing French fries intake and French fries plate waste in an on-campus restaurant setting. More specifically, a portion size reduction by 20.9% resulted in a reduction by 9.1% in total French fries intake and a reduction by 66.4% for total French fries plate waste. Satiety of the consumers did not change and no dietary compensation effects were observed. A large part of French fries consumers noticed the reduced portion size. Although the majority thought that the portion size was sufficient, only a minority agreed with a permanent implementation. Changing portion size is a relatively easy and promising environmental strategy which may lead to a more balanced/healthier food intake.

Abbreviations

BMI: Body mass index; SLIM: Satiety Labelled Intensity Magnitude

Acknowledgements

The authors thank Philippe Merckx (manager of the university restaurant) and Leen Cleymans (university restaurant dietician), together with all other kitchen staff, for their contributions to this study. We also thank the two nutrition and dietetics students involved in this study for their help with data collection as well as the job students working in the tray return area. Finally, we thank all students and employees participating in this study.

Authors' contributions
MV, MS, PM, ED, BD, PC and TD conceived and designed the experiments. MV, TD and W performed the experiments. MV and TD analysed the data. MV wrote the manuscript. W, MS, PM, ED, BD, PC and TD reviewed the manuscript critically. All authors read and approved the final manuscript.

Competing interests
The authors declare that they have no competing interests.

Author details
[1]Department of Movement and Sport Sciences, Vrije Universiteit Brussel, Pleinlaan 2, 1050 Brussels, Belgium. [2]Department of Interdisciplinary Social Sciences, Utrecht University, Heidelberglaan 1, 3584 CS Utrecht, Netherlands. [3]Department of Psychological Assessment and Health Psychology, University of Konstanz, Universitätsstraße 10, D-78464 Konstanz, Germany. [4]International Prevention Research Institute (iPRI), 15 chemin du Saquin, 69130 Ecully (Lyon), France. [5]Department of Public Health, Ghent University, De Pintelaan 185, 9000 Ghent, Belgium.

References

1. Hanks AS, Just DR, Smith LE, Wansink B. Healthy convenience: nudging students toward healthier choices in the lunchroom. J Public Health (Oxf). 2012;34(3):370–6.
2. Hubbard KL, Bandini LG, Folta SC, Wansink B, Eliasziw M, Must A. Impact of a Smarter Lunchroom intervention on food selection and consumption among adolescents and young adults with intellectual and developmental disabilities in a residential school setting. Public Health Nutr. 2015;18(2):361–71.
3. Miller N, Reicks M, Redden JP, Mann T, Mykerezi E, Vickers Z. Increasing portion sizes of fruits and vegetables in an elementary school lunch program can increase fruit and vegetable consumption. Appetite. 2015;91:426–30.
4. Mobley CC, et al. Effect of nutrition changes on foods selected by students in a middle school-based diabetes prevention intervention program: the HEALTHY experience. J Sch Health. 2012;82(2):82–90.
5. Van Kleef E, Vrijhof M, Polet IA, Vingerhoeds MH, de Wijk RA. Nudging children towards whole wheat bread: a field experiment on the influence of fun bread roll shape on breakfast consumption. BMC Public Health. 2014;14(1):906.
6. Thomas LN, Hill TF, Gaines A, Dollahite JS. Implementing Smarter Lunchrooms Makeovers in New York state middle schools: an initial process evaluation. Arch Public Health. 2016;74(1):41.
7. Roy R, Kelly B, Rangan A, Allman-Farinelli M. Food environment interventions to improve the dietary behavior of young adults in tertiary education settings: a systematic literature review. J Acad Nutr Diet. 2015;115(10):1647–81.
8. Meiklejohn S, Ryan L, Palermo C. A systematic review of the impact of multi-strategy nutrition education programs on health and nutrition of adolescents. J Nutr Educ Behav. 2016;48(9):631–646.e1.
9. Vadeboncoeur C, Townsend N, Foster C. A meta-analysis of weight gain in first year university students: is freshman 15 a myth? BMC Obes. 2015; 2(February):22.
10. Fedewa MV, Das BM, Evans EM, Dishman RK. Change in weight and adiposity in college students: a systematic review and meta-analysis. Am J Prev Med. 2014;47(5):641–52.
11. Sharma M. Using multitheory model to predict initiation and sustenance of small portion size consumption among college students. Health Promot Perspect. 2016;6(3):137–44.
12. Deforche B, Van Dyck D, Deliens T, De Bourdeaudhuij I. Changes in weight, physical activity, sedentary behaviour and dietary intake during the transition to higher education: a prospective study. Int J Behav Nutr Phys Act. 2015;12(1):16.
13. Deliens T, Clarys P, Van Hecke L, De Bourdeaudhuij I, Deforche B. Changes in weight and body composition during the first semester at university. A prospective explanatory study. Appetite. 2013;65:111–6.
14. Steenhuis I, Van Assema P, Van Breukelen G, Glanz K, Kok G, De Vries H. The impact of educational and environmental interventions in Dutch worksite cafeterias. Health Promot Int. 2004;19(3):335–43.
15. Donohoe CM, Mas M, Mph MDM. Insights in public health promoting healthy snack and beverage choices in Hawaii worksites : the Choose Healthy Now! pilot project. Hawaii J Med Public Health. 2014;73(11):365–71.
16. Vermeer WM, Steenhuis IHM, Leeuwis FH, Heymans MW, Seidell JC. Small portion sizes in worksite cafeterias: do they help consumers to reduce their food intake? Int J Obes. 2011;35(9):1200–7.
17. Dubbert PM, Johnson WG, Schlundt DG, Montague NW. The influence of caloric information on cafeteria food choices. J Appl Behav Anal. 1984;17(1): 1307920.
18. Engbers LH, van Poppel MN, Chin A Paw M, van Mechelen W. The effects of a controlled worksite environmental intervention on determinants of dietary behavior and self-reported fruit, vegetable and fat intake. BMC Public Health. 2006;6(1):253.
19. Holdsworth M, Raymond NT, Haslam C. Does the Heartbeat Award scheme in England result in change in dietary behaviour in the workplace? Health Promot Int. 2004;19(2):197–204.
20. Sorensen G, et al. Work-site nutrition intervention and employees' dietary habits: the treatwell program. Am J Public Health. 1992;82(6):877–80.
21. Vyth EL, Steenhuis IHM, Heymans MW, Roodenburg AJC, Brug J, Seidell JC. Influence of placement of a nutrition logo on cafeteria menu items on lunchtime food Choices at Dutch work sites. J Am Diet Assoc. 2011;111(1):131–6.
22. Williams C, Poulter J. Formative evaluation of a workplace menu labelling scheme. J Hum Nutr Diet. 1991;4(4):251–62.
23. Thorndike AN, Riis J, Sonnenberg LM, Levy DE. Traffic-light labels and choice architecture: promoting healthy food choices. Am J Prev Med. 2014;46(2): 143–9.
24. Kroese FM, Marchiori DR, De Ridder DTD. Nudging healthy food choices: a field experiment at the train station. J Public Health (Oxf). 2016;38(2):e133–7.
25. Kallbekken S, Sælen H. "Nudging" hotel guests to reduce food waste as a win-win environmental measure. Econ Lett. 2013;119(3):325–7.
26. Olstad DL, Goonewardene LA, McCargar LJ, Raine KD. Choosing healthier foods in recreational sports settings: a mixed methods investigation of the impact of nudging and an economic incentive. Int J Behav Nutr Phys Act. 2014;11(1):6.
27. Kongsbak I, et al. Increasing fruit and vegetable intake among male university students in an ad libitum buffet setting: a choice architectural nudge intervention. Food Qual Prefer. 2016;49:183–8.
28. Service O, et al. EAST four simple ways to apply behavioural insights. Nesta. 2014:53.
29. Grieger JA, Wycherley TP, Johnson BJ, Golley RK. Discrete strategies to reduce intake of discretionary food choices: a scoping review. Int J Behav Nutr Phys Act. 2016;13(1):57.
30. Rolls BJ, Roe LS, Meengs JS. The effect of large portion sizes on energy intake is sustained for 11 days. Obesity (Silver Spring). 2007;15(6):1535–43.
31. Rolls BJ, Roe LS, Meengs JS. Reductions in portion size and energy density of foods are additive and lead to sustained decreases in energy intake. Am J Clin Nutr. 2006;83(1):11–7.
32. Vermeer WM, Steenhuis IHM, Poelman MP. Small, medium, large or supersize? The development and evaluation of interventions targeted at portion size. Int J Obes. 2014;38(S1):S13–8.
33. Freedman MR, Brochado C. Reducing portion size reduces food intake and plate waste. Obesity (Silver Spring). 2010;18(9):1864–6.
34. Rolls BJ, Roe LS, Kral TVE, Meengs JS, Wall DE. Increasing the portion size of a packaged snack increases energy intake in men and women. Appetite. 2004; 42(1):63–9.
35. Jeffery RW, Rydell S, Dunn CL, Harnack LJ. Effects of portion size on chronic energy intake. Int J Behav Nutr Phys Act. 2007;4:61–71.
36. Lewis HB, et al. Effect of reducing portion size at a compulsory meal on later energy intake, gut hormones, and appetite in overweight adults. Obesity. 2015;23(7):1362–70.
37. WHO. Diet, nutrition and the prevention of chronic diseases. World Health Organ Tech Rep Ser. 2003;916:i–viii-1-149-backcover.
38. Rodríguez-Arauz G, Ramírez-Esparza N, Smith-Castro V. Food attitudes and well-being: the role of culture. Appetite. 2016;105:180–8.
39. Rozin P, Fischler C, Imada S, Sarubin A, Wrzesniewski A. Attitudes to food and the role of food in life in the U.S.A., Japan, Flemish Belgium and France: possible implications for the diet-health debate. Appetite. 1999;33(2):163–80.
40. Frankenfeld CL, Poudrier JK, Waters NM, Gillevet PM, Xu Y. Dietary intake measured from a self-administered, online 24-hour recall system compared with 4-day diet records in an adult US population. J Acad Nutr Diet. 2012; 112(10):1642–7.

19

Association of maternal omega-6 fatty acid intake with infant birth outcomes: Korean Mothers and Children's Environmental Health (MOCEH)

Eunjung Lee[1,2], Hyesook Kim[1], Hyejin Kim[1], Eun-Hee Ha[3] and Namsoo Chang[1*]

Abstract

Background: Maternal fatty acids (FAs) intake has an effect on birth weight, birth length, and gestational age, as fetal development is entirely dependent on the maternal essential FA supply. This study aimed to identify the association between the maternal intake of FAs and birth outcomes among pregnant women who participated in the Mothers and Children's Environmental Health (MOCEH) prospective cohort study in South Korea.

Methods: A total of 1407 pregnant women, aged 30.2 ± 3.7 years, at 12 to 28 weeks' gestation were recruited between August 2006 and December 2010. Their dietary intake during pregnancy was investigated by the 1-day 24-h dietary recall method. The pregnancy outcome data—namely infant's gestational age, birth weight, and birth length—were analyzed for their associations with their mothers' intake of FAs.

Results: When adjusted for confounding factors, multiple regression analysis revealed adverse effects on birth weight ($P = 0.031$) and birth length ($P = 0.025$) with high maternal intake of omega-6 FAs. In the multiple logistic regression analysis, the odds ratio (OR) for the risk of being below the 10th percentile for birth weight was higher in the highest quintile (Q5) compared to the lowest quintile (Q1) of omega-6 FA intake levels (OR = 2.444; 95% CI = 1.038–5.751; P for trend = 0.010). Also, the OR for being above the 90th percentile of birth length was lower in the highest quintile (Q5) compared to that in the lowest quintile (Q1) of omega-6 FA intake (OR = 0.432; 95% CI = 0.211–0.884; P for trend = 0.020). However, the maternal intake of omega-3 FAs was not related to gestational age, birth weight, or birth length.

Conclusions: A high maternal omega-6 FA intake was negatively associated with birth weight and birth length.

Keywords: Pregnancy outcome, Omega-6 fatty acids, Pregnant women, Birth weight

Background

Many studies have demonstrated a link between maternal fatty acids (FAs) intake and pregnancy outcomes, including infant's birth weight and birth length. Despite these findings, the mechanisms underlying the correlation between maternal FAs intake and fetal size have not been fully elucidated. Nevertheless, deficiencies in the levels of the mothers' FAs intake could have negative outcomes on the birth weight, birth length, and gestational age of the infant, as fetal development is entirely dependent on the maternal supply of essential FAs [1]. Long-chain polyunsaturated fatty acids (LCPUFAs), such as docosahexaenoic acid (DHA; 22:6 *n*-3) and arachidonic acid (ARA; 20:4 *n*-6), are important for the development of the fetus during pregnancy [2–4].

Omega-3 FAs have received considerable attention in exploring the correlations of maternal FAs intake with birth weight. Several studies have indicated that gestational age, birth weight, and birth length increase when the consumption of omega-3 FAs during pregnancy increases [5–11]. However, other studies have shown conflicting results [12–14].

Nonetheless, few investigations have focused on the relationship between maternal omega-6 FAs intake and

* Correspondence: nschang@ewha.ac.kr
[1]Department of Nutritional Science and Food Management, Ewha Womans University, Seoul, South Korea
Full list of author information is available at the end of the article

birth outcomes, with only one literature report, to date, which pertained to pregnant women in India. It found that the birth weight was low at both low and high intakes of maternal linoleic acid (LA; 18:2 *n*-6), suggesting an inverted U–shaped relationship [15]. In addition, infants born to the group whose maternal diet had a higher omega-6/omega-3 ratio had lower birth weights, and vice versa. Other researchers have noted that higher levels of omega-6 FAs and ARA in maternal blood significantly lowered birth weight in early pregnancy and that elevated levels of ARA in late pregnancy were also associated with decreasing birth weight [16, 17]. Furthermore, Meher and coworkers observed that total omega-6 FA and ARA levels in maternal erythrocytes were higher in mothers delivering low-birth-weight babies (< 2. 5 kg) than those whose newborns weighed more than 2. 5 kg [18].

The preceding examples suggest that there is a high correlation between maternal FAs intake and fetal weight but, except for the assessment of pregnant women for FAs intake, there have been no in-depth studies of Korean women in this regard [19]. Also, the only study that measured total omega-3 and omega-6 FAs intake among pregnant women in Korea was limited, owing to the lack of an FA database for estimation of FA intake levels in the Korean population, at that time.

Therefore, the purpose of this study was to estimate the FAs intake of pregnant Korean women and to investigate the relationship between FAs intake and pregnancy outcomes, using a prospective sample from the Mothers and Children's Environmental Health (MOCEH) study [20].

Methods

Study design and participants

Study subjects were 1751 midstage (12–28 weeks of gestation) pregnant women enrolled in the MOCEH study [20] between August 2006 and December 2010. Of these 1751 women, 69 were excluded from our study (31 who were carrying twins, 35 who had had a miscarriage and/or were carrying a fetus with a congenital anomaly, and 3 who had an intrauterine growth restriction). Of the remaining 1682 women, 39 more were excluded (38 who had complications such as hypertension or/and diabetes and 1 had dropped out and whose pregnancy outcome data were not available). Among the remaining 1643 women, 236 more were excluded (229 whose dietary intake data were not collected and 7 whose total energy consumption was less than 500 or more than 4000 kcal per day). Therefore a total of 1407 women were finally included in the analysis. The study protocols and consent forms were approved by the three institutional review boards at the Ewha Womans University School of Medicine, the Dankook University Hospital, and the Ulsan University Hospital. All subjects provided informed consent to participate in the study, and they were questioned by trained interviewers.

General information on demographic factors, socioeconomic factors, and health-related behaviors was collected at a regular midtrimester checkup through an individual interview. Detailed data included subject's age, height, weight, parity, education level, family monthly income, dietary supplement use, smoking behavior, and alcohol. Pre-pregnancy body mass index (BMI) was calculated as weight (kg) divided by height (m^2) by employing self-reported height and weight values before conception. Education levels were categorized as less than high school graduation, university level graduation, or higher than university level graduation. Family monthly income was categorized as less than US$2000, US$2000 to US$4000, and greater than US$4000. Cigarette smoking was classified as current smoker or nonsmoker, and alcohol drinking was categorized into current drinker or nondrinker. Exposure to secondhand smoke was defined as living with someone who smoked or working in an environment where smoking was permitted. Smoking and drinking were assessed by self-report.

Dietary assessment

Dietary intake data at midpregnancy were collected by 24-h recall for intake the day before the participant's visit to the center. For the 24-h recall method, experienced, well-trained dietary interviewers asked the respondents to recall and describe all the foods and beverages they had consumed over the preceding 24 h. The food items most frequently mentioned were pictured on a chart which was shown to the participants to help them report more accurately. These nutrients in these dietary intakes were assessed using a computerized nutrient intake assessment software program (CAN-Pro 4.0, Korean Nutrition Society, Seoul, Korea) [21]. For the assessment of maternal FA intake, the CAN-Pro 4.0 FA database was supplemented by the step of database development [22], which covered about 93% of total FA intake of the 24-h recall method of the subjects.

Infant birth outcome

Information on neonates such as gestational age, birth weight, birth length, and gender was obtained from birth records. Gestational age at delivery was counted from the last menstrual period and examined by ultrasound.

Statistical analysis

General characteristics of the pregnant women and their neonates were expressed as means with standard deviations or as numbers with percentages. Multiple linear regression analysis was performed to evaluate the association between maternal FA intake and pregnancy outcome, such as birth weight and birth length. Multiple logistic regression analysis was also performed to estimate the odds ratios (ORs) and 95% confidence intervals (CIs) for the risk of less than 10th percentile or more than 90th percentile for birth weight and length across dietary FA intake level (quintiles). The covariates included maternal age [23], pre-pregnancy BMI [24–28], level of education, neonate's gender [29], log-transformed maternal urinary cotinine level (ln) [30], gestational age at delivery [31, 32], and energy intake. In analyzing the association between maternal FA intake and birth length, vitamin C intake was included among the covariates because it has been reported that maternal vitamin C intake is associated with birth length [33]. All the statistical analyses were conducted using SAS 9.4 software (SAS Institute Inc., Cary, NC, USA); the level of significance was set at $P < 0.05$.

Results

General characteristics

The mean (SD) maternal age at study enrollment was 30.2 ± 3.7 years, and prepregnancy BMI was 21.3 ± 3. 1 kg/m^2 (Table 1). Approximately 56.9% of subjects took nutritional supplements. The average energy and fat intakes of the women were respectively 1760.4 ± 494. 9 kcal and 46.2 ± 23.7 g per day.

Fatty acid intake of subjects

The average total FA intake of subjects was 43.5 ± 25.5 g per day. Saturated, monounsaturated, and polyunsaturated FA intakes were respectively 14.8 ± 10.0 g, 16.6 ± 11.2 g, and 11.9 ± 6.7 g per day. Total omega-3 FA intake was 1.47 ± 1.45 g per day, and the intake of DHA was 0.30 ± 0.83 g per day. Total omega-6 FA intake was 10.73 ± 6.34 g per day. The ratio of omega-6 to omega-3 FAs was 9.82 ± 7.00 (Table 2).

Relationship between fatty acid intake and birth outcome

In a multiple regression analysis (Table 3)—after adjusting for maternal age, prepregnancy BMI, education level, neonatal gender, log-transformed maternal urinary cotinine level, gestational age at delivery, energy intake, and vitamin C intake (only for birth length)—total maternal omega 6 FA intake was negatively associated with birth weight ($\beta = -0.161$; $P = 0.031$) and length ($\beta = -0.033$; $P = 0.025$).

As shown in Table 4, the multiple logistic regression analysis with covariates revealed that the odds ratio for a lower birth weight (below the 10th percentile) was significantly high in the 5th quintile compared with that in the 1st quintile of total omega-6 FA intake (OR = 2.444; 95% CI = 1.308–5.751; P for trend = 0.010). In addition, the odds ratio for a greater birth length (above the than 90th percentile) was significantly low in the 5th quintile compared with that in the 1st quintile of total omega-6 FA intake (OR = 0.432; 95% CI = 1.308–5.751; P for trend = 0. 020). When we further analyzed the relationship between the %E of n-6 FA intakes and birth weight and length, no significant association was found in multiple regressions. However, when we based our analysis on the recommended level of n-6 FA intakes for Korean (4–10%E), the odds ratio (OR) for the risk of being below the 10th percentile for birth weight was higher in the > 10%E (Q5) than in the < 4%E for omega-6 FA intake levels (OR; 4.013 CI; 1.199–3.432) (data not shown).

Discussion

In our study, fetal growth was inversely associated with maternal omega-6 FA intake, because, after confounding variables were corrected, birth weight decreased with increasing maternal omega-6 FAs intake during pregnancy. In addition, when the maternal omega-6 FA intake was divided into quintiles, the odds ratio for a birth weight below the 10th percentile was significantly higher in the 5th quintile (Q5), which represents a higher intake of omega-6 FAs than in the 1st quintile (OR = 2.444; 95% CI = 1.308–5.751; P for trend = 0.010). Maternal omega-3 FAs intake and omega-6/omega-3 ratio, however, were not associated with birth weight or length.

The results of our study, showing that maternal omega-6 FAs intake is inversely related to birth weight, are quite unlike those of other studies; therefore it was difficult to find similar results. However, a recent report from India states that maternal intake of LA, which accounts for a large proportion of omega-6 FAs, is inversely related to birth weight. In that study (although not statistically significant but similar to our study), the birth weight was low when the maternal LA intake was high. In addition, birth weight was lower in the low maternal LA intake group, indicating an inverted U–shaped relationship between maternal LA intake and birth weight [15]. In our study, the relationship between maternal LA intake and birth weight was not statistically significant but showed a weakly negative relationship ($P = 0.061$), similar to the study in India.

Western diets are typically high in omega-6 FAs and low in omega-3 FAs, while the average intake of omega-3 FAs among our subjects was significantly higher. Therefore, omega-6 FAs may have different effects on pregnancy outcomes. Previous studies have also reported that birth weight is affected by race [34, 35]. The Danish study reported that pregnant women who consumed a Western diet that contained high omega-6 FAs had a high SGA baby birth rate, suggesting that omega-6 FAs intake may also influence the birth weight among Western people [36]. However, several studies [6, 37, 38] that reported increased birth size due to supplementation of omega-3 FAs showed that omega-3 FAs intake in Western populations plays an important role in pregnancy outcomes. Maternal increased intake of omega-6 FAs at

Table 1 General characteristics of study subjects

	n	Mean ± SD		Range
Pregnant women				
Age, y	1326	30.2 ± 3.7		18–45
Height, cm	1300	161.2 ± 4.8		146–180
Weight, kg				
Pre-pregnancy	1316	55.3 ± 8.5		39–94
Pregnancy	1258	59.6 ± 9.3		37–117
Body mass index, kg/m^2				
Pre-pregnancy	1292	21.3 ± 3.1		15.8–42.8
Pregnancy	1248	22.9 ± 3.4		15.8–43.5
Parity	1138			
Primigravida, *n*(%)			638(56.1)	
Multigravida, *n*(%)			500(43.9)	
Education, *n*(%)	1276			
≤ High school			342(26.8)	
≤ University			852(66.8)	
≥ Graduate school			82(6.4)	
Family monthly income(USD), *n*(%)	1253			
< 2000			339(27.1)	
2000 ≤ and < 4000			675(53.9)	
≥ 4000			239(19.1)	
Supplement user, *n*(%)	1405		799(56.9)	
Cigarette smoker, current, *n*(%)	1315		12(0.9)	
Secondhand smoking exposer, *n*(%)	1237		179(14.5)	
Urinary cotinine, μg/g creatinine	1323	45.3 ± 312.1		0–5882
Alcohol drinker, current, *n*(%)	1237		67(5.4)	
Daily dietary intake	1407			
Energy, kcal/day		1760.4 ± 494.9		
Fat, g/day		46.2 ± 23.7		
Neonates				
Gestational age at delivery, days	1262	274.8 ± 10.3		191–294
Birth weight, g	1291	3262.5 ± 427.0		500–4650
Birth length, cm	1201	50.5 ± 2.5		26–38.5
Gender	1296			
Boys, *n*(%)			674(52.0)	
Girls, *n*(%)			622(48.0)	

high levels of omega-3 FAs intake among our subjects resulted in low birth weight, and that involved different conditions from previous studies for Western women.

The mechanisms of the relationship between maternal intake of omega-6 FAs and infant birth weight is not well established. However, some investigators have indeed found that pregnant women who had higher levels of total omega-6 FAs and ARA in their blood at late pregnancy delivered low-birth-weight babies [18, 39]. In addition, others have observed an association between higher levels of omega-6 FAs and ARA with reduced birth weight in early pregnancy [1, 17]. The elongation and desaturation of omega-6 and omega-3 FAs involve the same enzyme [40], indicating that high levels of omega-6 FAs can inhibit the conversion of omega-3 FAs. The mechanism of omega-3 FAs in improving fetal growth may be related to its effect on the endothelium [41]. The omega-3 LCPUFAs improves membrane fluidity [42] and receptor activity by increasing flow-mediated vasodilation in young adults [43], so it is

Table 2 Daily maternal fatty acids intake (*n* 1407)

	Mean ± SD*	Range*
TFAs, g	43.51 ± 25.53	0.48–205.36
SFAs, g	14.78 ± 9.99	0.07–85.37
MUFAs, g	16.60 ± 11.15	0.12–90.11
PUFAs, g	11.90 ± 6.70	0.29–54.82
Total n-3 FAs, g	1.47 ± 1.45	0.04–11.88
18:3 *n*-3, g	1.05 ± 0.78	0.02–8.06
20:4 *n*-3, g	0.00 ± 0.02	0.00–0.00
20:5 *n*-3, g	0.14 ± 0.35	0.00–3.43
22:5 *n*-3, g	0.01 ± 0.03	0.00–1.00
22:6 *n*-3, g	0.30 ± 0.83	0.00–9.76
Total *n*-6 FAs, g	10.73 ± 6.34	0.44–50.88
18:2 *n*-6, g	9.99 ± 6.09	0.03–49.79
20:2 *n*-6, g	0.07 ± 0.12	0.00–1.00
20:3 *n*-6, g	0.09 ± 0.08	0.00–1.00
20:4 *n*-6, g	0.06 ± 0.10	0.00–0.85
22:5 *n*-6, g	0.02 ± 0.10	0.00–1.00
n-6/*n*-3	9.82 ± 7.00	0.31–63.00

TFAs, Total fatty acids; SFAs, saturated fatty acids; MUFAs, mono unsaturated fatty acids; PUFAs, poly unsaturated fatty acids; FAs, fatty acids
*All intakes are rounded to the second decimal place

possible that these FAs may increase the fetal growth rate by increasing placental blood flow and decreasing blood viscosity through the production of omega-3 FAs metabolite, such as prostacyclin and thromboxane [44]. This suggests that the decrease in birth weight when omega-6 FAs intake was high may be related to the inhibition of the positive effects of omega-3 FAs on fetal growth. Among our subjects, n-3 FAs intake and the omega-6/omega-3 ratio in fifth quintile were 2.86 ± 1.75 g and 9.12 ± 3.41, respectively, which were within FAO/WHO recommendations. However, the subtype of omega-3 FAs intake was mainly alpha-linolenic acid (ALA) among our subjects (Table 2). Theoretically, ALA, which is the essential fatty acid, is synthesized to DHA in the liver [45], but since ALA is hardly converted to DHA in young women [46, 47], it is doubtful whether the adequate DHA supply for fetal development was efficient. An intervention study [48] reported that the addition of ALA in the maternal diet did not increase the DHA level for the baby, suggesting that maternal direct intake of DHA would be more beneficial to the fetus. Our subjects had a high intake of omega-3 FAs but mostly ALA as mentioned, so it seemed difficult to show the positive effects of DHA or EPA in pregnancy outcomes. In addition, the average intake of omega-6 FAs in the fifth quintile was 21.35 ± 5.75 g, which was approximately 50% of the total fat intake, suggesting that excessive omega-6 FAs intake may be related to the inhibition of fatty acids synthesis such as DHA and EPA, consequently suppressing the positive effects of DHA in fetal growth.

Our study did not show any association between maternal intake of omega-3 FAs and birth weight. Some studies relating maternal intake of omega-3 FAs during pregnancy with birth outcome report a positive association between maternal omega-3 FAs intake and birth size [14, 49–51], while others have found no association [12, 52] or a negative association [53]. The study of

Table 3 Coefficients from multiple regression analysis between maternal fatty acids intakes with birth weight and birth length

	Birth weight(*n* 1291)						Birth length(*n* 1201)					
	Unadjusted			Adjusted[a]			Unadjusted			Adjusted[b]		
	β	SE	*P* value	*β*	SE	*P* value	*β*	SE	*P* value	*β*	SE	*P* value
TFAs	−0.009	0.463	0.985	−0.243	0.575	0.673	0.000	0.003	0.981	−0.001	0.004	0.806
SFAs	0.452	1.180	0.702	0.336	1.359	0.805	0.003	0.007	0.711	0.003	0.009	0.719
MUFAs	−0.057	1.059	0.957	−0.478	1.252	0.703	0.001	0.006	0.903	−0.001	0.008	0.951
PUFAs	−1.196	1.774	0.501	−2.847	2.109	0.177	−0.010	0.011	0.340	−0.017	0.014	0.199
Total *n*-3 FAs	0.965	8.785	0.913	−0.075	8.679	0.993	−0.058	0.052	0.261	−0.061	0.053	0.249
18:3 *n*-3	−12.306	15.416	0.425	−17.617	15.971	0.270	−0.131	0.092	0.155	−0.152	0.100	0.129
20:5 *n*-3	43.365	34.607	0.210	31.952	33.022	0.334	0.016	0.206	0.938	0.064	0.206	0.754
22:6 *n*-3	14.954	14.550	0.304	10.818	13.442	0.421	0.017	0.091	0.350	0.005	0.089	0.957
Total *n*-6 FAs	−2.946	2.076	0.156	−5.161	2.394	0.031*	−0.017	0.012	0.158	−0.033	0.015	0.025*
18:2 *n*-6	−2.315	1.953	0.236	−4.246	2.266	0.061	−0.011	0.012	0.332	−0.018	0.015	0.209
20:4 *n*-6	2.887	125.055	0.982	−67.266	121.643	0.580	0.002	0.760	0.998	−0.433	0.782	0.580
n-6/*n*-3	0.117	2.489	0.963	−0.439	2.437	0.857	0.013	0.015	0.398	0.015	0.015	0.304

TFAs, Total fatty acids; SFAs, saturated fatty acids; MUFAs, mono unsaturated fatty acids; PUFAs, poly unsaturated fatty acics
$*P < 0.05$
[a]adjusted for maternal age, pre-pregnancy BMI, level of education, neonatal gender, maternal urinary cotinine level (ln), gestational age and energy intake
[b]adjusted for maternal age, pre-pregnancy BMI, level of education, neonatal gender, maternal urinary cotinine level (ln), gestational age, energy and vitamin C intake

Table 4 Odds ratio (OR) and 95% confidence interval (CI) of birth weight and birth length with quintile of omega 6 intakes in the subjects

		n-6 FA intakes, quintiles (range, g/d)					*P* for trend
		Q1 (0.44–5.70)	Q2 (5.70–8.07)	Q3 (8.07–10.76)	Q4 (10.76–15.16)	Q5 (15.16–47.57)	
Birth weight (*n* 1078)							
For below 10th% (*n* 111)							
Unadjusted	OR	1.00	0.797	0.717	0.728	1.554	0.424
	95% CI		0.420–1.510	0.371–1.383	0.377–1.405	0.885–2.730	
Adjusted[a]	OR	1.00	0.666	0.680	0.939	2.444	0.010*
	95% CI		0.302–1.468	0.293–1.574	0.418–2.108	1.038–5.751	
For above 90th% (*n* 116)							
Unadjusted	OR	1.00	1.026	0.834	0.725	0.611	0.078
	95% CI		0.583–1.807	0.462–1.507	0.393–1.338	0.326–1.146	
Adjusted[a]	OR	1.00	0.974	0.633	0.716	0.539	0.109
	95% CI		0.517–1.836	0.316–1.268	0.350–1.465	0.237–1.224	
Birth length (*n* 1008)							
For below 10th% (*n* 100)							
Unadjusted	OR	1.00	0.951	0.994	0.476	0.968	0.593
	95% CI		0.508–1.779	0.531–1.861	0.224–1.010	0.521–1.799	
Adjusted[b]	OR	1.00	0.694	1.163	0.501	1.300	0.597
	95% CI		0.320–1.503	0.546–2.476	0.200–1.250	0.534–3.165	
For above 90th% (*n* 184)							
Unadjusted	OR	1.00	0.917	0.963	0.921	0.509	0.015*
	95% CI		0.563–1.493	0.591–1.570	0.562–1.509	0.296–0.874	
Adjusted[b]	OR	1.00	0.985	0.902	0.910	0.432	0.020*
	95% CI		0.559–1.735	0.501–1.655	0.501–1.655	0.211–0.884	

*$P < 0.05$
[a]Adjusted for maternal age, pre-pregnancy BMI, level of education, neonatal gender, maternal urinary cotinine level (ln), gestational age and energy intake
[b]Adjusted for maternal age, pre-pregnancy BMI, level of education, neonatal gender, maternal urinary cotinine level (ln), gestational age, energy and vitamin C intake

pregnant women in India reported that birth weight was greater with a high intake of omega-3 FAs [15], suggesting the importance of omega-3 FAs intake for pregnant women in India. Our results, which showed no relationship between the maternal intake of omega-3 FAs and fetal growth, are probably explained by the relatively high intake of omega-3 FAs (mean intake 1470 mg per day, range from 40 to 11,880 mg) among our subjects. By comparison, the intake of omega-3 FAs by pregnant women was 11.49 mg per day in India [54] and 147 mg per day in the United Kingdom [12], both significantly lower than those in our study. Therefore it is important to determine whether the extremely low omega-3 FA intake among pregnant women in Korea is related to negative pregnancy outcomes.

The average fat intake of our subjects was 43.5 g (23.6% of the energy intake, EI), which is lower than the 71.8 g (31.9% of EI) in the United States [55], 99.1 g (29% of EI) in Mexico [56], and 74 g (31% of EI) in Denmark [57]; otherwise the fat intake in India (24% of EI) was similar [15]. Also, our subjects consumed 5.2% and 0.8% of energy in the form of omega-6 and omega-3 FAs respectively, which is within the range for omega-6 and omega-3 FAs recommended for pregnant women by the Food and Agriculture Organization/World Health Organization [58]. Our subjects in Q5 (comprising those with the highest intake of the omega-6 FAs), incidentally, consumed more than 10% (range from 7.7% to 24.3%) of their energy as omega-6 FAs. The mean omega-6/omega-3 ratio of our subjects was 9.8; it was 27.5 among pregnant women in India [15] and 12.3 among those in Mexico [56], indicating the omega-6/omega-3 ratios in our study were lower than those in other countries. However, this is explained by the fact that the omega-3 FAs intake of pregnant women in other countries is very low, while that of pregnant women in Korea is high. Nevertheless the omega-6/omega-3 ratio of our subjects was somewhat high when compared with the recommended standards [59]; therefore we concluded that it would be important to improve the dietary patterns of pregnant women in Korea.

This study has several limitations. First, it was difficult to accurately reflect the daily intake because the dietary intake of pregnant women was measured by a 1-day 24-h recall survey. However, in order to improve the accuracy of this method, we conducted a dietary survey employing trained dietitians using standard protocols, which helped the subjects reflect on their daily diets in detail, and we asked subjects whether their meal on the day of the dietary survey was the same as usual to reduce within-person variations. In addition, a study that was part of the Korean Health and Nutrition Survey showed that the values of fat intake obtained in each interview did not differ much from those of an additional one-day, 24-h recall and the original one-day diet interview, which was 2.5% [60]. Second, the results of FAs supplementation in our study were not available owing to the lack of data on omega-3 FAs– and omega-6 FAs–related products that might be consumed by our subjects. In our study, more than 50% of our subjects were taking supplements, and 57% of the supplements were folate supplements and iron supplements. Also, 36% of the supplements included prenatal multi supplements. Among the supplement users, only 3% of the pregnant women were consuming supplements containing omega FAs. Considering the fact that supplementation of omega-3 FAs such as DHA can affect pregnancy outcomes, further studies are needed to investigate the intake of omega-3 FAs through supplements. Finally, we lacked the data on omega-3 FAs and omega-6 FAs in the plasma, which could have substantiated the relationship observed between maternal omega-6 FAs nutrition and birth weight due to the limited availability of samples for other measurements (environmental heavy metals, toxins, etc.). Measuring the plasma PUFAs levels and analyzing their relationship with pregnancy outcomes is important to further support the results of our study. Therefore, we will consider measuring plasma FAs for the future studies. Nevertheless these limitations, this study is the first, comprising a large cohort, to examine FAs intake among pregnant women in Korea and the relationship of FAs intake with pregnancy outcome. Based on this study, future studies are needed to elucidate how an excessive intake of omega-6 FAs is related to pregnancy outcome. It will also be important to suggest ways in which to limit the consumption of omega-6 FAs among pregnant women in Korea.

Conclusion

This study was the first to investigate the relationship between the intake of FAs and pregnancy outcome among pregnant women in Korea. Despite adequate levels of omega-3 FAs, women who had high levels of omega-6 FAs tended to have lower birth weight infants. Therefore, reducing excessive omega-6 FAs intake of pregnant women in Korea will improve maternal nutritional status and also have more positive outcomes of pregnancy.

Abbreviations

ARA: Arachidonic acid; DHA: docosahexaenoic acid; FAs: Fatty acids; LA: Linoleic acid; LC-PUFAs: Long-chain polyunsaturated fatty acids; MOCEH: Mothers' and Children's Environmental Health; MUFAs: Mono unsaturated fatty acids; n-6/n-3: Ratio of n-6-to-n-3 polyunsaturated fatty acids; PUFAs: Polyunsaturated fatty acids SFAs: Saturated fatty acids; TFAs: Total fatty acids

Acknowledgements

This study was supported by MOCEH (Mothers and Children's Environmental Health) project of the National Institute of Environmental Research, Republic of Korea.

Funding

This research was supported by the Ministry of Environment and by Brain Korean 21 Plus.

Author's contributions

NC and EHH designed the research protocols; EL, HK, and HK conducted the research; EL and HK analyzed the data; EL and NC wrote the manuscript, and NC was primarily responsible for the final contents. All the authors read and approved the final manuscript.

Competing interests

All authors, E Lee, H Kim, H Kim, EH Ha, and N Chang, declare that they have no competing interests.

Author details

[1]Department of Nutritional Science and Food Management, Ewha Womans University, Seoul, South Korea. [2]Department of Nutrition Consultation, Seoul National University Hospital, Healthcare System Gangnam Center, Seoul, South Korea. [3]Department of Occupational and Environmental Medicine, Ewha Womans University, College of Medicine, Seoul, South Korea.

References

1. Smits LJ, Elzenga HM, Gemke RJ, Hornstra G, van Eijsden M. The association between interpregnancy interval and birth weight: what is the role of maternal polyunsaturated fatty acid status? BMC Pregnancy Childbirth. 2013; 13:23.
2. Martinez M. Tissue levels of polyunsaturated fatty acids during early human development. J Pediatr. 1992;120:S129–33.
3. Rustan AC, Drevon CA. Fatty acids: structures and properties. Hoboken: John Wiley & Sons, Ltd.; 2001.
4. Al MD, Hornstra G, van der Schouw YT, Eulstra-Ramakers MT, Huisjes HJ. Biochemical EFA status of mothers and their neonates after normal pregnancy. Early Hum Dev. 1990;24:239–48.
5. Makrides M, Gibson RA. Long-chain polyunsaturated fatty acid requirements during pregnancy and lactation. Am J Clin Nutr. 2000;71:307s–11s.
6. Olsen SF, Sorensen JD, Secher N, Hedegaard M, Henriksen TB, Hansen HS, Grant A. Randomised controlled trial of effect of fish-oil supplementation on pregnancy duration. Lancet. 1992;339:1003–7.

7. Smuts CM, Huang M, Mundy D, Plasse T, Major S, Carlson SE. A randomized trial of docosahexaenoic acid supplementation during the third trimester of pregnancy. Obstet Gynecol. 2003;101:469–79.
8. Makrides M, Duley L, Olsen SF. Marine oil, and other prostaglandin precursor, supplementation for pregnancy uncomplicated by pre-eclampsia or intrauterine growth restriction. Cochrane Database Syst Rev. 2006; 3(Cd003402).
9. Ramakrishnan U, Stein AD, Parra-Cabrera S, Wang M, Imhoff-Kunsch B, Juarez-Marquez S, Rivera J, Martorell R. Effects of docosahexaenoic acid supplementation during pregnancy on gestational age and size at birth: randomized, double-blind, placebo-controlled trial in Mexico. Food Nutr Bull. 2010;31:S108–16.
10. Harris MA, Reece MS, McGregor JA, Wilson JW, Burke SM, Wheeler M, Anderson JE, Auld GW, French JI, Allen KG. The effect of Omega-3 docosahexaenoic acid supplementation on gestational length: randomized trial of supplementation compared to nutrition education for increasing n-3 intake from foods. Biomed Res Int. 2015;2015:123078.
11. Olsen SF, Hansen HS, Sorensen TI, Jensen B, Secher NJ, Sommer S, Knudsen LB. Intake of marine fat, rich in (n-3)-polyunsaturated fatty acids, may increase birthweight by prolonging gestation. Lancet. 1986;2:367–9.
12. Rogers I, Emmett P, Ness A, Golding J. Maternal fish intake in late pregnancy and the frequency of low birth weight and intrauterine growth retardation in a cohort of British infants. J Epidemiol Community Health. 2004;58:486–92.
13. Thorsdottir I, Birgisdottir BE, Halldorsdottir S, Geirsson RT. Association of fish and fish liver oil intake in pregnancy with infant size at birth among women of normal weight before pregnancy in a fishing community. Am J Epidemiol. 2004;160:460–5.
14. Olsen SF, Grandjean P, Weihe P, Viderø T. Frequency of seafood intake in pregnancy as a determinant of birth weight: evidence for a dose dependent relationship. J Epidemiol Community Health. 1993;47:436–40.
15. Mani I, Dwarkanath P, Thomas T, Thomas A, Kurpad AV. Maternal fat and fatty acid intake and birth outcomes in a south Indian population. Int J Epidemiol. 2016;45:523–31.
16. Much D, Brunner S, Vollhardt C, Schmid D, Sedlmeier EM, Bruderl M, Heimberg E, Bartke N, Boehm G, Bader BL, et al. Effect of dietary intervention to reduce the n-6/n-3 fatty acid ratio on maternal and fetal fatty acid profile and its relation to offspring growth and body composition at 1 year of age. Eur J Clin Nutr. 2013;67:282–8.
17. van Eijsden M, Hornstra G, van der Wal MF, Vrijkotte TG, Bonsel GJ. Maternal n-3, n-6, and trans fatty acid profile early in pregnancy and term birth weight: a prospective cohort study. Am J Clin Nutr. 2008;87:887–95.
18. Meher A, Randhir K, Mehendale S, Wagh G, Joshi S. Maternal fatty acids and their association with birth outcome: a prospective study. PLoS One. 2016; 11:e0147359.
19. Kwon SK, Lim SJ, Shin JS, Jang SH, Ahn HS. Comparison of maternal fatty acid intake and fatty acid composition of serum phospholipids between singleton and twin pregnancies. Korean J Community Nutr. 2008;13:555–64.
20. Kim BM, Ha M, Park HS, Lee BE, Kim YJ, Hong YC, Kim Y, Chang N, Roh YM, Kim BN, et al. The mothers and Children's environmental health (MOCEH) study. Eur J Epidemiol. 2009;24:573–83.
21. Center KNI. Computer aided nutritional analysis program for professionals. 4. 0 edition. Seoul: The Korean Nutrition Society; 2011.
22. Yoon MO, Kim KR, Hwang JY, Lee HS, Son TY, Moon HK, Shim JE. Development of a fatty acids database using the Korea National Health and nutrition examination survey data. J Nutr Health. 2014;47:435–42.
23. Delbaere I, Verstraelen H, Goetgeluk S, Martens G, De Backer G, Temmerman M. Pregnancy outcome in primiparae of advanced maternal age. Eur J Obstet Gynecol Reprod Biol. 2007;135:41–6.
24. Hindmarsh PC, Geary MP, Rodeck CH, Kingdom JC, Cole TJ. Intrauterine growth and its relationship to size and shape at birth. Pediatr Res. 2002;52:263–8.
25. Lagiou P, Tamimi RM, Mucci LA, Adami HO, Hsieh CC, Trichopoulos D. Diet during pregnancy in relation to maternal weight gain and birth size. Eur J Clin Nutr. 2004;58:231–7.
26. Okubo H, Miyake Y, Sasaki S, Tanaka K, Murakami K, Hirota Y, Kanzaki H, Kitada M, Horikoshi Y, Ishiko O, et al. Maternal dietary patterns in pregnancy and fetal growth in Japan: the Osaka maternal and child health study. Br J Nutr. 2012;107:1526–33.
27. Loy SL, Marhazlina M, Azwany YN, Hamid Jan JM. Higher intake of fruits and vegetables in pregnancy is associated with birth size. Southeast Asian J Trop Med Public Health. 2011;42:1214–23.
28. Ronnenberg AG, Wang X, Xing H, Chen C, Chen D, Guang W, Guang A, Wang L, Ryan L, Xu X. Low preconception body mass index is associated with birth outcome in a prospective cohort of Chinese women. J Nutr. 2003;133:3449–55.
29. Catalano PM, Drago NM, Amini SB. Factors affecting fetal growth and body composition. Am J Obstet Gynecol. 1995;172:1459–63.
30. Shu XO, Hatch MC, Mills J, Clemens J, Susser M. Maternal smoking, alcohol drinking, caffeine consumption, and fetal growth: results from a prospective study. Epidemiology. 1995;6:115–20.
31. Rum P, Hornstra G. The n-3 and n-6 polyunsaturated fatty acid composition of plasma phospholipids in pregnant women and their infants. Relationship with maternal linoleic acid intake. Clin Chem Lab Med. 2002;40:32–9.
32. Baack ML, Puumala SE, Messier SE, Pritchett DK, Harris WS. What is the relationship between gestational age and docosahexaenoic acid (DHA) and arachidonic acid (ARA) levels? Prostaglandins Leukot Essent Fatty Acids. 2015;100:5–11.
33. Chang W. Relationship of maternal vitamin C nutrition and GSTM1/GSTT1 polymorphisms to fetal and infant growth. Master Dissertation. Ewha Womans University; 2014.
34. Fulda KG, Kurian AK, Balyakina E, Moerbe MM. Paternal race/ethnicity and very low birth weight. BMC Pregnancy Childbirth. 2014;14:385.
35. Barron SL. Birthweight and ethnicity. Br J Obstet Gynaecol. 1983;90:289–90.
36. Knudsen VK, Orozova-Bekkevold IM, Mikkelsen TB, Wolff S, Olsen SF. Major dietary patterns in pregnancy and fetal growth. Eur J Clin Nutr. 2008;62:463–70.
37. Makrides M, Gibson RA, McPhee AJ, Yelland L, Quinlivan J, Ryan P. Effect of DHA supplementation during pregnancy on maternal depression and neurodevelopment of young children: a randomized controlled trial. JAMA. 2010;304:1675–83.
38. Szajewska H, Horvath A, Koletzko B. Effect of n-3 long-chain polyunsaturated fatty acid supplementation of women with low-risk pregnancies on pregnancy outcomes and growth measures at birth: a meta-analysis of randomized controlled trials. Am J Clin Nutr. 2006;83:1337–44.
39. Dirix CE, Kester AD, Hornstra G. Associations between neonatal birth dimensions and maternal essential and trans fatty acid contents during pregnancy and at delivery. Br J Nutr. 2009;101:399–407.
40. Arterburn LM, Hall EB, Oken H. Distribution, interconversion, and dose response of n– 3 fatty acids in humans. Am J Clin Nutr. 2006;83:S1467–1476S.
41. Shimokawa H, Vanhoutte PM. Dietary cod-liver oil improves endothelium-dependent responses in hypercholesterolemic and atherosclerotic porcine coronary arteries. Circulation. 1988;78:1421–30.
42. Goode GK, Garcia S, Heagerty AM. Dietary supplementation with marine fish oil improves in vitro small artery endothelial function in hypercholesterolemic patients: a double-blind placebo-controlled study. Circulation. 1997;96:2802–7.
43. Leeson CP, Mann A, Kattenhorn M, Deanfield JE, Lucas A, Muller DP. Relationship between circulating n-3 fatty acid concentrations and endothelial function in early adulthood. Eur Heart J. 2002;23:216–22.
44. Makila UM, Jouppila P, Kirkinen P, Viinikka L, Ylikorkala O. Placental thromboxane and prostacyclin in the regulation of placental blood flow. Obstet Gynecol. 1986;68:537–40.
45. Sprecher H, Luthria DL, Mohammed B, Baykousheva SP. Reevaluation of the pathways for the biosynthesis of polyunsaturated fatty acids. J Lipid Res. 1995;36:2471–7.
46. Pawlosky RJ, Hibbeln JR, Novotny JA, Salem N Jr. Physiological compartmental analysis of alpha-linolenic acid metabolism in adult humans. J Lipid Res. 2001;42:1257–65.
47. Williams CM, Burdge G. Long-chain n-3 PUFA: plant v. Marine sources. Proc Nutr Soc. 2006;65:42–50.
48. de Groot RH, Hornstra G, van Houwelingen AC, Roumen F. Effect of alpha-linolenic acid supplementation during pregnancy on maternal and neonatal polyunsaturated fatty acid status and pregnancy outcome. Am J Clin Nutr. 2004;79:251–60.
49. Olsen SF, Secher NJ. Low consumption of seafood in early pregnancy as a risk factor for preterm delivery: prospective cohort study. BMJ. 2002;324:447.
50. Larque E, Gil-Sanchez A, Prieto-Sanchez MT, Koletzko B. Omega 3 fatty acids, gestation and pregnancy outcomes. Br J Nutr. 2012;107(Suppl 2):S77–84.
51. Carlson SE, Colombo J, Gajewski BJ, Gustafson KM, Mundy D, Yeast J, Georgieff MK, Markley LA, Kerling EH, Shaddy DJ. DHA supplementation and pregnancy outcomes. Am J Clin Nutr. 2013;97:808–15.

52. Olsen SF, Hansen HS, Secher NJ, Jensen B, Sandstrom B. Gestation length and birth weight in relation to intake of marine n-3 fatty acids. Br J Nutr. 1995;73:397–404.
53. Oken E, Kleinman KP, Olsen SF, Rich-Edwards JW, Gillman MW. Associations of seafood and elongated n-3 fatty acid intake with fetal growth and length of gestation: results from a US pregnancy cohort. Am J Epidemiol. 2004;160:774–83.
54. Muthayya S, Dwarkanath P, Thomas T, Ramprakash S, Mehra R, Mhaskar A, Mhaskar R, Thomas A, Bhat S, Vaz M. The effect of fish and ω-3 LCPUFA intake on low birth weight in Indian pregnant women. Eur J Clin Nutr. 2009; 63:340–6.
55. Crume TL, Brinton JT, Shapiro A, Kaar J, Glueck DH, Siega-Riz AM, Dabelea D. Maternal dietary intake during pregnancy and offspring body composition: the healthy start study. Am J Obstet Gynecol. 2016;215:609–e601.
56. Parra-Cabrera S, Stein AD, Wang M, Martorell R, Rivera J, Ramakrishnan U. Dietary intakes of polyunsaturated fatty acids among pregnant Mexican women. Matern Child Nutr. 2011;7:140–7.
57. Maslova E, Rytter D, Bech BH, Henriksen TB, Olsen SF, Halldorsson TI. Maternal intake of fat in pregnancy and offspring metabolic health–a prospective study with 20 years of follow-up. Clin Nutr. 2016;35:475–83.
58. Organization FA. Fat and fatty acids in human nutrition – report of an expert consultation. Geneva: Food Agriculture Organization; 2008.
59. Welfare MoHa. Dietary Reference Intakes for Koreans 2015. Sejong: Ministry of Health and Welfare; 2015. 2015
60. Korea Centers for Disease Control and Prevention. Report presentation of the Korea National Health and nutrition examination survey (KNHANES) IV. Seoul: Ministry of Health and Welfare; 2009. 2010

20

Probiotic fruit beverages with different polyphenol profiles attenuated early insulin response

Jie Xu[1*], Tommy Jönsson[2], Merichel Plaza[3,4], Åsa Håkansson[5], Martin Antonsson[6], Irini Lazou Ahrén[7], Charlotta Turner[4], Peter Spégel[4] and Yvonne Granfeldt[5]

Abstract

Background: Consumption of polyphenol-rich fruits and vegetables may improve postprandial glucose and insulin levels and hence promote well-being. Previously it has been observed that consumption of bilberry decreases the postprandial insulin demand. The intention with the present study was to compare the impact of different supplements with various polyphenol profiles, on the postprandial glucose and insulin responses in healthy young adults.

Methods: In a randomized, controlled, crossover study the postprandial glycemic and insulin responses were observed in eleven healthy adults after intake of five different beverages containing bilberry (European blueberry), blackcurrant, beetroot, mango and rose hip, respectively; all drinks were enriched with the same composition of fermented oatmeal and probiotics. The control was a glucose drink. The profile and content of the polyphenols in the different beverages were determined by HPLC-DAD analysis. The antioxidative capacity of the different beverages were measured by TEAC and DPPH assays.

Results: Beverages containing bilberry, blackcurrant, mango or rose hip significantly attenuated the early postprandial insulin response (0–90 min), but showed no effect on glucose response. Drinks with bilberry or rose hip reduced the insulin response from the very early phase (0–30 min), and had significantly lower insulin index compared with the control. The efficiency of the bilberry and rose hip to decrease early postprandial insulin responses correlated with higher phenolic contents.

Conclusions: Supplements with bilberry, blackcurrant, mango or rose hip in the tested probiotic and oatmeal enriched beverage attenuated early-phase insulin response, but had no effect on the postprandial glycemic response. The improved ability of bilberry and rose hip to lower the very early phase of insulin response seems to be due to a higher phenolic content.

Keywords: Bilberries, Blackcurrant, Mango, Rose hip, Beetroot, Postprandial insulin response

* Correspondence: jie.xu@liu.se
[1]Department of Clinical and Experimental Medicine, Linköping University, Linköping, Sweden
Full list of author information is available at the end of the article

Background

Postprandial hyperglycemia contributes to the development of cardiovascular diseases and type 2 diabetes [1, 2]; both diseases lay burden on the healthcare systems, globally [3]. Postprandial hyperglycemia is a condition that can be improved through lifestyle and diet modifications. In functional food research, dietary polyphenols have shown potential to improve the postprandial glucose and insulin responses and promote well-being via several postulated underlying mechanisms: 1) inhibition of carbohydrate digestion and the subsequent glucose absorption, 2) stimulation of insulin secretion from pancreatic β-cells, 3) modulation of hepatic glucose output, 4) activation of insulin receptors and glucose uptake in insulin-sensitive tissues, and 5) modulation of intracellular signaling pathways and gene expression [4–6].

Fruits, berries, vegetables, tea and coffee are the common sources of dietary polyphenols [7]. Decreased postprandial blood glucose and insulin responses have been reported in healthy adults after consumption of freeze-dried fruits (apple peel, blackberry, blackcurrant and strawberry) with green tea [8], beetroot juice [9], and blackcurrants and lingonberries [10]. In healthy adults, an attenuated postprandial insulin response, but not glucose response was also reported in some studies with extract of baobab fruit [11] and berries [12]. Similar effects were observed in obese and insulin-resistant male volunteers after intake of black tea, but not after intake of beetroot juice [13]. Although the polyphenol-rich fruits and vegetables have showed improving effects on postprandial glycemic and/or insulin responses, the efficacy of the dietary polyphenols in improving postprandial glucose and insulin responses seems to be influenced by multiple factors such as source of polyphenols, dose and sort of polyphenols. For example, the postprandial response was more efficiently decreased after consumption of blackcurrant than of lingonberries [10]. It was speculated that the difference in polyphenol compositions between the two berries could be the contributing factor. However, in another study performed by the same group, no correlation could be found between the insulin lowering effect and the polyphenol composition of the berries [12].

In a previous study [14], we observed that intake of a drink containing oatmeal fermented by the probiotic strain *Lactobacillus plantarum* 299v and supplemented with bilberry (European blueberry) induced a lower postprandial insulin response compared with the white bread control. The lowered acute insulin demand was more profound with higher dose of bilberries. In addition, a corresponding drink supplemented with rose hip decreased the insulin response to some extent, however, not to a statistically significant level. Thus, it is important to clarify the relationship between dietary polyphenols and insulin response.

In the present study, we hypothesized that polyphenol rich beverages enriched with fruits (bilberry, blackcurrant, rose hip and mango) and vegetable (beetroot) can attenuate postprandial glycemic and insulin responses. The presence of a probiotic strain with polyphenol splitting ability in the drink may enhance the physiological availability of the phenolics [15]. The acute postprandial glycemic and insulin responses as well as the polyphenol content and antioxidative capacity of the tested beverages were measured. The relation between the polyphenol content and the postprandial glycemic and insulin responses were examined with multivariate data analysis.

Methods

Study design and participants

The study was a randomized, controlled, crossover study with the aim to investigate and compare the postprandial glycemic and insulin responses after consuming five different probiotic fruit or vegetable beverages. Twelve healthy young adults, 6 men and 6 women (median age 23.5 years with interquartile range [IQR] 23–29.5 years) with body mass index (BMI) 24.3 ± 2.4 kg/m^2 (mean ± SD) were recruited in the study. The inclusion criteria were healthy adult individuals (18–65 years) with no medication, no diagnosed allergy, and having BMI between 20 and 30 kg/m^2 with a stable body weight (less than 5% weight change in the last three months before the inclusion).

The study was performed at the clinical research center at Skåne University Hospital (Lund, Sweden) and was completed within 6 weeks. Every participant visited the study center once a week (~ 3 h per visit; about every 7th day). The evening (9–10 pm) before each test, the participants were asked to eat a standardized meal consisting of two pieces of white bread and were thereafter only allowed to drink a small amount of water. On the test day, venous blood from the left arm was sampled and within the following 15 min participants were given one of the five test products or the reference drink, in a randomized order. A randomized table with weekly intervention for each individual was generated before the start of the study using an online random number generator (https://www.random.org). Thereafter, 3 and 3.5 ml of blood samples were taken at 15, 30, 45, 60, 90 and 120 min to analyze postprandial glucose and insulin responses, respectively. The beverage was served from newly opened packages.

Study products

The test products with the trade name ProViva® were provided by ProViva AB (Solna, Sweden). It is a fruit drink containing fermented oatmeal and live *Lactobacillus plantarum* 299v (DSM 9843; Probi AB, Lund, Sweden). The test products were supplemented with different fruits or vegetables: 1) 10% bilberry (Bilberry), 2) 25% blackcurrant (Blackcurrant), 3) 15% beetroot (Beetroot), 4) 6.5% mango (Mango), and 5) 14% rose hip (Rose hip). The amount of the beverages was standardized to contain 30 g of the available carbohydrates. The amount of the test products served to the participants were: Bilberry, 244 g; Blackcurrant, 262 g; Beetroot, 272 g; Mango, 288 g; and Rose hip 285 g. The reference glucose drink was prepared by dissolving 30 g of the glucose in 270 g of water. To note, we also included another control drink based on only fermented oatmeal with added sugar which was later excluded for analysis when we realized that the added sugar was not in correct amount.

Analyses of blood samples

Venous blood samples were taken through a venous catheter in the morning between 09:00 and 12:00 h after fasting for 10 h. Whole blood were drained into 5 ml of serum and plasma separation tubes. Plasma glucose and serum insulin were analyzed by standard methods at the Department of Clinical Chemistry, Skåne University Hospital, Lund, Sweden.

Viable count of lactobacilli

Samples taken from the five test products were serially diluted, and 100 μl from each dilution were plated on MRS agar and incubated anaerobically for 24–72 h at 37 °C prior to counting of colony forming units (CFU).

Sample preparation for analysis of phenolic compounds and antioxidant capacity determination

The five test beverages were centrifuged for 10 min. The supernatant was then filtrated through Teflon filter (0.2 μm) (VWR International, West Chester, PA, USA) prior to the analysis without further clean up.

Analysis of phenolic compounds during shelf life

Batch and inter-day variations were investigated for the five test products when stored in unopened packages at + 4 °C. Two different batches of the four test products (Bilberry, Blackcurrant, Mango and Rose hip) were analyzed during the study time. The first batch was analyzed on the first day of the intervention and 4 weeks later (shelf life). The second batch was analyzed in the week 5 and 6 (completion of the study). Three batches were analyzed for Beetroot. The first batch was analyzed on the first day of the intervention and 2 weeks later (shelf life). The second batch was analyzed in the week 3 and 5. The third batch was analyzed in week 4 and 6 of the study. Analysis of phenolic compounds in the five probiotic drinks was determined by HPLC-DAD method according to a previous work [16] with some modifications. Separation was carried out with porous-shell fused core Ascentis Express C18 analytical column (150 mm × 2.1 mm, 2.7 μm) from Supelco (Bellefonte, PA, USA). The mobile phases consisted of (A) water with 5% of formic acid, and (B) methanol with 5% of formic acid in a gradient elution analysis programmed as follows: 0 min, 5% (B); 0–5 min, 5% (B); 5–35 min, 40% (B); 35–40 min, 40% (B); with 10 min of post-time for column conditioning at a flow rate of 300 μl/min. The column temperature was set at 50 °C, the injection volume was 2 μl and the vial tray was held at 4 °C. Three wavelengths 280 nm, 350 nm and 520 nm were selected for identification of phenolic acids, flavonols and anthocyanins/betalains, respectively.

Total phenolic content

The total phenolic content of the test products was determined by the Folin-Ciocalteu (FC) assay [17]. The volume of the reaction mixture was miniaturized to 1 ml. 10 μl of sample were mixed, to which 50 μl of undiluted Folin-Ciocalteu reagent was subsequently added. After 1 min, 150 μl of 2% (*w*/*v*) Na_2CO_3 and 790 μl of water were added. After 2 h of incubation at 25 °C, 300 μl of the mixture was transferred into a well of the microplate, the absorbance was measured at 760 nm in a microplate spectrophotometer reader (Multiskan GO, Thermo Fisher, Germering, Germany) and compared to a gallic acid calibration curve (0.025–2.000 mg/ml) elaborated in the same manner. Three different packages of each beverage were analyzed and each package was analyzed in triplicate. The total phenolic content was estimated as gallic acid equivalents (GAE), expressed as mg gallic acid/ml of test drink.

Total antioxidant capacity

Trolox equivalent antioxidant capacity (TEAC) assay and DPPH assay were used to determine the total antioxidant capacity.

The TEAC assay employed was described by Re et al. [18] with some modifications. ABTS radical cation ($ABTS^{\cdot+}$) was produced by reacting 7 mM ABTS with 2.45 mM potassium persulfate and allowing the mixture to stand in the dark at room temperature for 12–16 h before use. The aqueous $ABTS^{\cdot+}$ solution was diluted with 5 mM phosphate buffer (pH = 7.4) to an absorbance of 0.70 (± 0.02) at 734 nm. Ten microliters of test beverages (four different dilutions) were added to 1 ml of diluted $ABTS^{\cdot+}$ radical solution. After 50 min at 30 °C, 300 μl of the mixture were transferred into a well of the microplate, and the absorbance was measured at 734 nm in a microplate spectrophotometer reader (Thermo Fisher). Trolox was used as a reference standard and results were expressed as TEAC values (mmol Trolox/l of test beverage). These values were obtained from at least four different dilutions of each test product in the assay giving a linear response between 20 and 80% of the initial absorbance. Three different packages of each product were analyzed and each package was analyzed in triplicate.

The DPPH radical scavenging assay was used [19]. Briefly, a solution was prepared by dissolving 23.5 mg of DPPH in 100 ml of methanol. This stock solution was further diluted with methanol 1:10. Both solutions were stored at 4 °C until use. Four different dilutions of each beverage were tested. 25 µl of these solutions were added to 975 µl of DPPH diluted solution to complete the final reaction medium (1 ml). After 4 h at room temperature, 300 µl of the mixture were transferred into a microplate well and the absorbance was measured at 516 nm in a microplate spectrophotometer reader (Multiskan GO, Thermo Fisher). DPPH-methanol solution was used as a reference sample. The DPPH concentration remaining in the reaction medium was calculated from a calibration curve. Three different packages of each beverage were analyzed and each package was analyzed in triplicate. The results are presented as DPPH radical inhibition (%).

Data treatment and statistical analysis

All univariate statistical analyses were conducted in RStudio Version 0.99.902 [20]. The incremental areas under the curves (IAUCs) were calculated for blood glucose and serum insulin using the trapezoidal rule and ignoring the area below the baseline. Glycemic index (GI) and insulin index (II) were calculated from the IAUCs obtained after the intake of test products divided by the IAUCs obtained after intake of the reference glucose drink with each participant as his/her own control. GI and II were calculated for both 0–90 min and 0–120 min. In a few cases of hemolysis, missing data were substituted by mean values calculated from the same time point but different weeks. Three participants did not complete one test occasion each (one for mango, one for bilberry and one for blackcurrant) and were hence excluded from the data analysis of the corresponding group. Incremental blood glucose and serum insulin data were not normally distributed, thus Skillings-Mack test (equivalent to Friedman test but with the possibility to handle missing data) [21] was used to detect differences between the six beverage groups. When significant differences were detected, Conover post hoc test was performed for pairwise comparisons with false discovery rate (FDR) *P*-value adjustment. Comparisons of glycemic and insulin indices were performed using Wilcoxon signed rank test and *P* values were corrected for multiple comparisons. Multivariate data analyses were performed with SIMCA-P+ 12.0.1 (Umetrics, Umeå, Sweden). $P < 0.05$ was considered statistically significant.

The study was approved by the Ethics Committee of the Faculty of Medicine at Lund University, Sweden (Dnr 2014/435).

Results

One participant discontinued due to personal reasons after two test occasions, and was removed from the study. Thus the study is based on eleven participants.

Viable count

The lactobacilli counts in the five probiotic drinks were stable during the storage period, and between the different batches ($3–5 \times 10^7$ CFU/ml).

Glycemic response

The incremental blood glucose response after intake of the Bilberry, Blackcurrant, Beetroot, Mango, Rose hip products and the reference glucose drink are shown in Fig. 1. No significant differences regarding the incremental blood glucose concentrations were found between the groups at any of the time points, and the same was true for the glycemic responses measured by IAUCs (Table 1).

Insulin response

The incremental serum insulin response after intake of the test products and the reference glucose drink are shown in Fig. 2. A significant difference ($P = 0.03$) in the serum insulin concentrations between the six groups was seen after 30 min. Pairwise comparisons showed that Bilberry and Rose hip groups had significantly lower increase in serum insulin levels compared with the Beetroot group ($P = 0.02$ and P = 0.02, respectively). Blackcurrant also showed a tendency of lower serum insulin elevation compared with Beetroot ($P = 0.05$). No significant differences were detected between the groups at other time points.

Comparisons of the IAUCs at different time periods are presented in Table 2. The IAUCs (0–30 min) were significantly different (P = 0.03) between the groups. Pairwise comparisons showed that Bilberry and Rose hip had significantly lower values of IAUCs compared to the reference Glucose group ($P = 0.032$ and P = 0.032, respectively). Additionally, in comparison to Bilberry and Rose hip, Beetroot and Mango showed significantly higher values of IAUCs (Beetroot vs. Bilberry, $P = 0.033$; Beetroot vs. Rose hip, P = 0.033; Mango vs. Bilberry P = 0.032; and Mango vs. Rose hip, P = 0.032). A similar pattern was observed for IAUCs (0–45 min). A significant difference was detected in the overall comparisons ($P = 0.01$). Compared to Glucose, Bilberry and Rose hip showed significantly lower IAUCs ($P = 0.007$ and P = 0.007, respectively). In addition, Blackcurrant also showed a lower value of IAUC compared with the

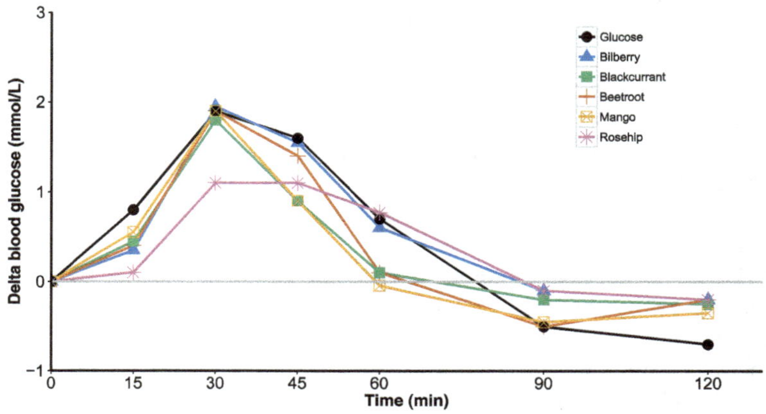

Fig. 1 Incremental blood glucose response curve during the two-hour postprandial period. The change in blood glucose concentration was calculated by deducting the basal level from the blood glucose level measured after intake of the test drinks and was represented as delta blood glucose. Median values were plotted

reference Glucose although slightly above the statistical significance threshold ($P = 0.053$). Moreover, in comparison to the Bilberry and Rose hip, Beetroot showed a significantly higher value of IAUC (P = 0.007 and P = 0.007, respectively). In the period of 0–60 min, there was a significant difference among the groups ($P = 0.019$). Pairwise comparisons showed that Bilberry had a significantly lower value of IAUC compared to the reference Glucose ($P = 0.021$). Rose hip also showed a lower IAUC compared to Glucose but did not reach statistical significance ($P = 0.086$). In comparison to Bilberry and Rose hip, Beetroot had a significantly higher value of IAUCs ($P = 0.01$ and $P = 0.035$, respectively). In the period of 0–90 min, a significant difference was found among the six groups (P = 0.02). Pairwise comparisons showed that except for the Beetroot, the other four probiotic fruit drinks had significantly lower IAUCs compared to the reference Glucose (Bilberry vs. Glucose, $P = 0.006$; Blackcurrant vs Glucose, P = 0.03; Mango vs. Glucose, P = 0.03; and Rose hip vs. Glucose, P = 0.03). In the period of 0–120 min, no significant difference was found among the six groups ($P = 0.07$).

Glycemic and insulin indices

Glycemic and Insulin indices were calculated using IAUCs at 90 and 120 min (Table 3). The five test products did not have significantly different glycemic indices compared to the reference Glucose at either time duration. Insulin indices calculated at 90 min showed that Bilberry and Rose hip had significantly lower value than the reference Glucose (P = 0.01 and $P = 0.012$, respectively). Blackcurrant also had significantly lower insulin index compared to Glucose ($P = 0.037$), however, after P-value adjustment the difference was no longer significant ($P = 0.06$). Comparisons of insulin indices that were calculated at 120 min showed that Bilberry and Rose hip had significantly lower values than the reference Glucose ($P = 0.02$ and P = 0.02, respectively).

Polyphenol profiles

The analysis of phenolics (Table 4) showed that the highest values of the total phenolic compounds (280 nm) and flavonols (350 nm) were found in Bilberry whereas Mango had the lowest. The highest values of total anthocyanins/betalains (520 nm) were found in Bilberry and Beetroot, while these families of

Table 1 Incremental area under two-hour blood glucose response curve

Tested products	IAUC(0–15 min) (mmol min/L)	IAUC(0–30 min) (mmol min/L)	IAUC(0–45 min) (mmol min/L)	IAUC(0–60 min) (mmol min/L)	IAUC(0–90 min) (mmol min/L)	IAUC(0–120 min) (mmol min/L)
Glucose ($n = 11$)	6.0 (3.4–7.9)	26.3 (17.6–36.0)	45.0 (37.6–67.5)	63.0 (44.7–91.5)	71.7 (48.9–112.1)	71.7 (48.9–117)
Bilberry ($n = 10$)	2.6 (0.8–4.5)	19.1 (13.5–24.8)	44.3 (33.8–52.5)	50.6 (45.8–73.5)	58.6 (47.5–82.5)	61.5 (47.5–82.5)
Blackcurrant (n = 10)	3.4 (1.5–6.8)	23.3 (13.5–30.0)	44.6 (31.5–63.8)	55.5 (39.0–71.3)	57.6 (40.5–101.3)	57.6 (45.1–111.8)
Beetroot (n = 11)	3.0 (0.8–3.0)	20.3 (15.8–22.1)	40.5 (33.0–64.9)	53.3 (34.3–93.4)	54.2 (34.3–118.6)	54.2 (35.0–123.2)
Mango (n = 10)	4.1 (0–6.0)	24.4 (11.3–29.3)	42.2 (28.5–53.3)	46.7 (33.8–66.1)	50.0 (34.0–66.1)	54.0 (34.0–66.1)
Rose hip (n = 11)	0.8 (0–2.3)	12.0 (5.2–16.9)	29.6 (16.8–42.0)	46.8 (26.7–65.6)	48.0 (29.9–88.2)	51.3 (30.0–96.4)

Data are presented as median (IQR)

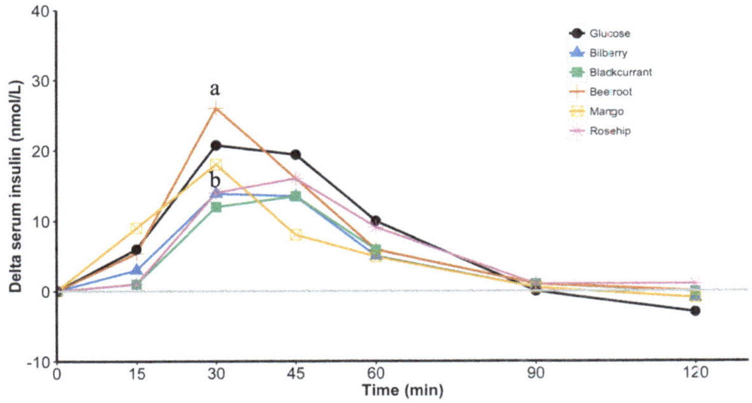

Fig. 2 Incremental serum insulin response curve during the two-hour postprandial period. The change in serum insulin concentration was calculated by deducting the basal level from the insulin level measured after intake of the test drinks and was represented as delta serum insulin. Median values were plotted. Median values with different letters denote significant differences between Beetroot and Bilberry, and between Beetroot and Rose hip ($P < 0.05$)

polyphenols were not detected in either mango or rose hip. Chromatograms corresponding to the HPLC-DAD analysis of the five test products are presented in supplementary figures (see Additional file 1: Figure S1 to S5). Regarding the analysis of the total phenolic measured by FC assay and total antioxidant capacity measured by DPPH and TEAC assays (Table 5), Rose hip beverage was the one with the highest phenolic content and the highest antioxidant capacity. Mango presented the lowest phenolic content and antioxidant capacity.

Multivariate data analysis with PCA and OPLS-DA

Among the five tested drinks, Bilberry and Rose hip formed clusters separated from the Glucose when analyzing the data of postprandial responses using OPLS-DA (Fig. 3). The pronounced differences in polyphenol profiles of the five drinks were revealed by PCA analysis (Additional file 2: Figure S6). Based on the distinct clusterings of Bilberry and Rose hip that were observed with postprandial responses data and phenolics contents, we performed OPLS-DA by setting Bilberry and Rose hip as one class (Bil_Rose) and the other three products as the second class. The difference between the two classes was explained by 31.6% of the variance (Fig. 4a) and Bil_Rose class had higher levels of phenolics and antioxidant capacities (Fig. 4b).

Discussion

Consumption of the polyphenol rich probiotic fruit and vegetable beverages did not affect postprandial glycemic responses, but the four fruit drinks supplemented with bilberry, blackcurrant, mango and rose hip significantly attenuated the insulin response in the early postprandial period (0–90 min).

Among the four fruit drinks, Bilberry showed the most profound insulin lowering effect at the 30 min postprandial and this effect was maintained throughout the early postprandial period. Rose hip showed similar efficiency in attenuating postprandial insulin response. Except for the postprandial period 0–60 min, Rose hip led to a decreased insulin response during the 30, 45 and 90 min of postprandial period. GI calculated at 90 and 120 min postprandial were not significantly different between the groups. However, Bilberry and Rose hip had significantly lower II compared with Glucose during both time periods (Table 3). These results from Bilberry and Rose hip are in agreement with our previous study [14], where we found that the bilberry drink attenuated postprandial

Table 2 Incremental area under two-hour serum insulin response curve

Tested products	IAUC(0–15 min) (nmol min/L)	IAUC(0–30 min) (nmol min/L)	IAUC(0–45 min) (nmol min/L)	IAUC(0–60 min) (nmol min/L)	IAUC(0–90 min) (nmol min/L)	IAUC(0–120 min) (nmol min/L)
Glucose (*n* = 11)	45.0 (30.0–82.5)^{a}	245.6 (191.3–333.8)^{ac}	502.5 (465.0–622.5)^{a}	735.0 (706.6–930.0)^{a}	907.5 (807.1–1140.1)^{a}	907.5 (807.2–1155.9)^{a}
Bilberry (*n* = 10)	22.5 (15.0–45.0)^{a}	157.1 (104.1–210.0)^{b}	340.4 (292.5–405.0)^{b}	465.0 (405.9–562.5)^{b}	505.0 (457.5–915.0)^{b}	598.1 (477.5–1020.0)^{a}
Blackcurrant (*n* = 10)	7.5 (0–45.0)^{a}	201.9 (79.5–322.5)^{abc}	368.0 (279.0–600.0)^{abc}	507.2 (450.8–600.0)^{abc}	645.4 (592.5–877.5)^{b}	697.5 (592.5–907.5)^{a}
Beetroot (*n* = 11)	40.5 (18.0–60.0)^{a}	234.0 (183.8–363.8)^{ac}	525.0 (446.3–652.5)^{ac}	684.4 (645.0–764.3)^{ac}	900 (705.2–952.5)^{ab}	998.5 (846.5–1083.8)^{a}
Mango (*n* = 10)	67.5 (0–90.0)^{a}	285 (112.9–427.5)^{c}	465.0 (320.2.0–810.0)^{abc}	583.9 (487.5–1095.0)^{abc}	684.1 (517.5–1202.6)^{b}	684.1 (532.5–1210.1)^{a}
Rose hip (*n* = 11)	7.5 (0–26.3)^{a}	180 (81.3–210.0)^{b}	375.0 (253.8–551.3)^{b}	682.5 (335.7–750.0)^{abc*}	801.1 (441.9–993.8)^{b}	765.0 (593.3–1068.8)^{a}

Superscripted data are presented as median (IQR). Groups that do not share the same letter are significantly different. *only different from Beetroot not Glucose

Table 3 Glycemic and insulin indices

Tested products	Glycemic index (0–90 min) (%)	Glycemic index (0–120 min) (%)	Insulin index (0–90 min) (%)	Insulin index (0–120 min) (%)
Glucose ($n = 11$)	100	100	100[a]	100[a]
Bilberry ($n = 10$)	88.9 (66.0–101.3)	95.3 (70.6–102.1)	65.7 (54.1–86.7)[b]	63.8 (56.5–86.7)[b]
Blackcurrant ($n = 10$)	75.1 (45.1–141.1)	75.4 (45.1–141.1)	73.8 (61.2–101.6)[b#]	76.9 (59.2–105.0)[ab]
Beetroot ($n = 11$)	85.9 (39.7–112.4)	91.0 (39.1–113.7)	86.9 (74.7–112.9)[ab]	86.5 (73.2–114.6)[ab]
Mango ($n = 10$)	68.4 (43.2–128.9)	68.4 (43.2–129.1)	67.6 (61.2–89.6)[ab]	68.9 (59.3–89.6)[ab]
Rose hip ($n = 11$)	63.5 (41.1–111.3)	58.2 (41.1–112.6)	72.3 (58.1–87.7)[b]	70.8 (62.6–93.6)[b]

Superscripted data are presented as median (IQR). Groups that do not share the same letter are significantly different. [#]Before P value adjustment $P = 0.034$, after adjustment $P = 0.062$

insulin response in two separate studies and the same rose hip drink showed an insulin attenuating tendency. In addition, in the present study, Bilberry and Rose hip showed higher efficiencies in lowering the early phase insulin responses in comparison to the other test products. This was linked to their higher levels of the phenolic contents (Fig. 4). The different efficiencies in improving postprandial responses have earlier been observed between blackcurrants and lingonberries that containing different subclasses of polyphenols [10].

In the present study, Blackcurrant also led to a reduced early phase postprandial insulin response with a moderate rate compared to Bilberry and Rose hip. At the same time, Bilberry had highest amounts of phenolics, followed by the Blackcurrant (Table 4). Anthocyanins account for the major polyphenols in bilberries [22]. It has been reported that consumption of a bilberry extract containing 36% (*w*/w) anthocyanins, reduced both postprandial glycemic and insulin responses in the individuals with type 2 diabetes [23]. Furthermore, anthocyanins have been reported to be capable of modulating insulin and AMP-activated protein kinase (AMPK) signaling pathways [24, 25]. Thus, a lower level of anthocyanins in Blackcurrant may have contributed to the different efficacies in reducing insulin response. On the other hand, the observed effect from Rose hip indicates that anthocyanins could not be the sole bioactive compound accounting for the attenuated insulin response. Since the seeds were removed from the rose hip fruits, Rose hip drink did not contain any anthocyanins. On the other hand, Rose hip had the highest amount of total phenolic content. It should be noted that FC assay reagent is nonspecific to phenolic compound, instead it measures the total antioxidant capacity. Therefore, high amount of vitamin C and carotenoids in Rose hip [26, 27] could have contributed to the observed highest antioxidant capacity. The highest antioxidant capacity of Rose hip was also confirmed by the TEAC and DPPH assays. Rose hips have been used in traditional medicine for treating multiple illnesses [28]. Consumption of the rose hip extract significantly reduced hyperglycemia in diabetic rats. It was speculated that the antioxidant property of the rose hip extract led to a reduction in the oxidative stress, which helped preserving the pancreatic β-cell integrity and finally led to insulinotrophic action [29]. In a recent study in vitro, rose hip extract enhanced the pancreatic β-cell proliferation [30]. In an animal study, it was reported that intake of rose hip extract led to increased insulin sensitivity via downregulation of hepatic lipogenesis [31]. Although the bioactive compounds in rose hip contributing to the observed effects were not identified, these findings suggest that rose hip could have multiple mechanisms of action leading to an improved insulin response.

Interestingly, despite the lowest values determined for total phenolic content, total flavonols and total antioxidant capacity in Mango we observed a decreased postprandial insulin response at 90 min. It has been reported that a major phenolic compound in mango, mangiferin

Table 4 Quantification of polyphenol contents by HPLC

Products	Total phenolic compounds (280 nm) (mAU*min)	Total flavonols (350 nm) (mAU*min)	Total anthocyanins (520 nm) (mAU*min)
Bilberry	74.34 (7.70)	13.59 (9.73)	89.56 (9.07)
Blackcurrant	47.29 (7.66)	8.69 (8.0)	30.98 (9.15)
Beetroot	43.40 (4.36)	6.69 (7.52)	74.6 (6.89)
Mango	23.18 (7.17)	0.8 (6.42)	ND[#]
Rose hip	26.35 (6.32)	3.56 (4.27)	ND[#]

Values are presented as Mean (relative standard deviation %). [#]ND means not detected

Table 5 Quantification of phenolic content and total antioxidant capacity

Products	FC assay (mg gallic acid/ml drink)	TEAC assay (mmol trolox/l)	DPPH scavenging activity (%) (dilution factor)
Bilberry	0.41 ± 0.03	16.38 ± 0.68	74.2 ± 3.2 (4)
Blackcurrant	0.61 ± 0.04	45.55 ± 2.0	41.2 ± 1.8 (100)
Beetroot	0.4 ± 0.01	11.22 ± 0.94	54.2 ± 1.4 (4)
Mango	0.18 ± 0.03	8.48 ± 0.39	52.7 ± 1.6 (4)
Rose hip	1.37 ± 0.22	137.9 ± 13.84	76.9 ± 3.0 (100)

Values are presented as Mean ± SD

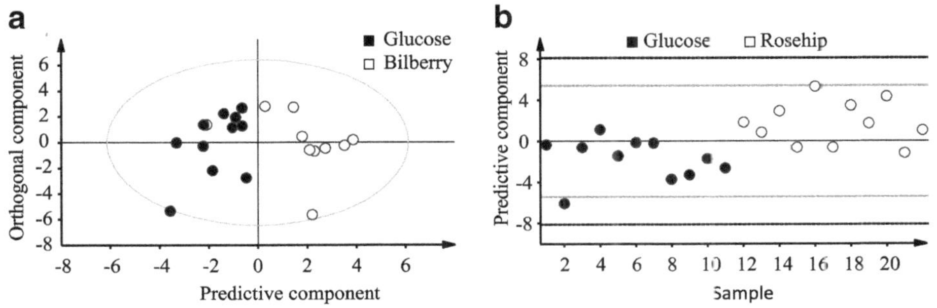

Fig. 3 Orthogonal projections to latent structures discriminant analysis (OPLS-DA) score plots of postprandial responses data. **a** Model calculated to discriminate between Bilberry and Glucose (described response variation, $R^2Y = 0.63$; predicted response variation, $Q^2Y = 0.48$). **b** Model discriminating between Rose hip and Glucose ($R^2Y = 0.43$, $Q^2Y = 0.32$). The x-axis in (**b**) consists of the 22 analyzed samples. Grey dashed line shows 1.04376*(±2SD) and the black dashed line 1.04376*(±3SD)

[32] could improve glucose and insulin profiles in high fat fed mice [33]. Also, other bioactive compounds such as carotenoids, vitamin C and dietary fiber in mango may affect the blood glucose and insulin metabolism [34]. On the contrary, the high polyphenol content in Beetroot was not associated with such a beneficial effect. Again, this indicates that the polyphenol content or antioxidant capacity itself could not be directly linked to the insulin attenuating effects of the present test products. To note, Beetroot had the second highest value of anthocyanin content, which should be from the betalains (pigment compound of beetroot) sharing structural similarities with anthocyanins. Although the retention times of the peaks from Beetroot were different from those of Bilberry and Blackcurrant, we could not distinguish between anthocyanin and betalain with the current HPLC analysis settings due to lack of standard and subsequent mass spectrometry analysis for identification. A degradation product of betalain, neobetanin was associated with a reduced early phase postprandial (0–60 min) insulin response [9]. However, in the present study we did not observe beneficial effects from Beetroot. We postulated that the postprandial glycemic and insulin improving effects could be linked to the polyphenol content. The high efficiency of Bilberry and Rose hip in attenuating early postprandial insulin responses were correlated with higher phenolic contents. However, phenolic levels alone were not directly linked to the insulin lowering effect. It cannot be ruled out that specific phenolic components could serve as the contributing factors for the observed insulin attenuating effect in the four fruit supplemented test products. Moreover, other bioactive compounds present in the test products may have contributed in a synergistic manner when decreasing insulin demand.

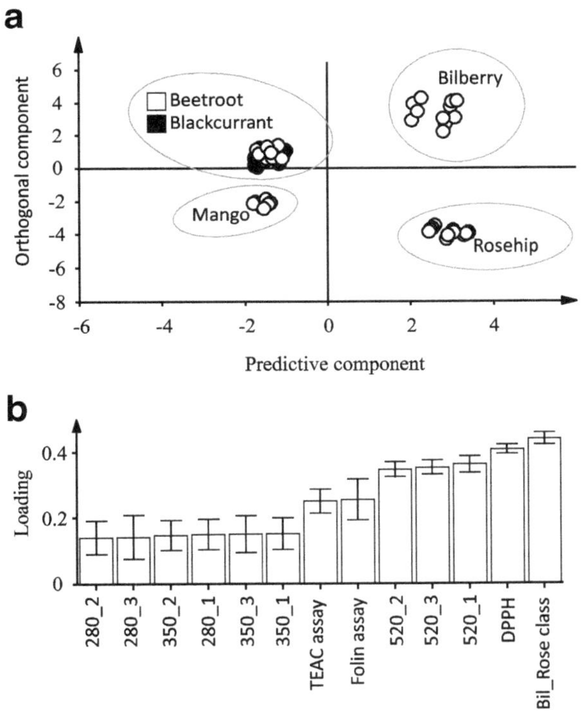

Fig. 4 Orthogonal projections to latent structures discriminant analysis (OPLS-DA) model calculated on polyphenol profiles and discriminating between Bilberry and Rose hip (Bil_Rose class) and other tested beverages (described response variation, $R^2Y = 0.977$; predicted response variation, $Q^2Y = 0.973$). The difference between the two classes of berries was explained by 31.6% of the variation in polyphenol data. **a** Score scatter plot. **b** Loadings bar plot showing the driving forces for the observed cluster separation. The Bil_Rose class had higher levels of phenolics as compared to the other berries

There are limitations in the current study that could be improved in the future research. We intended to investigate and compare the effects of test products with a baseline product containing only fermented oatmeal besides the glucose control group. Unfortunately, we had to exclude the fermented oatmeal group from the data analysis due to improper carbohydrate compensation, and could not assess the impact of probiotic fermented oatmeal per se. Although not evaluated in the current study, beneficial effects of probiotic bacteria in managing glycemic control have been demonstrated in multiple animal models and human studies [35, 36]. Further research efforts are needed to discover the underlying mechanisms.

Conclusions

Consistent with the previous study [14], we found an inconsistency between the early glycemic and the insulin responses. The intake of test products containing bilberry, rose hip, blackcurrant or mango did not affect the postprandial glycemic response, but attenuated early stage postprandial (0–90 min) insulin responses. The higher efficiency of bilberry and rose hip drinks in lowering insulin responses was associated with amounts of phenolics. The health-related relevance of our findings is that consumption of food products that induce a lower insulin response may enhance insulin sensitivity.

Additional files

Additional file 1: Figure S1. Chromatograms corresponding to the HPLC-DAD analysis of bilberry beverage at 280 nm, 350 nm and 520 nm. P, phenolic compounds; F, flavonols; and A, anthocyanins. **Figure S2.** Chromatograms corresponding to the HPLC-DAD analysis of blackcurrant beverage at 280 nm, 350 nm and 520 nm. P, phenolic compounds; F, flavonols; and A, anthocyanins. **Figure S3.** Chromatograms corresponding to the HPLC-DAD analysis of Rose hip beverage at 280 nm, 350 nm and 520 nm. P, phenolic compounds; and F, flavonols. **Figure S4.** Chromatograms corresponding to the HPLC-DAD analysis of Mango beverage at 280 nm, 350 nm and 520 nm. P, phenolic compounds; and F, flavonols. **Figure S5.** Chromatograms corresponding to the HPLC-DAD analysis of beetroot beverage at 280 nm, 350 nm and 520 nm. P, phenolic compounds; F, flavonols; and B, betalains.

Additional file 2: Figure S6. PCA score plot of data from phenolic analysis of the five tested drinks. PC1 and PC2 explained 60.4 and 25.2% of the variance in the data respectively.

Acknowledgements

We thank the clinical trial unit at Skåne Univeristy Hospital for their assistance with collecting samples and Ms. Eleonor Gautier for her enthusiastic support with statistical analyses as part of her internship at ProViva AB. We also thank Prof. Göran Molin for proofreading and valuable feedbacks.

Funding

We would like to thank TvärLivsprogrammet and Vinnova for the financial support.

Authors' contributions

JX analyzed the glucose and insulin responses data and was a major contributor in drafting the manuscript. TJ, MP, ÅH, MA, ILA, CT and YG participated in the design of the study and statistical analyses. MP conducted polyphenol analysis and PS performed multivariate data analysis. All authors contributed to the writing and revising of the manuscript. All authors read and approved the final manuscript.

Competing interests

The author MA is employed at ProViva AB and ILA is employed at Probi AB.

Author details

[1]Department of Clinical and Experimental Medicine, Linköping University, Linköping, Sweden. [2]Center for Primary Health Care Research, Lund University, Skåne University Hospital, Malmö, Sweden. [3]Department of Analytical Chemistry, Physical Chemistry and Chemical Engineering, Faculty of Biology, Environmental Sciences and Chemistry, Universidad de Alcalá, Ctra. Madrid-Barcelona Km. 33.600, Alcalá de Henares, Madrid, Spain. [4]Department of Chemistry, Lund University, Lund, Sweden. [5]Department of Food Technology, Engineering and Nutrition, Lund University, Lund, Sweden. [6]ProViva AB, Lunnarp, Sweden. [7]Probi AB, Lund, Sweden.

References

1. Aryangat AV, Gerich JE. Type 2 diabetes: postprandial hyperglycemia and increased cardiovascular risk. Vasc Health Risk Manag. 2010;6:145–55.
2. Ceriello A, Genovese S. Atherogenicity of postprandial hyperglycemia and lipotoxicity. Rev Endocr Metab Disord. 2016;17:111–6.
3. World Health O. Noncommunicable diseases fact sheet. Geneva: World Health Organization; 2013.
4. Hanhineva K, Torronen R, Bondia-Pons I, Pekkinen J, Kolehmainen M, Mykkanen H, Poutanen K. Impact of dietary polyphenols on carbohydrate metabolism. Int J Mol Sci. 2010;11:1365–402.
5. Mirmiran P, Bahadoran Z, Azizi F. Functional foods-based diet as a novel dietary approach for management of type 2 diabetes and its complications: a review. World J Diabetes. 2014;5(3):267–81.
6. Coe S, Ryan L. Impact of polyphenol-rich sources on acute postprandial glycaemia: a systematic review. J Nutr Sci. 2016;5:e24.
7. Scalbert A, Williamson G. Dietary intake and bioavailability of polyphenols. J Nutr. 2000;130:2073S–85S.
8. Nyambe-Silavwe H, Williamson G. Polyphenol- and fibre-rich dried fruits with green tea attenuate starch-derived postprandial blood glucose and insulin: a randomised, controlled, single-blind, cross-over intervention. Br J Nutr. 2016;116:443–50.
9. Wootton-Beard PC, Brandt K, Fell D, Warner S, Ryan L. Effects of a beetroot juice with high neobetanin content on the early-phase insulin response in healthy volunteers. J Nutr Sci. 2014;3:e9.
10. Torronen R, Kolehmainen M, Sarkkinen E, Mykkanen H, Niskanen L. Postprandial glucose, insulin, and free fatty acid responses to sucrose consumed with blackcurrants and lingonberries in healthy women. Am J Clin Nutr. 2012;96:527–33.
11. Coe S, Ryan L. White bread enriched with polyphenol extracts shows no effect on glycemic response or satiety, yet may increase postprandial insulin economy in healthy participants. Nutr Res. 2016;36:193–200.
12. Torronen R, Kolehmainen M, Sarkkinen E, Poutanen K, Mykkanen H, Niskanen L. Berries reduce postprandial insulin responses to wheat and rye breads in healthy women. J Nutr. 2013;143:430–6.
13. Fuchs D, Nyakayiru J, Draijer R, Mulder TP, Hopman MT, Eijsvogels TM, Thijssen DH. Impact of flavonoid-rich black tea and beetroot juice on postprandial peripheral vascular resistance and glucose homeostasis in obese, insulin-resistant men: a randomized controlled trial. Nutr Metab (Lond). 2016;13:34.
14. Granfeldt YE, Bjorck IM. A bilberry drink with fermented oatmeal decreases postprandial insulin demand in young healthy adults. Nutr J. 2011;10:57.
15. Rodriguez H, Curiel JA, Landete JM, de las Rivas B, Lopez de Felipe F, Gomez-Cordoves C, Mancheno JM, Munoz R. Food phenolics and lactic acid bacteria. Int J Food Microbiol. 2009;132:79–90.
16. Plaza M, Batista AG, Cazarin CB, Sandahl M, Turner C, Ostman E, Marostica Junior MR. Characterization of antioxidant polyphenols from Myrciaria jaboticaba peel and their effects on glucose metabolism and antioxidant status: a pilot clinical study. Food Chem. 2016;211:185–97.
17. Koşar M, Dorman HJD, Hiltunen R. Effect of an acid treatment on the phytochemical and antioxidant characteristics of extracts from selected Lamiaceae species. Food Chem. 2005;91:525–33.
18. Re R, Pellegrini N, Proteggente A, Pannala A, Yang M, Rice-Evans C. Antioxidant activity applying an improved ABTS radical cation decolorization assay. Free Radic Biol Med. 1999;26:1231–7.

19. Brand-Williams W, Cuvelier M-E, Berset C. Use of a free radical method to evaluate antioxidant activity. LWT-Food Sci Technol. 1995;28:25–30.
20. Team R: RStudio: integrated development for R. *RStudio, Inc, Boston, MA URL http://www RStudio com/ide* 2014.
21. Chatfield M, Mander A. The Skillings-Mack test (Friedman test when there are missing data). Stata J. 2009;9:299–305.
22. Koponen JM, Happonen AM, Mattila PH, Torronen AR. Contents of anthocyanins and ellagitannins in selected foods consumed in Finland. J Agric Food Chem. 2007;55:1612–9.
23. Hoggard N, Cruickshank M, Moar KM, Bestwick C, Holst JJ, Russell W, Horgan G. A single supplement of a standardised bilberry (Vaccinium Myrtillus L.) extract (36% wet weight anthocyanins) modifies glycaemic response in individuals with type 2 diabetes controlled by diet and lifestyle. J Nutr Sci. 2013;2:e22.
24. Takikawa M, Inoue S, Horio F, Tsuda T. Dietary anthocyanin-rich bilberry extract ameliorates hyperglycemia and insulin sensitivity via activation of AMP-activated protein kinase in diabetic mice. J Nutr. 2010;140:527–33.
25. Singh S, Netticadan T, Ramdath DD. Expression of cardiac insulin signalling genes and proteins in rats fed a high-sucrose diet: effect of bilberry anthocyanin extract. Genes Nutr. 2016;11:8.
26. Ercisli S. Chemical composition of fruits in some rose (Rosa spp.) species. Food Chem. 2007;104:1379–84.
27. Roman I, Stanila A, Stanila S. Bioactive compounds and antioxidant activity of Rosa Canina L. biotypes from spontaneous flora of Transylvania. Chem Cent J. 2013;7:73.
28. Chrubasik C, Roufogalis BD, Muller-Ladner U, Chrubasik S. A systematic review on the Rosa Canina effect and efficacy profiles. Phytother Res. 2008;22:725–33.
29. Taghizadeh M, Rashidi AA, Taherian AA, Vakili Z, Sajadian MS, Ghardashi M. Antidiabetic and antihyperlipidemic effects of ethanol extract of rosa canina L. fruit on diabetic rats: an experimental study with Histopathological evaluations. J Evid Based Complement Altern Med. 2016;21(4):NP25-NP30.
30. Fattahi A, Niyazi F, Shahbazi B, Farzaei MH, Bahrami G. Antidiabetic mechanisms of Rosa Canina fruits: an in vitro evaluation. J Evid Based Complement Altern Med. 2017;22(1):127-33.
31. Andersson U, Henriksson E, Strom K, Alenfall J, Goransson O, Holm C. Rose hip exerts antidiabetic effects via a mechanism involving downregulation of the hepatic lipogenic program. Am J Physiol Endocrinol Metab. 2011;300:E111–21.
32. Masibo M, He Q. Major mango polyphenols and their potential significance to human health. Compr Rev Food Sci Food Saf. 2008;7:309–19.
33. Apontes P, Liu Z, Su K, Benard O, Youn DY, Li X, Li W, Mirza RH, Bastie CC, Jelicks LA, et al. Mangiferin stimulates carbohydrate oxidation and protects against metabolic disorders induced by high-fat diets. Diabetes. 2014;63:3626–36.
34. Lucas EA, Li W, Peterson SK, Brown A, Kuvibidila S, Perkins-Veazie P, Clarke SL, Smith BJ. Mango modulates body fat and plasma glucose and lipids in mice fed a high-fat diet. Br J Nutr. 2011;106:1495–505.
35. Ruan Y, Sun J, He J, Chen F, Chen R, Chen H. Effect of probiotics on glycemic control: a systematic review and meta-analysis of randomized, controlled trials. PLoS One. 2015;10:e0132121.
36. Razmpoosh E, Javadi M, Ejtahed HS, Mirmiran P. Probiotics as beneficial agents in the management of diabetes mellitus: a systematic review. Diabetes Metab Res Rev. 2016;32:143–68.

21

A school-based intervention improved dietary intake outcomes and reduced waist circumference in adolescents: a cluster randomized controlled trial

Angélica Ochoa-Avilés[1*], Roosmarijn Verstraeten[2,3], Lieven Huybregts[4], Susana Andrade[1], John Van Camp[3], Silvana Donoso[1], Patricia Liliana Ramírez[1], Carl Lachat[3], Lea Maes[5] and Patrick Kolsteren[3]

Abstract

Background: In Ecuador, adolescents' food intake does not comply with guidelines for a healthy diet. Together with abdominal obesity adolescent's inadequate diets are risk factors for non-communicable diseases. We report the effectiveness of a school-based intervention on the dietary intake and waist circumference among Ecuadorian adolescents.

Methods: A pair-matched cluster randomized controlled trial including 1430 adolescents (12–14 years old) was conducted. The program aimed at improving the nutritional value of dietary intake, physical activity (primary outcomes), body mass index, waist circumference and blood pressure (secondary outcomes). This paper reports: (i) the effect on fruit and vegetable intake, added sugar intake, unhealthy snacking (consumption of unhealthy food items that are not in line with the dietary guidelines eaten during snack time; i.e. table sugar, sweets, salty snacks, fast food, soft drinks and packaged food), breakfast intake and waist circumference; and, (ii) dose and reach of the intervention. Dietary outcomes were estimated by means of two 24-h recall at baseline, after the first 17-months (stage one) and after the last 11-months (stage two) of implementation. Dose and reach were evaluated using field notes and attendance forms. Educational toolkits and healthy eating workshops with parents and food kiosks staff in the schools were implemented in two different stages. The overall effect was assessed using linear mixed models and regression spline mixed effect models were applied to evaluate the effect after each stage.

Results: Data from 1046 adolescents in 20 schools were analyzed. Participants from the intervention group consumed lower quantities of unhealthy snacks (−23.32 g; 95% CI: −45.25,-1.37) and less added sugar (−5.66 g; 95% CI: −9.63,-1.65) at the end of the trial. Daily fruit and vegetable intake decreased in both the intervention and control groups compared to baseline, albeit this decrease was 23.88 g (95% CI: 7.36, 40.40) lower in the intervention group. Waist circumference (−0. 84 cm; 95% CI: −1.68, 0.28) was lower in the intervention group at the end of the program; the effect was mainly observed at stage one. Dose and reach were also higher at stage one.

Conclusions: The trial had positive effects on risk factors for non-communicable diseases, i.e. decreased consumption of unhealthy snacks. The program strategies must be implemented at the national level through collaboration between the academia and policy makers to assure impact at larger scale.

Trial registration: ClinicalTrial.gov-NCT01004367.

Keywords: Health promotion, Dietary intake, Andes, Cluster randomized controlled trial

* Correspondence: angelica.ochoa@ucuenca.edu.ec
[1]Departmento de Biociencias, Grupo Nutrición Alimentación y Salud, Facultad de Ciencias Químicas, Universidad de Cuenca, Avenida 12 de Abril y Avenida Loja, 0101168 Cuenca, Ecuador
Full list of author information is available at the end of the article

Background

In the last decades (since 1980 until 2013), overweight and obesity prevalence has increased around 47% among children and adolescents; affecting both high and low- and middle-income countries [1]. Overweight-obese children show higher mortality rates and are more likely to become obese adults [2]. The risk of obesity and other non-communicable diseases (NCDs) is attenuated by reducing blood pressure, increasing physical activity, supporting diets rich in fruit, vegetables, grains and nuts, and restricting the intake of sugared beverages and sweets [3–7]. In Ecuador, type 2 diabetes, hypertension and stroke are leading causes of death [8], with a larger disease burden in the urban areas [9]. Overweight, obesity and dyslipidemia [10], together with a diet poor in fiber, fruit and vegetables, and high in added sugar, refined grains and processed food are prevalent among Ecuadorian adolescents [11].

Prevention is needed to tackle this increasing burden of NCDs [12]. Interventions focusing on education and improvements of the food environment have proven to be effective to reduce the risk of NCDs [12–14]. Schools are suitable settings to implement preventive interventions for adolescents as they deal with environmental drivers [14] with respect to dietary intake and its determinants [13]. However, school-based lifestyle interventions in LMICs have methodological and conceptual flaws i.e. they are often not theory- and evidence-based or adapted to the specific context [13]. In Latin America, only a few school-based interventions targeting healthy eating and/or physical activity have been implemented [13, 15, 16]. The available programs in the region are usually short term, target small samples and/or at risk populations [13, 16], and showed deficiencies in their designs and evaluations [13, 16, 17]. Unfortunately, school-based interventions have not been performed in Andean States such as Colombia, Bolivia, Ecuador and Perú, where the ethnic, cultural and social context differs in comparison with other Latin American countries [18, 19]. This is especially important as health promotion success rates rely on context considerations [20].

We conducted a school-based cluster randomized controlled trial with parental involvement called "ACTIVITAL", aimed at improving the nutritional value of dietary intake and physical activity in a sample of school-going Ecuadorian adolescents. To our knowledge, the ACTIVITAL trial is innovative in its setting as it (i) was tailored to the local context using a theoretical framework and participatory approaches and (ii) targeted multiple populations (i.e. adolescents, school staff, and parents) and dietary risk factors for NCDs as well as physical activity. This paper reports: (i) the overall effect of the trial after three consecutive school years on dietary intake (primary outcome) and waist circumference, (ii) the effect of the trial after the first 17 months and the last 11 months of implementation, as well as (ii) the dose and reach of the strategies implemented. The effect on physical activity and body mass index was reported elsewhere [21].

Methods

Setting and context

The study targeted 12–14 year-old adolescents and was conducted in the urban area of Cuenca, the third largest city of Ecuador. At the time of the study, the Ecuadorian school system was comprised of four levels: elementary school (3–5 year-old children), primary school (1st-7th grade; 6–11 year-old children), middle school (8th to 10th grade; 12–14-year-old adolescents) and high school (1st-3rd year high school; 15–17 year-old adolescents). Within the education system, there are both private and public schools. Students attend school either in the morning (7:00–13:00) or in the afternoon (12:00–18:00), with one break of approximately 30 min. A school year in Cuenca runs from September to June. Most adolescents (73%) regularly attend school in the urban area of Cuenca [22]. All schools must follow a standard curriculum and use government issued learning materials.

A la carte foods (e.g. pre-packaged snacks, hot meals and soft drinks) are offered by private on-site school food kiosks. These operators function independently but are regulated by the Ministries of Health and Education. Adolescents also have easy access to street food near the schools.

Study design and sample size

This study was conducted in 20 schools. A pair-matched cluster randomized controlled trial was designed with the schools (clusters) as units of randomization. To reach the desired sample size of 70 students per school, schools were eligible if they (i) were located in the urban area of Cuenca, and (ii) had at least 90 students enrolled in the 8th and 9th grade. The schools' selection process is described in Fig. 1: 28 schools were matched by size (total number of students; no more than a 15% difference), type (public-private), school gender (single gender or co-ed. schools) and socioeconomic status (monthly fee; no more than 30% difference) into 14 pairs. The best ten matching pairs were selected. From the ten allotted pairs, each school was randomly assigned to either the treatment group or the control group, using random numbers in Stata 12.0 by a researcher who was not directly involved in the implementation. Adolescents and school staff were not aware about the existence of a counterfactual school.

In each school, two 8th and two 9th grades were randomly selected. All adolescents from these grades were invited to participate and 70 students were selected at

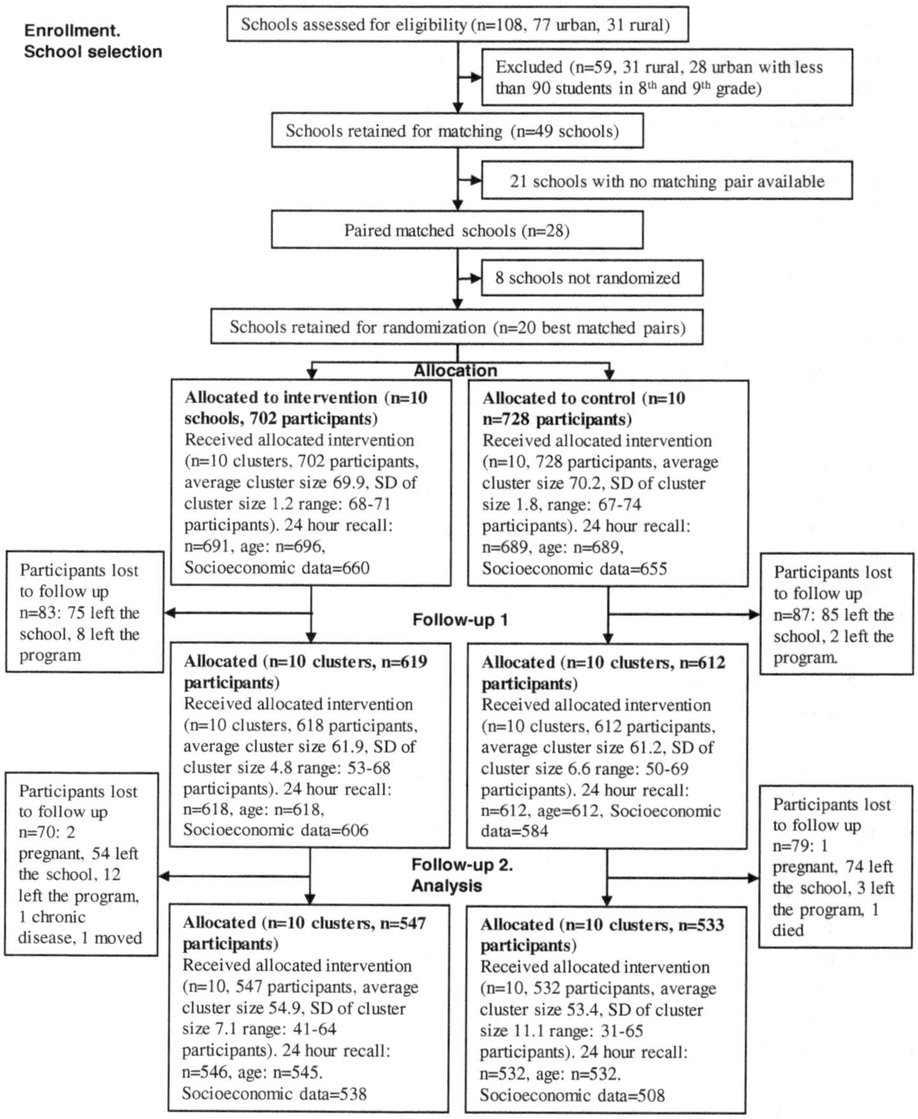

Fig. 1 Flow chart of progress

random. A total of 10 matched pairs of schools including an average sample of 65 children per school considering a Type I error of 5%, a coefficient of between-cluster variation (K_m) of 0.15 and a power of 80% [23], allowed for the detection of a decrease in 10% of the energy percentage derived from fat. This corresponded to a total sample size of 1300 adolescents in 20 schools. Considering an expected 10% drop-out we sampled 1430 adolescents.

Intervention development

Figure 2 summarizes the intervention development process. A needs assessment, including both qualitative [24] and quantitative [10, 11] data, was performed to ensure appropriateness of the program. Focus group discussions identified the following factors as influencing dietary intake: lack of knowledge about nutrition quality and healthy eating, less healthy eating habits at high school, and greater accessibility to pocket money used to buy tasty yet unhealthy food [24]. A dietary assessment prior to the study showed that the study population consumed insufficient fiber, fruit and vegetables, and an excess of added sugar, refined grains and processed foods during snacking [11]. These data served to define the intervention objectives and strategies using the Intervention Mapping (IM) [25] and the Comprehensive and Participatory Planning and Evaluation (CPPE) approach [26]. The possible intervention strategies identified during the CPPE were combined with the IM techniques to define the final intervention strategies [27]. This process

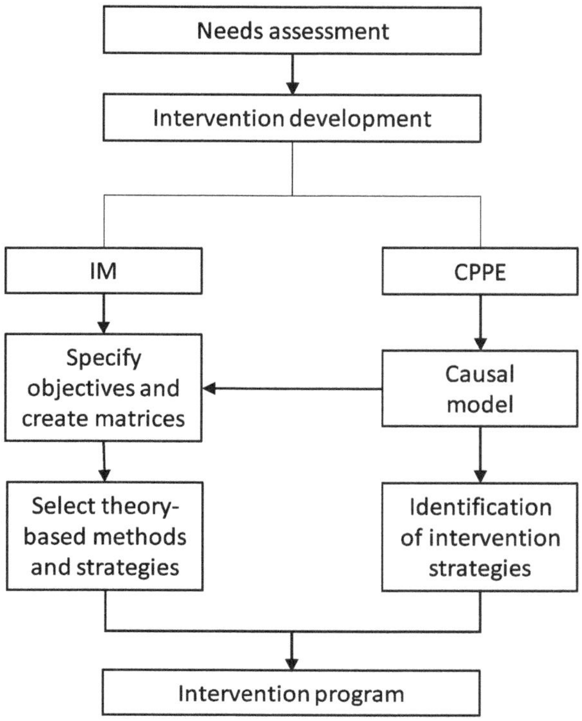

Fig. 2 Description of the intervention development process. IM: Intervention mapping, CPPE: Comprehensive and Participatory Planning and Evaluation

resulted in the development of the intervention program named ACTIVITAL with the following intervention objectives: adolescents (i) decrease their sugar intake, (ii) increase their daily fruit and vegetable intake, (iii) decrease their unhealthy snack intake, (iv) increase their healthy breakfast intake, and (v) school food kiosks increase the offer of healthy food. Separate matrices of change objectives for adolescents, parents and school staff were generated. Finally, different effective theoretical methods were identified from literature [25, 28] to translate the objectives into intervention strategies.

Intervention strategies and components

Intervention strategies were integrated into a curriculum-based (educational toolkits) and an environment-based (workshops and social events) component implemented in two different intervention stages (Table 1).

In the intervention schools, the ACTIVITAL program was implemented. The first stage was comprised of three activities: (i) participatory workshops with school staff and adolescents to increase ownership of the intervention and to revise the implementation strategy, (ii) introductory workshops on eating healthily with school staff and adolescents, and (iii) the implementation of intervention package one. Stage two only included the implementation of intervention package two (Table 1 and Fig. 3). In the control schools, no additional activities other than the existing national curriculum followed in health science lectures were included.

Outcomes

The nutritional value of dietary intake was a primary outcome and included the following variables: added sugar intake, fruit and vegetables intake, unhealthy snacking in general, consumption of unhealthy school snacks and breakfast intake. Energy contribution from fat per day was also included as a primary outcome (%). Waist circumference was a secondary outcome. All outcome measurements were performed by trained health related professionals at baseline and after stage one and two, at 17 and 28 months, respectively (Fig. 3). All the outcomes are analyzed at individual level.

Dietary intake

Dietary intake was estimated by means of two 24-h dietary recalls conducted on two randomly chosen weekdays. The average of the 2 days was used for the final analysis to estimate mean group intake [29]. Portion sizes and food consumption were estimated using standardized local utensils (measuring cups or graduated cylinders filled with water). If detailed information was missing for ingredients and/or cooking methods, we obtained these from recipes which were prepared in triplicate by local volunteering housewives.

In the absence of an Ecuadorian food composition table, the United States (USDA, 2012), Mexican (INNSZ, 1999), Central American (INCAP/OPS, 2012) and the Peruvian (CENAN/INS, 2008) databases were searched. For data that was still unavailable, food labels and the results of local proximal analysis were used. In the case of the latter, 12 samples per food item were randomly taken from local markets and then mixed to form a composite sample. One analytical portion was analyzed in triplicate for moisture and dry matter, ash, total fat by Weibull, total nitrogen by the Kjeldahl method and total carbohydrates were determined by difference [30].

Added sugar included artificially added sugars to processed or prepared food [31]. Sugar content was unavailable in the searched food composition tables for 271 of the total 872 food items reported. Data on added sugar for these food items were obtained from food labels (n = 175 food items), by extrapolating the sugar content from food items with similar nutritional characteristics ($n = 73$ food items) or by using the information of the standardized recipes ($n = 23$ food items). Added sugar intake is reported as g/day.

Fruit intake included raw fruit and fruit used in juices or any other preparation. Vegetables included dark green, red and orange vegetables, either raw or boiled. Beans or starchy vegetables were not included as they

Table 1 The ACTIVITAL intervention packages, components and strategies to improve the nutritional value of dietary intake

Stage	IP	Component/Strategy	Content of the session	Responsible	Target population	Support material
Stage one	IP1	Curriculum-based component/ Interactive educational toolkit: Classes every two weeks	1. Food pyramid 2. Healthy eating (introduction) 3. Healthy breakfast 4. Healthy snacking 5. Sugary drinks 6. Game. Financial autonomy	Life science school teachers or external teachers	Adolescents (8th -9th grades)	Booklets, games, didactic material
	IP1	Environment-based component/ School food kiosks staff workshops	1. Identification of needs and problems 2. Prioritization of needs and problems 3. Introduction to food safety 4. HACCP and recipe development 5. Food pyramid 6. Cooking skills 7. Food preparation 8. Breakfast, snacks, sugary drink and fruit and vegetable preparation 9. National legislation, adaptation and implementation 10. Management of the food kiosk	ACTIVITAL staff	Food kiosks staff	Recipes, leaflets, books, food.
	IP1	Environment-based component/ Parental workshops	1. Food pyramid 2. Breakfast, snacks and sugary drinks 3. Healthy eating and physical activity	ACTIVITAL staff	Parents	Booklets based on the curriculum based component
	IP1	Environment-based component/ Preparation of a healthy breakfast	Students prepare a healthy breakfast at school in small groups	Teachers, ACTIVITAL staff	Adolescents (8th - 9th grades)	Books, food, utensils, blackboards.
Stage two	IP2	Curriculum-based component/ Interactive educational toolkit: Classes every two weeks	1. Nutrients 2. Food labels 3. Portion sizes 4. Fruit and vegetables 5. Healthy lunch and dinner 6. Advertisements	Life science school teachers or external teachers	Adolescents (10th and 1st bachelor grades)	Booklets, games, didactic material
	IP2	Environment-based component/ School food kiosks staff workshops	1. Portion sizes and nutritional guidelines 2. Healthy menu planning 3. Analysis, evaluation and discussion of implanting healthy menus	ACTIVITAL staff	Food kiosks staff	Recipes, leaflets, books, food.
	IP2	Environment-based component/ Parental workshops	1. Portion sizes 2. Food labels and advertisements	ACTIVITAL staff	Parents	Booklets based on the curriculum based component

HACCP hazard analysis and critical control points, *IP* intervention package, *IP1* intervention package one (September 2010 – February 2011), *IP2* intervention package two (September 2011 – February 2012)

were not the main target in the educational toolkit. Fruit and vegetables were classified as one food group reported as g/day consumed.

Unhealthy snacking is defined as the consumption of "unhealthy foods" eaten during snack time. Snack times - including morning, afternoon, and evening snacks - were defined according to the schools' schedules (morning or afternoon) and the day of the week. In the case of weekdays, the times were set as follows: in the morning schools, morning snack was set between 7:00–13:00 and afternoon snack from 16:00–18:00. For afternoon schools, the timings were morning snack from 8:00–11:00 and afternoon snack from 12:00–18:00. Night snacks were set equally for the whole sample at any hour later than 21:00. The timing during weekend was similar for all the participants: morning snack from 9:00–12:00, afternoon snack from 15:00–18:00 and night snack at any hour later than 21:00. Secondly, all the "unhealthy"

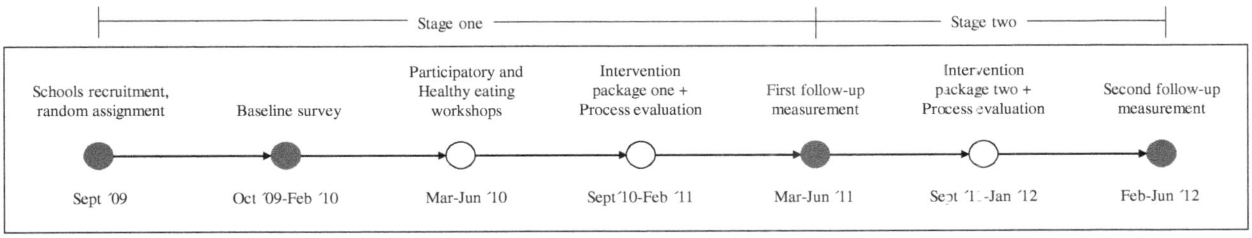

Fig. 3 Timeline and measurements of the ACTIVITAL trial. •Activities performed in both, intervention and control schools. ○ Activities performed in the intervention schools only

food items rich in sodium, fat or added sugar but low in nutrition value (usually available in vending machines, cafeterias and food kiosks [32]) consumed during these snack times were identified. These items comprised: (a) table sugar and sweets (honey, candies, chocolates, ice creams, sweet cookies, traditional sweet desserts and sugar added to juices, coffee, etc.), (b) salty snacks and fast food (packaged salty snacks, salty crackers, French fries, pizza, hamburgers) (c) soft drinks (soda, artificial sweetened juices, energy drinks) and (d) other packaged food (ketchup, packaged soups, gelatine). Finally, the intake of unhealthy foods per day during all the snack times was calculated. Unhealthy snacking is reported as g/day.

Unhealthy snacking at school was defined by identifying consumers of unhealthy foods prepared at school according to the following procedure: (i) from the list of recipes classified as unhealthy foods, we identified those prepared at school; next (ii) the participants were classified as 0 = non-consumers, if they had not reported any of the school-prepared items in the 24-h recalls, and 1 = consumers if at least one of the school-prepared item was reported in any recall.

Breakfast time was defined following a similar approach as the snack timing definition. For morning schools, breakfast time was set between 5:00–7:00 and for afternoon schools from 5:00–8:00. Breakfast intake is reported as a dichotomous variable (0 = non-consumers; 1 = consumers).

Energy from fat was calculated by dividing the daily energy of fat by the total energy intake per day (E%/day).

Other measurements

Waist circumference was measured in duplicate by two trained interviewers using standardized procedures. Waist circumference was measured twice at the midpoint between the last rib and the iliac-crest.

Socio-economic characteristics were assessed at baseline using the Integrated Social Indicator System tool for Ecuador [33]. Poverty was defined using the definition of Unsatisfied Basic Needs (UBN). This system categorizes a household as poor if one or more deficiencies in access to education, health, housing, water, electricity and employment are reported. Adolescents were allocated to one of two groups: 'Poor' if at least one deprivation was present or 'Better-off' if none was reported. The following extra questions based on the national census [34] about remittances and snack allowance were asked: 'Does the family receive remittances from abroad?' 'Does the adolescent receive a daily snack allowance?' and 'How much does the adolescent receive for his/her snack allowance?' Age was obtained from the reported date of birth.

Dose and reach of the intervention

Dose and reach of the intervention strategies were evaluated for different audiences (adolescents, parents and school staff) using field notes and attendance signed forms. For "dose", the number of activities performed (i.e. classes, workshops, events) was divided by those scheduled. For "reach", the number of participants (i.e. adolescents, parents and school staff) attending all the classes/workshops was divided by the number of invited participants.

Data management and data analysis

Waist circumference and socio-economic data was entered in duplicate into Epidata (Epidata Association, Odense, Denmark) by two independent researchers. Any discrepancy was corrected using the original forms. Food intake data was entered using an online software designed to analyze 24-h recall data (Lucille software 0.1, 2010, Ghent University; www.foodintake.ugent.be). Data management and statistical analysis were conducted using Stata 12.0 (Stata Corporation, Texas, USA). Statistical significance was set at 5% and all tests were two-sided.

Descriptive data are reported as proportions, means with SD, or medians with 25th and 75th percentile using all the available data per follow-up time point after adjustment for the cluster design.

Outcome differences at baseline between dropout and data retained for analysis were assessed using linear regression models adjusted for treatment allocation matching pairs and cluster design. Absolute differences in outcomes at baseline between the intervention and the control group were calculated and highlighted when they were larger than 5%.

An intention-to-treat analysis was performed to evaluate the intervention effect at the end of the program and after each intervention stage. The overall effect after the full intervention period was assessed using linear mixed models. The models were adjusted for baseline differences between the treatment and the control group [35]. The models comprised the school pair and participants as random effect. The treatment allocation was nested as a random slope within each pair. Adolescent's sex and UBN at baseline were included as fixed effects. The effect of the intervention was evaluated by testing the interaction term between follow-up time (in months) and treatment allocation. The results of the interaction term between the treatment groups with time (in months) were multiplied by 28 (duration of the trial) to calculate the overall intervention effect. Therefore, the reported differences between the intervention and the control group correspond to the effect after the whole program implementation and indicates the mean differences for continuous dependent variables and the proportion difference for dichotomous outcomes between the treatment and the control group [36]. The Akaike Information Criteria (AIC) and Schwartz's Bayesian Information Criteria (BIC) were used to select the optimal covariance structure for the models.

As intervention stages one (17 months) and two (11 months) were considerably different in timing as well as in strategies and content (Fig. 3 and Table 1), the intervention effect was estimated separately. Regression spline mixed effects models were used for this purpose, accounting for the effects of clustering by individual and school. One knot (the point of time where the slope of the linear function changes) was defined at the mean time (in months) of the first follow-up data collection (17 months). The Stata command "mkspline" was used to create two auxiliary variables (t1 = time in months one and t2 = time in months two). The models were adjusted for baseline differences between the treatment and the control group [35] and were built with the same random effects, random slope and fixed effects as the linear mixed models. The effect of the intervention was evaluated by testing the interaction term between time1 and treatment allocation and then again time2 and treatment allocation. The Beta coefficients of these interaction terms were multiplied by 17 for the effect after the first stage and by 11 for the second stage, corresponding to the respective duration of both stages. Therefore, the reported differences between the intervention and the control group correspond to the effect after each intervention stage and indicates the mean differences for continuous dependent variables and the proportion difference for dichotomous outcomes between the treatment and the control group [36].

Sensitivity analysis

We assessed the influence of missing data on the outcomes with a $P < 0.1$. For this purpose, we used a multiple imputation strategy using chained equations ($n = 50$ imputations) to impute the missing outcome data under the assumption of 'missing at random. Predictors for the regression models for the imputation were adolescent's sex, UBN and Body Mass Index z-score at baseline.

Results

A total of 1430 adolescents from 20 schools were recruited (Fig. 1). There were relatively more girls than boys (66% vs. 59%) in the intervention group (Table 2). More participants in the intervention group received remittances from abroad (24% vs. 17%). Outcome data at baseline and the two follow-up periods are reported in Table 3. At baseline, adolescents from the intervention group consumed (7%) more fruit and vegetables than those in the control group (median (IQR) intake: 204.6 g (119.1–337.0) for the intervention and 191.5 (104.1–304.2) for the control group). Whilst adolescents in the control group consumed 11% more unhealthy foods during snacking (median (IQR) intake: 94.5 g (27.5–220.0) for the intervention and 97.5 g (40.0–258.0) for the control group).

The sample size retained for analysis of all the dietary intake outcomes included 1046 adolescents in 20 schools; 538 (78% of the sample at baseline) in the intervention and 508 (74% of the sample at baseline) in the control group. Sample sizes for the other outcomes differed slightly (Fig. 1) but the attrition rate was similar for both groups (22 and 20% for the intervention and control group respectively, $P = 0.55$). No significant differences in primary and secondary outcomes at baseline were found between participants who dropped out and those retained for analysis.

Overall effect

The effect of the program after 28 months is presented in Table 4. Participants from the intervention group consumed lower quantities of unhealthy snacks (−23.32 g; 95% CI: −45.25,1.37) and less added sugar (−5.66 g; 95% CI: −9.63, 1.65) at the end of the trial. Daily fruit and vegetable intake decreased in both the intervention and control groups compared to baseline (Table 3), but the decrease was 23.88 g (95% CI: 7.36, 40.40) lower among the intervention group. Waist circumference (−0.84 cm; 95% CI: −1.68, 0.28) was lower in the intervention group at the end of the program (Table 4).

Effect according to intervention stage

The effect was higher during the first stage (Table 4). The effect on fruit and vegetables intake (29.2 g; 95% CI: 10.4, 47.6) and on waist circumference (−1.68 cm; 95% CI: −2.38, 1.02) was in favor of the intervention

Table 2 Baseline characteristics at individual and cluster level[a]

	Intervention group		Control Group	
Individual level	n	Mean ± SD or %	n	Mean ± SD or %
Age (y)	696	12.9 ± 0.8	692	12.9 ± 0.8
Girls (%)	702	66.2	699	58.2
Better off (%)	670	68.2	655	67.5
Remittances from abroad (%)	643	23.8	636	16.5
Snack allowance (%)	651	82.5	643	82.9
Amount of snack allowance ($)	642	0.9 ± 0.6	653	0.9 ± 0.6
Education of the father (years)	568	12.1 ± 4.8	571	12.2 ± 4.9
Education of the mother (years)	611	11.8 ± 4.7	613	11.5 ± 4.8
Cluster level	n	Median (25th–75th) or %	n	Median (25th–75th) or %
Students per school (n)	10	751 (335–1169)	10	787 (326–1335)
Public schools (%)	10	50.0	10	50.0
Co-ed. schools (%)	10	70.0	10	70.0
Monthly fee ($)	10	7.00 (0.0–68.3)	10	6.50 (0.0–81.8)
Morning schools (%)	10	60.0	10	60.0

[a]Summary statistics adjusted for the cluster design

Table 3 Primary and secondary outcomes at baseline and at follow-up measurements by treatment group[a]

	Measurement	Intervention group		Control group	
		n	Median (25th–75th) or %	n	Median (25th–75th) or %
Fruit and vegetables (g/d)	Baseline	691	204.6 (119.1–337.0)	689	191.5 (104.1–304.2)
	First follow-up	618	176.7 (111.0–274.3)	612	164.4 (99.0–247.8)
	Second follow-up	546	150.6 (101.2–248.1)	532	153.1 (48.6–181.9)
Added sugar (g/d)	Baseline	691	68.2 (48.1–92.7)	689	68.9 (84.2–240.4)
	First follow-up	618	58.1 (42.7–77.5)	612	60.3 (44.6–82.9)
	Second follow-up	546	57.1 (41.7–75.2)	532	62.8 (42.9–85.0)
Total fat (E %/d)	Baseline	691	25.5 (22.0–29.0)	689	25.3 (21.6–29.2)
	First follow-up	618	25.5 (21.7–29.3)	612	26.3 (22.4–30.2)
	Second follow-up	546	25.9 (22.1–30.5)	532	26.2 (22.5–30.5)
Unhealthy snacking[b](g/d)	Baseline	691	94.5 (27.5–220.0)	689	97.5 (40.0–258.0)
	First follow-up	618	63.8 (0.00–184.6)	612	81.5 (12.6–204.6)
	Second follow-up	546	60.0 (0.00–180.0)	532	98.1 (16.3–233.8)
Unhealthy snacking at school (% of consumers)	Baseline	691	18.4	689	20.6
	First follow-up	618	18.1	612	31.4
	Second follow-up	546	26.5	532	32.3
Breakfast intake (% of consumers)	Baseline	691	78.4	689	75.6
	First follow-up	618	79.3	612	77.3
	Second follow-up	546	74.0	532	80.8
Waist circumference (cm)	Baseline	691	68.9 (9.0)	692	68.3 (8.1)
	First follow-up	615	68.3 (8.0)	607	69.4 (7.6)
	Second follow-up	543	71.1 (8.4)	530	71.2 (7.9)

[a]Summary statistics using all the available individual data at baseline and follow-up points adjusted for the cluster design
[b]Consumption of unhealthy foods eaten during snack time; i.e. table sugar, sweets, salty snacks, fast food, soft drinks and packaged food

Table 4 Intervention effect at the end of the intervention and by intervention stage

	n	Effect at the end of the intervention (28 months)[a]			Effect after stage 1 (17 months)[b]		Effect after stage 2 (11 months)[b]		
		Diff[c] (95% CI)	P[d]	ICC[e]	Diff[c](95% CI)	P[d]	Diff (95% CI)	P[d]	ICC[f]
Added sugar (g/d)	1046	−5.66 (−9.63;-1.65)	0.006	0.36	−2.72 (−6.97; 1.36)	0.20	−4.07 (−8.47; 0.44)	0.07	0.35
Fruit and vegetables (g/d)	1046	23.88 (7.36; 40.40)	0.005	0.26	29.2 (10.4; 47.6)	0.002	−13.4 (−37.4; 10.2)	0.27	0.26
Unhealthy snacking (g/d)[g]	1046	−23.32 (−45.25;-1.37)	0.04	0.16	−9.35 (−32.1; 13.4)	0.42	−18.5 (−44.8; 7.81)	0.17	0.17
Unhealthy snacking at school (PD[h])	1046	−0.03 (−0.08; 0.06)	0.49	0.10	−0.15 (−0.20;-0.08)	<0.001	0.11 (0.08; 0.50)	0.005	0.11
Breakfast intake (PD[h])	1046	−0.03 (−0.06; 0.03)	0.39	0.42	0.03 (−0.005; 0.085)	0.11	−0.07 (−0.13;-0.02)	0.011	0.44
Fat (E%/d)	1046	−0.45 (−1.20; 0.31)	0.25	0.22	−0.51 (−1.36; 0.24)	0.17	0.11 (−0.77; 1.10)	0.74	0.21
Waist circumference (cm)	1079	−0.84 (−1.68;-0.28)	0.005	0.77	−1.68 (−2.38;-1.02)	<0.001	0.66 (−0.07; 1.21)	0.08	0.78

[a]Results obtained from mixed effects models accounting for the effects of clustering by individual and school. These models were adjusted for sex, UBN and differences at baseline (excluding the treatment group main effect) [35]
[b]Results obtained from regressions spline mixed effects models. One knot was defined at the mean time of the first follow up data collection (17 months)
[c]Mean differences
[d]*P* value
[e]Intraclass correlation coefficient of mixed effects models
[f]Intraclass correlation coefficient of regression spline mixed effects models
[g]Consumption of unhealthy foods eaten during snack time; i.e. table sugar, sweets, salty snacks, fast food, soft drinks and packaged food
[h]Proportion difference

group and reached statistical significance only after stage one (Table 4). The proportion of consumers of unhealthy snacks prepared at school decreased by 15% (95% CI: −20.0,-8.0) after stage one, but increased by 11% (95% CI: 8.0, 50.0) after stage two in the intervention schools when compared with the control schools. During stage two, the percentage of breakfast consumers also decreased in the intervention schools (−7%; 95% CI: −13.0, −2.0) compared with the control group. On the other hand, the intake of unhealthy snacks decreased largely at stage two but did not reach statistically significance at any stage (−9.35 g; 95% CI: −32.1, 13.4 at stage one and −18.5 g; 95% CI: −44.8, 7.81 at stage two).

Dose and reach

Dose and reach are reported in Table 5. While 99% of the classes were delivered in stage one, this percentage decreased to 91% in stage two (Table 5). This decrease is explained by the fact that half of the participants reached high school; in the Ecuadorian school system, at high school, adolescents are distributed into different specializations according to their preferences, the last implies that more classrooms had to be included to involve all the sampled adolescents. A higher proportion of schoolteachers implemented the classes themselves in stage one (70%) compared to stage two (31%).

All the workshops with the food kiosks staff and with parents were performed in both intervention stages. In total, 70% of the schools attended at least 80% of the food kiosks staff workshops at stage one and 60% at stage two. One private school was absent in all the workshops as the school owner operated the food kiosk and considered that the nutritional quality was adequate. Similarly, more parents attended the workshops in stage one vs. stage two (20% vs. 11%).

Table 5 Dose and Reach of ACTIVITAL by intervention stage

Intervention component	Process evaluation element	Output	Overall (%)	Stage 1 (%)	Stage 2 (%)
The curriculum-based component	Dose delivered	% of classes delivered	94	99	91
	Reach	% of classes delivered by school teachers	46	70	31
The environment-based component/ Food kiosks staff workshops	Dose delivered	% of workshops delivered	100	100	100
	Reach	% of schools that attended to at least 80% of the workshops	65	70	60
The environment-based component/ Parental workshops	Dose delivered	% of workshops delivered	100	100	100
	Reach	% of parents reached	15	20	11

Sensitivity analysis

The overall intervention effect did not change considerably after imputing missing values, the effect on unhealthy snacks was no longer significant ($P = 0.092$) and the coefficient decreased from −23.3 to −18.3 g/day (95% CI: 39.5, 2.54). The effect on fruit and vegetables (20 g; 95% CI: 2.24, 37.2), added sugar (−6.7 g; 95% CI: −0.97,-12.5) and waist circumference (−1 cm; 95% CI: −1.64,-0.39) remained significant and with similar coefficients.

Discussion

The ACTIVITAL trial positively influenced unhealthy snacking, added sugar intake and waist circumference while attenuating the decrease in fruit and vegetables intake in the intervention group. This study adds value to the current literature as it provides a comprehensive school-based intervention designed by means of a theoretical and participative approach able to target multiple populations and risk factors among adolescents living in an Andean upper middle-income country.

At the end of the intervention, fruit and vegetable intake decreased in both the intervention and control groups, but this decrease was lower in the intervention group. Although the intervention was unable to increase the fruit and vegetable intake, it effectively attenuated the decrease of fruit and vegetable intake during adolescence. Still, the intake in the intervention group in the present study remained below the recommended intake of 400 g of fruits and vegetables per day [37] and the effect is lower compared to other school-based health promotion programs in this age group [38, 39]. However, the latter programs, included fruit and vegetables as the only outcome.

We report a decrease of 23 g/d in unhealthy snack intake and a decrease of 15% in the proportion of consumers of unhealthy snacks prepared at school in the intervention group after the first stage. Previous research has demonstrated that multicomponent programs involving parents, aiming at the food sources both in and outside of school and focusing on a variety of unhealthy food items seem to be less likely to fail [40]. The decrease in the fraction of consumers of unhealthy food at school during stage one suggests improvements in the food prepared at school as it concurs with a higher staff response.

Our reductions of 1 cm of waist circumference is comparable to previous studies [41]. Diets high in fruit and vegetables, low in fast food and soda, and improvements in physical fitness were previously found inversely correlated with waist circumference. The ACTIVITAL trial also had important effects on both physical activity and physical fitness [21]. The proportion of adolescents reaching the recommended moderate to vigorous physical activity decreased less in the intervention group, the proportion of adolescents spending more than 3 h in front of a screen decreased in the intervention group during weekdays, performance on the vertical jump test was better among the intervention participants, and finally, participants in the control group performed worse on the speed shuttle run test [21].

The effect on fruit and vegetable intake, unhealthy snacking and waist circumference was larger during stage one of the intervention. Differences in program implementation between stage one and two can explain this. In contrast to stage two, (i) participatory workshops were performed, (ii) dose and reach were higher (iii) and more workshops with the food kiosks staff were implemented during stage one. Previous studies have shown how participatory approaches [42] and parental support are important factors for school-based health promotion [43]. The low parental response could be the consequence of the lack of parents' recognition of their responsibility in their children's eating behavior according with qualitative data obtained in the same population [24]. Future studies should identify the most effective strategies to involve parents in diet-oriented health promotion programs implemented in LMICs. Previous reports from high-income countries have documented the difficulty of reaching parents even after adapting interventions to their requirements [44]. The latest research suggests that there is still insufficient evidence on how to engage and reach parents in these kinds of programs.

Cluster randomized controlled trials should have both internal and external validity to enable generalizability [45]. Although our sample size retained for analysis was smaller than expected, there are several reasons to conclude that ACTIVITALs' internal validity was fairly acceptable: (i) analysis of missing values did not provide different results, (ii) outcome differences between the dropouts and the sample retained for analysis were small, (iii) the cluster nature of the study was considered in both the sample size calculations and data analyses, and, (v) the participants in the intervention and the control group were selected at random.

External validity could be evaluated by the adoption, i.e. the extent to which the setting is representative to the wider population, and the evaluation of the implementation of the program [45]. Regarding adoption, the findings of ACTIVITAL are mainly applicable to urban areas. The program may not be effective among rural adolescents as the needs assessment showed that determinants of healthy eating and physical activity were substantially different between both areas [24, 46]. Even though some urban schools were not considered for randomization in the pair-matching process because they either had very few students or an unavailable matching pair, this selection does not influence the adoption of the program in the urban area. In recent years, the Ecuadorian school system was reformed. Currently, all the schools have become co-ed., and an important proportion of the small schools have closed [47].

We acknowledge a number of limitations. The 24-h recalls were applied only during weekdays. Although the average of two recalls is appropriate to estimate mean group intake [29], it does not allow estimating usual individual intake and the proportion of individuals at risk of inadequate intake [29]. The main purpose of the study however, was to assess differences between the intervention vs. control group. Data on differences between the adolescents who agreed to participate and those who did not was not collected. The causes of the differential effect between stage one and two remain to be confirmed using an effectiveness study comparing a highly controlled intervention with an intervention implemented in usual school conditions [48]. This research would clarify if the attenuated effect is the consequence of a relapse of the program or the consequence of the lack of control in habitual conditions.

Conclusions

ACTIVITAL had positive effects on dietary risk factors for NCDs, i.e. fruit and vegetable intake and the consumption of unhealthy food items during snacking. Although still below the nutritional recommendations, the combined effect of the intervention is encouraging and promising [4, 38]. It suggests that school-based interventions can address various risk factors simultaneously in adolescents from LMICs. The program strategies must be implemented at the national level by collaboration between the academia and policy makers to assure impact at larger scale.

Abbreviations

AIC: Akaike Information Criteria; BIC: Schwartz's Bayesian Information Criteria; CPPE: Comprehensive and Participatory Planning and Evaluation; IM: Intervention mapping; NCDs: Non-communicable diseases; UBN: Unsatisfied basic needs

Acknowledgements

We acknowledge the cooperation of schools, directors, teachers, parents, adolescents, school food kiosks staff and any other school staff involved in the ACTIVITAL program. We especially appreciate the contribution from Johana Ortiz, Diana Andrade, Diana Córdova, Marlene Gia, Silvia Torres, Lourdes Jerves, María Cecilia Vintimilla, Cecilia Romero, Torcasa Hidalgo and Alexandra Shourds.

Funding

This work was supported by grant from VLIR-UOS and Nutrition Third World. Within the cooperation between the University of Ghent (Belgium) and University of Cuenca (Ecuador).

Authors' contributions

AOA, RV, LM and PK designed research. AOA, RV, SA, SD and PR conducted research. AOA, LH and SA analyzed data. AOA and RV wrote the paper. AOA had primary responsibility for the final content. All authors read and approved the final manuscript.

Consent for publication

Not applicable.

Competing interests

The authors declare that they have no competing interests.

Author details

[1]Departmento de Biociencias, Grupo Nutrición Alimentación y Salud, Facultad de Ciencias Químicas, Universidad de Cuenca, Avenida 12 de Abril y Avenida Loja, 0101168 Cuenca, Ecuador. [2]Independent researcher, Ghent, Belgium. [3]Department of Food Safety and Food Quality, Faculty of Bioscience Engineering, Ghent University, Coupure Links 653, B-9000 Ghent, Belgium. [4]Poverty, Health and Nutrition Division, International Food Policy Research Institute, 2033 K St, NW, Washington, DC, USA. [5]Department of Public Health, Ghent University, Ghent, Belgium.

References

1. Ng M, Fleming T, Robinson M, Thomson B, Graetz N, Margono C, Mullany EC, Biryukov S, Abbafati C, Abera SF. Global, regional, and national prevalence of overweight and obesity in children and adults during 1980–2013: a systematic analysis for the global burden of disease study 2013. Lancet. 2014;384:766–81.
2. Biro FM, Wien M. Childhood obesity and adult morbidities. Am J Clin Nutr. 2010;91:1499S–505S.
3. Juhola J, Magnussen CG, Berenson GS, Venn A, Burns TL, Sabin MA, Srinivasan SR, Daniels SR, Davis PH, Chen W. Combined effects of child and adult elevated blood pressure on subclinical atherosclerosis the international childhood cardiovascular cohort consortium. Circulation. 2013;128:217–24.
4. Lim SS, Vos T, Flaxman AD, Danaei G, Shibuya K, Adair-Rohani H, AlMazroa MA, Amann M, Anderson HR, Andrews KG, et al. A comparative risk assessment of burden of disease and injury attributable to 67 risk factors and risk factor clusters in 21 regions, 1990–2010: a systematic analysis for the global burden of disease study 2010. Lancet. 2012;380:2224–60.
5. Mente A, de Koning L, Shannon HS, Anand SS. A systematic review of the evidence supporting a causal link between dietary factors and coronary heart disease. Arch Intern Med. 2009;169:659–69.
6. Mozaffarian D, Appel LJ, Van Horn L. Components of a Cardioprotective diet: new insights. Circulation. 2011;123:2870–91.
7. Ortega F, Ruiz J, Castillo M, Sjöström M. Physical fitness in childhood and adolescence: a powerful marker of health. Int J Obes. 2007;32:1–11.
8. Instituto Nacional de Estadísticas y Censos. Anuario de Estadísticas Vitales - Nacimientos y Defunciones 2014. 2014. http://www.ecuadorencifras.gob.ec/documentos/web-inec/Poblacion_y_Demografia/Nacimientos_Defunciones/Publicaciones/Anuario_Nacimientos_y_Defunciones_2014.pdf. Accessed 29 Nov 2017.
9. Freire W RM, Belmont P, Mendieta M, Silva M, Romero N, Sáenz K, Piñeiros P, Gómez L, Monge R.: Resumen Ejecutivo Tomo I. Encuesta Nacional de Salud y Nutrición del Ecuador. Ministerio de Salud Pública INdEyC ed. Quito Ecuador; 2013.
10. Ochoa-Avilés A, Andrade S, Huynh T, Verstraeten R, Lachat C, Rojas R, Donoso S, Manuel-y-Keenoy B, Kolsteren P. Prevalence and socioeconomic differences of risk factors of cardiovascular disease in Ecuadorian adolescents. Pediatric Obesity. 2012;7:274–83.
11. Ochoa-Aviles A, Verstraeten R, Lachat C, Andrade S, Van Camp J, Donoso S, Kolsteren P. Dietary intake practices associated with cardiovascular risk in urban and rural Ecuadorian adolescents: a cross-sectional study. BMC Public Health. 2014;14:939.
12. Jamison DT, Summers LH, Alleyne G, Arrow KJ, Berkley S, Binagwaho A, Bustreo F, Evans D, Feachem RGA, Frenk J, et al. Global health 2035: a world converging within a generation. Lancet. 2013;382:1898–955.
13. Verstraeten R, Roberfroid D, Lachat C, Leroy JL, Holdsworth M, Maes L, Kolsteren PW. Effectiveness of preventive school-based obesity interventions in low- and middle-income countries: a systematic review. Am J Clin Nutr. 2012;96:415–38.
14. Story M, Nanney MS, Schwartz MB. Schools and obesity prevention: creating school environments and policies to promote healthy eating and physical activity. Milbank Q. 2009;87:71–100.
15. Cunha DB, BdSNd S, Pereira RA, Sichieri R. Effectiveness of a randomized school-based intervention involving families and teachers to prevent excessive weight gain among adolescents in Brazil. PLoS One. 2013;8:e57498.

16. Marshall SJ, Simoes EJ, Eisenberg CM, Holub CK, Arredondo EM, Barquera S, Elder JP. Weight-related child behavioral interventions in Brazil: a systematic review. Am J Prev Med. 2013;44:543–9.
17. Kain J, Cordero SH, Pineda D, de Moraes AF, Antiporta D, Collese T, de Oliveira Forkert EC, González L, Miranda JJ, Rivera J. Obesity prevention in Latin America. Curr Obes Rep. 2014;3:150–5.
18. Martínez R. Hambre y desigualdad en los países andinos: la desnutrición y la vulnerabilidad alimentaria en Bolivia, Colombia, Ecuador y Perú. Santiago de Chile: United Nations Publications; 2005.
19. Guerrero AL, Gallucci SS, Michalijos P, Visciarelli S: Países Andinos: aportes teóricos para un abordaje integrado desde las perspectivas geográfica y turística. 2011.
20. Sparks M. The changing contexts of health promotion; 2013. p. 28.
21. Andrade S, Lachat C, Ochoa-Avilés A, Verstraeten R, Huybregts L, Roberfroid D, Andrade D, Van Camp J, Rojas R , Donoso S, et al. A school-based intervention improves physical fitness in Ecuadorian adolescents: a cluster-randomized controlled trial. Int J Behav Nutr Phys Act. 2014;11:153.
22. Sistema Nacional de Información. Indicadores de Educación [http://app.sni.gob.ec/web/menu/]. Accessed 29 Nov 2017.
23. Hayes R, Bennett S. Simple sample size calculation for cluster-randomized trials. Int J Epidemiol. 1999;28:319–26.
24. Verstraeten R, Van Royen K, Ochoa-Avilés A, Penafiel D, Holdsworth M, Donoso S, Maes L, Kolsteren P. A conceptual framework for healthy eating behavior in Ecuadorian adolescents: a qualitative study. PLoS One. 2014;9:e87183.
25. Bartholomew LK, Parcel GS, Kok G, Gottlieb NH, Fernandez ME. Planning health promotion programs: an intervention mapping approach. San Francisco: Wiley; 2011.
26. Ndirangu M, Perkins H, Yadrick K, West JR, Bogle ML, Avis-Williams A, Santell R, Connell CL. Conducting needs assessment using the comprehensive participatory planning and evaluation model to develop nutrition and physical activity interventions in a rural community in the Mississippi Delta. Prog Community Health Partnersh. 2007;1:41–8.
27. Bartholomew LK, Parcel G, Kok G, Gottlieb N: Intervention mapping: designing theory–and evidence-based health promotion programs. 2001.
28. Abraham C, Michie S. A taxonomy of behavior change techniques used in interventions. Health Psychol. 2008;27:379.
29. Willett W. Nutritional epidemiology. New York: Oxford University Press; 2012.
30. Greenfield H, Southgate D. Food composition data. Production, management and use. Barking: Elsevier Applied Science; 2003.
31. Welsh JA, Sharma AJ, Grellinger L, Vos MB. Consumption of added sugars is decreasing in the United States. Am J Clin Nutr. 2011;94:726–34.
32. Fried E, Simon M. The competitive food conundrum: can government regulations improve school food? Duke Law J. 2007:1491–539.
33. Sistema Integrado de Indicadores Sociales del Ecuador S. Necesidades Básicas Insatisfechas. Ecuador: Siise: Sistema Integrado de Indicadores Sociales del Ecuador; 2012.
34. Instituto Nacional de Estadísticas y Censos. Encuesta de Estratificación del Nivel Socio-Económico. Ecuador: INEC; 2011.
35. Fitzmaurice GM, Laird NM, Ware JH. Applied longitudinal analysis. Hoboken: Wiley; 2012.
36. Hellevik O. Linear versus logistic regression when the dependent variable is a dichotomy. Qual Quant. 2009;43:59–74.
37. World Health Organization JC, FAO Expert. Diet, nutrition and the prevention of chronic diseases, WHO technical report series; 2003. p. 916.
38. Knai C, Pomerleau J, Lock K, McKee M. Getting children to eat more fruit and vegetables: a systematic review. Prev Med. 2006;42:85–95.
39. Thomson CA, Ravia J. A systematic review of behavioral interventions to promote intake of fruit and vegetables. J Am Diet Assoc. 2011;111:1523–35.
40. Jaime PC, Lock K. Do school based food and nutrition policies improve diet and reduce obesity? Prev Med. 2009;48:45–53.
41. Vandongen R, Jenner DA, Thompson C, Taggart AC, Spickett EE, Burke V, Beilin LJ, Milligan RA, Dunbar DL. A controlled evaluation of a fitness and nutrition intervention program on cardiovascular health in 10-year-old to 12-year-old children. Prev Med. 1995;24:9–22.
42. Lytle LA, Murray DM, Perry CL, Story M, Birnbaum AS, Kubik MY, Varnell S. School-based approaches to affect adolescents' diets: results from the TEENS study. Health Educ Behav. 2004;31:270–87.
43. Clarke J, Fletcher B, Lancashire E, Pallan M, Adab P. The views of stakeholders on the role of the primary school in preventing childhood obesity: a qualitative systematic review. Obes Rev. 2013;14:975–88.
44. Van Lippevelde W, Bere E, Verloigne M, van Stralen M, De Bourdeaudhuij I, Lien N, Vik F, Manios Y, Grillenberger M, Kovacs E, et al. The role of family-related factors in the effects of the UP4FUN school-based family-focused intervention targeting screen time in 10- to 12-year-old children: the ENERGY project. BMC Public Health. 2014;14:857.
45. Eldridge S, Ashby D, Bennett C, Wakelin M, Feder G. Internal and external validity of cluster randomised trials: systematic review of recent trials. BMJ. 2008;336:876–80.
46. Van Royen K, Verstraeten R, Andrade S, Ochoa-Aviles A, Donoso S, Maes L, Kolsteren P. Factors affecting physical activity in Ecuadorian adolescents: a focus group study. J Phys Act Health. 2015;12:340–8.
47. Larrea C, Warnars L. Ecuador's Yasuni-ITT initiative: avoiding emissions by keeping petroleum underground. Energy Sustain Dev. 2009;13:219–23.
48. Singal AG, Higgins PD, Waljee AK. A primer on effectiveness and efficacy trials. Clin Transl Gastroenterol. 2014;5:e45.
49. Campbell MK, Elbourne DR, Altman DG. CONSORT statement: extension to cluster randomised trials. BMJ. 2004;328:702–8.

Associations between fruit and vegetable, and antioxidant nutrient intake and age-related macular degeneration by smoking status in elderly Korean men

Eun-kyung Kim, Hyesook Kim, Aswathy Vijayakumar, Oran Kwon and Namsoo Chang*

Abstract

Background: Age-related macular degeneration (AMD) is one of the major causes of irreversible blindness. The objective of this study was to determine whether there is any relationship between dietary intake of fruits and vegetables (F&V) and antioxidant nutrients including carotenoids and AMD according to smoking status in elderly men.

Methods: We performed a cross-sectional analysis using nationally representative samples of elderly aged ≥ 65 years ($n = 1414$) from the Korea National Health and Nutrition Examination Survey (KNHANES, 2010–2012).

Results: The current smokers consumed less food in total, and, in particular, less cereals/potatoes/sugar products, fruits and vegetables than the nonsmokers and former smokers ($p < 0.05$). Intake of energy, thiamin, vitamin C, vitamin A, and β-carotene were significantly lower in the current smokers than in the nonsmokers and the former smokers. For current smokers, the ORs of the highest tertile compared with the lowest tertile were 0.36 (95% CI: 0.14–0.96, p for trend = 0. 0576) for F&V, 0.32 (95% CI: 0.12–0.85, p for trend = 0.0561) for vitamin C, 0.23 (95% CI: 0.08–0.67, p for trend = 0.0038) for α-carotene, 0.13 (95% CI: 0.04–0.46, p for trend = 0.0003) for β-carotene after adjusting for confounding factors. In contrast, there was no association between antioxidant nutrient intake and AMD among the nonsmokers and former smokers.

Conclusions: These results suggest that increased consumption of fruits and vegetables containing antioxidant components such as vitamin C, α-carotene, and β-carotene may have a protective effect on AMD. These effects may be more evident among current smokers.

Keywords: Age-related macular degeneration, Fruit and vegetables, Antioxidants, Elderly male smokers, KNHANES

Background

Age-related macular degeneration (AMD) is one of the major causes of irreversible blindness in older adults [1]. Several studies have identified risk factors for AMD, including age [2], family history [3], diabetes mellitus [4], alcohol consumption [5], cigarette smoking [6, 7] and dietary factors [8–11].

Smoking has been reported to be the strongest environmental risk factor for AMD [7, 12]. Toxins in cigarette smoke induce cellular oxidative damage secondary to dysfunction of the biological systems that detoxify reactive oxygen species (ROS) [13] and depletion of circulating antioxidants [14]. In particular, oxidative stress in the retinal pigment epithelium (RPE) is a major contributing factor in the etiology of AMD [15].

Among dietary factors, fruits and vegetables [16], dairy products [17], fish [18], n-3 fatty acid [19], antioxidant vitamins [16, 19, 20], and carotenoids, particularly β-carotene [19], lutein and zeaxanthin [21–23], are protective against AMD. Antioxidant vitamins protect cells from oxidative stress [24]. Carotenoids accumulate in the macular pigment and protect RPE cells from damage [25].

Most previous studies on the associations between diet and AMD have been conducted in Western countries, including America [26, 27], Europe [28, 29], and Australia [8, 9]. In Asia, several studies have been conducted in Japan [19, 30], China [31], and India [32]. Korea is expected to

* Correspondence: nschang@ewha.ac.kr
Department of Nutritional Science and Food Management, Ewha Womans University, Seoul 120-750, Republic of Korea

see a substantial increase in the number of elderly people in the next few decades and it has been estimated that the proportion of the population aged ≥ 60 years will be 41.5% by 2050 [33]. Therefore, age-related health complications are becoming more important. According to the Korea National Health Examination Survey (KNHANES) report, the prevalence of smoking among Korean men was 39.3% in 2015 [34]. In addition, Korea has the third highest number of smokers among the organization for economic cooperation and development (OECD) countries [35]. Knowledge on the epidemiology of AMD is essential to meeting future demands for eye health care and support for persons with AMD. Several studies have been carried out in an attempt to investigate the risk factors for AMD in the Korean population [2, 36]. However, the association between diet and AMD has never been studied.

Therefore, the aim of this study was to determine the relationship between F&V and antioxidant nutrient intake including carotenoids and AMD by cigarette smoking status in elderly men, using data from the Korea National Health and Nutrition Examination Survey (2010–2012).

Methods

Data source and study population

This study was based on data from the fifth KNHANES (2010–2012), a cross-sectional, nationally representative survey carried out by the Korea Centers for Disease Control and Prevention. The KNHANES uses a stratified, multi-stage sampling method and consists of a health interview survey, a health examination survey, and a nutrition survey. The response rates for each survey were 81.9, 80.4, and 80.0% in 2010–2012, respectively. This study was approved by the Institutional Review Board of the Korea Centers for Disease Control and Prevention (2010-02CON-21-C, 2011-02CON-06-C, 2012-01EXP-01-2C) and written informed consent was obtained from all subjects. Detailed information about the survey is available on the website (http://knhanes.cdc.go.kr) [37].

The study population comprised elderly men aged ≥ 65 years who responded to the 2010–2012 KNHANES ($n = 2031$). We excluded subjects without 24 h dietary recall data ($n = 122$); those without fundus photograph data ($n = 439$); and those lacking smoking status data ($n = 56$). A total of 1414 participants were included in the final analysis. General characteristics of the study subjects were not significantly different between those included and excluded from the study (data not shown).

Assessment of AMD

AMD was defined as per a diagnosis by an ophthalmologist in the health examination survey. The outcome used in this study was the presence of any AMD in at least 1 eye. The presence of early- and late-onset AMD was determined on the basis of the fundus photograph [38, 39]. All fundus photographs were graded twice using the International Age related Maculopathy Epidemiological Study Group grading system [40]. Preliminary grading was performed on the site by ophthalmologist. Detailed grading was later done by nine retina specialists experienced in grading early and late AMD. The decision on any inconsistencies between the preliminary and detailed grading was done by another reading specialist. When the fundus photograph for a participant's eyes were different in severity, the grade was defined based on the more advanced grade. When the fundus photograph for only one eye was available to be assessed, the grade was evaluated by that eye. Early AMD was defined by the following criteria: the presence of soft, indistinct drusen, or reticular drusen, and the presence of distinct drusen with pigmentary abnormalities in the absence of signs of late AMD. Participants were diagnosed with late AMD if they had neovascular AMD or geographic atrophy. Neovascular AMD was defined by either the detachment of the retinal pigment epithelium (RPE) or neurosensory retina, or the presence of hemorrhages in the sub-RPE or subretinal spaces. Geographic atrophy was identified by the presence of a discrete, circular depigmented area ≥ 175 μm in choroidal vessel diameter.

General characteristics and smoking behavior

The health interview survey and health examination survey were used to obtain the socio-demographic and lifestyle characteristics of the participants, such as age, body mass index (BMI), residential area, education, family income, alcohol consumption, dietary supplement use, and smoking behavior.

BMI was calculated as weight divided by height squared (kg/m^2). Residential area was categorized as urban or rural. Education level was categorized as less than high school or high school and above. Family income was categorized into 4 groups according to quartile. Alcohol consumption was assessed with 5 categories (never, ≤ 1 drink/mo, 2–4 drinks/mo, 2–3 drinks/wk., or ≥4 drinks/wk. within the last year). Dietary supplement use defined as a binary variable (yes or no), included the supplementation data of the study subjects for longer than 2 weeks during the previous year. Based on smoking status, the study subjects were divided into 3 groups, nonsmokers, former smokers or current smokers.

Dietary assessment and estimation of dietary intake of carotenoids

We assessed daily dietary intake using data from a single 24-h recall form recorded in the KNAHANES. Participants reported all food and drinks consumed during the previous day in a face-to-face interview.

The food items in this study were categorized into 9 food groups based on other previous study. The intake of foods, energy and 16 nutrients including vitamin and carotenoids were estimated. To estimate carotenoid intake, the carotenoid data was constructed based on the food items of KNHANES and the Carotenoid Content Database from the United States Department of Agriculture. A total of 2247 food items were included in the carotenoid database. The carotenoid database included 72% of all plant foods reported in the 24 h dietary recall method.

Statistical analysis

All statistical analyses were performed using SAS version 9.4 (SAS Institute, Cary, NC, USA). Distribution differences of the socio-demographic and lifestyle factors of the men grouped by smoking status were analyzed using the PROC SURVEYFREQ procedure. We analyzed the crude weighted mean and standard error of continuous variables by the PROC SURVEYMEAN procedure and statistical differences by smoking status were analyzed with the PROC SURVEYREG procedure. The PROC SURVEYLOGISTIC procedure was used to test our hypothesis about the relationships between fruits and vegetables, antioxidant nutrient intake, and AMD in nonsmokers and smokers. We estimated the odds ratios (ORs) and 95% confidence intervals (CIs) for AMD across the tertiles of fruit and vegetable, vitamin C, vitamin A, and β-carotene intake, where the lowest tertile was set as the reference. Model 1 was adjusted for socio-demographic factors (age, BMI, residential area, education level, and family income). Model 2 was adjusted for the variables in model 1 plus lifestyle factors (alcohol consumption, dietary supplement use, and total energy intake) and history of diseases (diabetes mellitus and hypertension). Further, for former smokers, the data on daily smoking amount and duration of smoking was included in model 2. For the current smokers, current daily smoking amount and duration of smoking were adjusted in model 2.

Results

Characteristics of the study population

The subjects' age, prevalence of AMD, residential area, dietary supplement use, and diabetes mellitus did not differ by smoking status (Table 1). However, the current smokers had lower BMI, educational status and lower family income than the nonsmokers and the former smokers. The ratio of subjects who had higher intake of alcohol was higher among current smokers than the nonsmokers and the former smokers. The ratio of subjects with hypertension was higher among former smokers than the nonsmokers and the current smokers. The subjects included in this study did not differ from excluded subjects in terms of their general characteristics (data not shown).

The current smokers consumed less food in total, and, in particular, less cereals/potatoes/sugar products, fruits and vegetables than did the nonsmokers and the former smokers (Table 2). Intake of energy, thiamin, vitamin C, vitamin A, and β-carotene were significantly lower in the current smokers than in the nonsmokers and the former smokers.

Relationship of F&V and antioxidant nutrient intake and smoking status with AMD

We further evaluated the relationship in separate smoking status (Table 3). As expected, for the current smokers, AMD was inversely associated with F&V [OR (95% CI) = 0.36 (0.14–0.96), p for trend = 0.0576], vitamin C [OR (95% CI) = 0.32 (0.12–0.85), p for trend = 0.0561], α-carotene [OR (95% CI) = 0.23 (0.08–0.67), p for trend = 0.0038] and β-carotene [OR (95% CI) = 0.13 (0.04–0.46), p for trend = 0.0003] intake after adjusted for confounding factors. For nonsmokers and former smokers, however, there was no association between intake of fruits and vegetables and antioxidant nutrients and AMD.

Discussion

We found significant inverse associations between F&V and antioxidant nutrient intake and AMD in smokers. The highest tertiles of F&V, vitamin C, α-carotene, and β-carotene intake were associated with significantly reduced odds ratios for AMD compared to the lowest tertiles. In contrast, no statistically significant associations were observed in nonsmokers.

We found that smokers consumed significantly less fruits and vegetables, and antioxidant nutrients, which is consistent with previous studies [41–44]. In this study, F&V intake was 23.3% lower in the current smokers (444.0 g/d) than in the nonsmokers (578.7 g/d). In the Food Habits of Canadians Survey, in adults aged 18–65 years, male smokers showed reduced intake of fruits and vegetables (4.0 servings/d vs. 5.6 servings/d) in comparison with nonsmokers [41]. In a national population-based cohort study conducted in the US, subjects in the highest quartile of fruit and vegetable consumption (29.62 times/week) were more likely to quit smoking and less likely to be heavy smokers than were those in the lowest quartile [42]. The China Seven Cities Study (CSCS) observed that smokers were 46–60% less likely to consume fruit at least once a day than were those who had never smoked [43].

Unlike in other studies [8, 16], no statistically significant associations were observed in nonsmokers and AMD. We found inverse associations between F&V and AMD in current smokers only. Several studies reported that high fruit and vegetable intake is inversely associated with AMD [8, 16]. A cross-sectional study conducted in

Table 1 Characteristics of participants by smoking status[a]

Variables	Nonsmokers ($n = 227$)	Former smokers ($n = 856$)	Current smokers ($n = 331$)	*p*-value
Age (y)	71.6 ± 0.4	72.1 ± 0.2	71.3 ± 0.3	0.1433
BMI (kg/m²)	23.6 ± 0.2	23.4 ± 0.1	22.7 ± 0.2	0.0009
AMD	35 (12.5)	115 (14.5)	56 (18.0)	0.3052
Residential area				
Urban	154 (66.0)	588 (67.5)	207 (62.3)	0.3489
Rural	73 (34.0)	268 (32.5)	124 (37.7)	
Education				
Less than high school	127 (57.3)	509 (64.0)	241 (74.9)	0.0005
High school and above	99 (42.7)	347 (36.0)	90 (25.1)	
Family income				
< 25th	88 (36.1)	373 (44.4)	182 (54.1)	0.0113
25th to 50th	76 (38.2)	251 (29.9)	76 (22.7)	
50th to 75th	38 (16.3)	129 (13.8)	40 (13.4)	
75th to 100th	24 (9.4)	96 (11.8)	30 (9.8)	
Alcohol consumption				
Never	88 (40.2)	281 (32.1)	83 (25.1)	0.0007
≤ 1 mo	41 (19.1)	162 (19.6)	51 (15.6)	
2–4/mo	42 (17.6)	138 (15.1)	52 (15.0)	
2–3/wk	35 (14.4)	124 (14.6)	55 (15.6)	
≥ 4 wk	20 (8.7)	148 (18.7)	89 (25.7)	
Dietary supplement use				
Yes	89 (36.1)	373 (42.2)	113 (34.4)	0.0940
Diabetes mellitus	35 (15.0)	162 (18.2)	68 (19.3)	0.5096
Hypertension	98 (42.2)	438 (52.4)	129 (40.2)	0.0028
Smoking behavior				
Daily smoking amount of former smokers (n/d)	–	29.8 ± 1.2	–	–
Duration of former smoking (y)	–	18.3 ± 0.5	–	–
Daily smoking amount of current smokers (n/d)	–	–	13.8 ± 0.5	–
Duration of smoking (y)	–	–	49.5 ± 0.5	–

Data availability was limited in the following categories: age ($n = 1414$); BMI ($n = 1414$); residential area ($n = 1414$); education ($n = 1413$); family income ($n = 1403$); alcohol consumption ($n = 1410$); dietary supplement use ($n = 1414$); diabetes mellitus ($n = 1414$); hypertension ($n = 1414$); daily smoking amount of former smokers ($n = 852$); duration of former smoking ($n = 855$); daily smoking amount ($n = 331$); duration of smoking ($n = 331$)

BMI body mass index, *AMD* age related macular degeneration

[a]Values are mean ± s.e. or n (%); $n = 1414$

Australia showed that the proportion of individuals who met the recommended daily intake of vegetables was lower amongst patients with late-stage AMD than in a population of age- and sex-matched controls with no signs of AMD (52.9% vs. 64.5%, $p = 0.0002$) [8]. Recent studies have assessed the associations between healthy dietary patterns, including high fruit and vegetable consumption, and AMD [45, 46]. In the Carotenoids in Age-Related Eye Disease Study (CAREDS), which used the Healthy Eating Index (HEI), subjects whose HEI scores were ranked in the highest quintile (median serving of 3.1 for fruits and 4.6 for vegetables) had a 46% lower risk of early-stage AMD compared to those in the lowest quintile (median serving of 1.5 for fruits and 3.0 for vegetables) [45]. In our study, the mean intake of fruits and vegetables was 578.7 g/d among nonsmokers, which is higher than what is observed in other elderly male populations (Chinese: 313.0 g/d [47], Malaysian: 2.51 svg/d [48], Swedish: 3.3 svg/d [49], American: 3.38 svg/d [50]). Furthermore, the prevalence of hypertension (52.4%), one of the risk factors for AMD, was higher in our study population compared to other study (35.6%) [51]. We presume that in our study, among Korean elderly male nonsmokers other risk factor for AMD will be more meaningful than intake of fruits and vegetables.

Table 2 Daily foods and nutrients intake by smoking status

	Nonsmokers (n = 227)	Former smokers (n = 856)	Current smokers (n = 331)	p-value	
				Model 1[a]	Model 2[b]
Foods					
Total foods (g)	1368.4 ± 62.0	1318.9 ± 31.7	1262.5 ± 47.2	0.2051	0.0049
Cereals/potatoes/sugar products (g)	401.5 ± 14.6	374.3 ± 7.7	358.2 ± 8.8	0.0128	0.0298
Beans/nuts/seeds (g)	41.6 ± 6.2	45.9 ± 3.0	35.6 ± 3.9	0.2132	0.1571
Meats and eggs (g)	70.7 ± 7.4	73.5 ± 5.3	80.9 ± 9.4	0.5601	0.3160
Fishes and shellfishes (g)	39.9 ± 4.9	47.1 ± 3.5	49.5 ± 5.1	0.3195	0.5066
Milk and dairy products (g)	48.3 ± 8.3	49.6 ± 4.7	35.8 ± 6.5	0.5836	0.6781
Fruits and vegetables (g)	578.7 ± 43.4	524.6 ± 19.2	444.0 ± 27.4	0.0020	0.0035
Fruits (g)	204.6 ± 32.8	156.0 ± 12.7	125.2 ± 23.4	0.0570	0.1301
Vegetables (g)	374.1 ± 22.5	368.7 ± 12.4	318.8 ± 12.6	0.0113	0.0062
Mushrooms (g)	4.6 ± 3.1	5.3 ± 1.7	1.5 ± 0.6	0.1014	0.1070
Seaweeds (g)	4.4 ± 1.1	5.1 ± 0.7	5.4 ± 1.9	0.8381	0.8973
Nutrients					
Energy (kcal)	2032.9 ± 67.7	1935.6 ± 36.1	1995.7 ± 47.5	0.5190	<.0001
Carbohydrate (g)	363.9 ± 12.2	340.8 ± 6.7	334.7 ± 7.6	0.0944	0.1450
Protein (g)	66.4 ± 2.5	63.6 ± 1.4	62.3 ± 2.0	0.6056	0.2334
Fat (g)	31.2 ± 2.0	29.0 ± 1.1	27.1 ± 1.4	0.4352	0.2659
Calcium (mg)	480.6 ± 23.9	496.4 ± 14.2	448.0 ± 19.2	0.1844	0.0732
Phosphorus (mg)	1228.6 ± 45.6	1134.1 ± 20.9	1108.8 ± 30.0	0.1332	0.1443
Iron (mg)	17.8 ± 2.0	15.1 ± 0.5	14.4 ± 0.7	0.2512	0.2554
Thiamin (mg)	1.4 ± 0.1	1.2 ± 0.0	1.2 ± 0.0	0.0522	0.0078
Riboflavin (mg)	1.1 ± 0.1	1.1 ± 0.0	1.0 ± 0.0	0.1723	0.1122
Niacin (mg)	15.9 ± 0.5	15.5 ± 0.4	15.3 ± 0.5	0.8700	0.2463
Vitamin C (mg)	105.6 ± 7.1	97.8 ± 3.4	78.7 ± 4.3	0.0003	0.0011
Vitamin A (μgRE)	729.2 ± 54.2	700.6 ± 28.0	601.1 ± 42.0	0.1100	0.0760
α-carotene (mg)	1.0 ± 0.2	0.8 ± 0.1	0.7 ± 0.1	0.1044	0.1323
β-carotene (mg)	4.9 ± 0.4	4.6 ± 0.2	3.6 ± 0.3	0.0148	0.0245
β-cryptoxanthin (mg)	0.6 ± 0.2	0.4 ± 0.0	0.4 ± 0.1	0.6031	0.7048
Lutein + zeaxanthin (mg)	2.9 ± 0.3	2.5 ± 0.2	2.4 ± 0.2	0.3354	0.5297
Lycopene (mg)	1.1 ± 0.3	1.3 ± 0.2	0.7 ± 0.2	0.0695	0.0755

[a]Adjusted for age, BMI, residential area, education level, and family income (n = 1401)
[b]Adjusted for age, BMI, residential area, education level, family income, alcohol consumption, dietary supplement use, diabetes mellitus, and hypertension, and total energy intake (n = 1397)

We also observed a significant inverse relationship between intake of antioxidant nutrients such as vitamin C, α-carotene, and β-carotene and AMD among current smokers. Major dietary sources of β-carotene include green leafy vegetables and yellow fruits and vegetables such as spinach, carrots, pumpkin, and sweet potato [52]. There has been no observational study showing the relationship of dietary intake and smoking with AMD. However, some experimental studies have shown the protective effects of micronutrients derived from fruits and vegetables, such as vitamin A (particularly β-carotene), vitamin C, vitamin E, folic acid, and phenolic compounds, against smoke-induced toxicity, via prevention of lipid peroxidation [53, 54]. Cigarette smoking causes a depletion of intrinsic antioxidant capacity and thus promotes lipid oxidation [53]. Cigarette smoke-induced free radical generation may be the first step in lipid peroxidation in the membrane of LDL particles. That is, lipid peroxidation of LDL may begin after depletion of intrinsic antioxidants such as vitamin E (α-tocopherol) and β-carotene [53]. These nutrients act as antioxidants, as they have the ability to scavenge free radicals and prevent membrane lipid peroxidation [53]. Hininger et al. reported in an intervention study, which involved increased

Table 3 Odds Ratios (95% CIs) for AMD according to dietary intake in nonsmokers and smokers

	Nonsmokers ($n = 227$)					Former smokers ($n = 856$)					Current smokers ($n = 331$)				
	n	AMD	Median	Model 1[a]	Model 2[b]	*n*	AMD	Median	Model 1[a]	Model 2[c]	*n*	AMD	Median	Model 1[a]	Model 2[d]
Fruits and vegetables (g/d)															
Tertile 1	75	8	194.1	1.00	1.00	285	43	195.3	1.00	1.00	110	22	159.6	1.00	1.00
Tertile 2	76	16	481.9	1.93 (0.73–5.12)	2.09 (0.70–6.29)	286	31	443.0	0.69 (0.38–1.25)	0.65 (0.37–1.16)	111	19	366.3	0.79 (0.33–1.86)	0.64 (0.26–1.60)
Tertile 3	76	11	925.1	1.38 (0.43–4.44)	1.28 (0.34–4.82)	285	41	834.2	1.23 (0.64–2.35)	1.17 (0.64–2.15)	110	15	639.1	0.65 (0.25–1.68)	0.36 (0.14–0.96)
P for trend				0.6838	0.9960				0.4561	0.4836				0.3844	0.0576
Vitamin C (mg/d)															
Tertile 1	75	11	40.8	1.00	1.00	285	42	34.5	1.00	1.00	110	21	28.5	1.00	1.00
Tertile 2	76	14	84.5	1.65 (0.59–4.63)	1.51 (0.53–4.29)	286	25	75.9	0.66 (0.37–1.19)	0.65 (0.35–1.19)	111	18	64.8	0.49 (0.21–1.14)	0.36 (0.15–0.86)
Tertile 3	76	10	159.8	1.15 (0.35–3.74)	0.76 (0.23–2.58)	285	48	160.6	1.59 (0.88–2.88)	1.57 (0.89–2.75)	110	17	132.6	0.64 (0.27–1.52)	0.32 (0.12–0.85)
P for trend				0.9692	0.5177				0.0770	0.0523				0.4130	0.0561
Vitamin A (μgRE/d)															
Tertile 1	75	10	221.0	1.00	1.00	285	44	196.8	1.00	1.00	110	22	156.5	1.00	1.00
Tertile 2	76	12	569.1	1.02 (0.34–3.11)	1.00 (0.31–3.25)	286	36	512.7	0.80 (0.43–1.46)	0.76 (0.42–1.37)	111	16	454.8	0.54 (0.23–1.27)	0.43 (0.17–1.07)
Tertile 3	76	13	1229.3	1.28 (0.44–3.68)	1.05 (0.32–3.41)	285	35	1228.4	0.97 (0.51–1.84)	0.92 (0.50–1.70)	110	18	968.2	0.47 (0.18–1.20)	0.37 (0.13–1.08)
P for trend				0.5544	0.8523				0.4956	0.9725				0.0689	0.0740
α-carotene (mg/d)															
Tertile 1	75	10	0.05	1.00	1.00	285	38	0.04	1.00	1.00	110	22	0.04	1.00	1.00
Tertile 2	76	11	0.25	1.38 (0.45–4.18)	1.47 (0.42–5.06)	286	43	0.17	1.24 (0.74–2.09)	1.28 (0.76–2.15)	111	23	0.14	0.65 (0.30–1.39)	0.53 (0.26–1.10)
Tertile 3	76	14	1.51	2.40 (0.81–7.10)	2.20 (0.67–7.21)	285	34	1.28	1.01 (0.53–1.92)	1.07 (0.56–2.03)	110	11	1.15	0.29 (0.12–0.73)	0.23 (0.08–0.67)
P for trend				0.1364	0.2745				0.7751	0.8183				0.0038	0.0038
β-carotene (mg/d)															
Tertile 1	75	10	1.30	1.00	1.00	285	46	1.00	1.00	1.00	110	25	0.88	1.00	1.00
Tertile 2	76	14	2.98	2.12 (0.72–6.22)	2.05 (0.69–6.13)	286	34	2.73	0.79 (0.47–1.35)	0.76 (0.45–1.29)	111	16	2.28	0.36 (0.16–0.82)	0.27 (0.11–0.63)
Tertile 3	76	11	7.41	1.36 (0.43–4.28)	1.16 (0.30–4.45)	285	35	7.19	0.94 (0.51–1.74)	0.91 (0.48–1.73)	110	15	5.76	0.24 (0.09–0.62)	0.13 (0.04–0.46)
P for trend				0.8311	0.8847				0.9707	0.9439				0.0028	0.0003

AMD age related macular degeneration, *BMI* body mass index

[a]Model 1 adjusted for age, BMI, residential area, education level, and family income

[b]Model 2 adjusted for age, BMI, residential area, education level, family income, alcohol consumption, dietary supplement use, and total energy intake

[c]Model 2 adjusted for age, BMI, residential area, education level, family income, alcohol consumption, dietary supplement use, total energy intake, daily smoking amount of former smokers, and duration of former smoking

[d]Model 2 adjusted for age, BMI, residential area, education level, family income, alcohol consumption, dietary supplement use, total energy intake, daily smoking amount of current smokers, and duration of smoking

fruit and vegetable consumption for two weeks providing additional 30 mg/day of carotenoids (10 mg β-carotene, 10 mg lycopene and 10 mg lutein) per day, that serum carotene concentrations in smokers are more susceptible to fluctuate compared to nonsmokers from the intervention study [55]. We presume that these mechanisms account for the clearer effect of high F&V consumption and high antioxidant intake among smokers.

We observed the extreme low values in OR for prevalence of AMD across the tertiles of β-carotene intake among smokers. This may be due to the relatively small number of subjects in the smoking-subgroups. A previous cross-sectional population-based study using the data from the National Health and Nutrition Examination Survey (NHANES) also found that subjects in the highest quintile category of carotenoid intake (lutein/zeaxanthin) had a

90% lower risk for AMD compared with those in the lowest quintile category [OR (95% CI) = 0.1 (0.0–0.9)] [56].

In our study, the smokers consumed fewer milk and dairy products and calcium than the nonsmokers. Although we did not observe any association between milk and dairy product intake and AMD, one recent study reported a significant linear trend, over a 15-year period between consumption of dairy foods and the incidence of late AMD [17]. Further research is needed to confirm these results.

The prevalence of AMD did not differ by smoking status in the current study. However, smoking strongly affect the onset and progression of AMD [7, 57]. Coleman et al. reported that, after 15-year of follow-up, the ORs for early-stage AMD among nonsmokers and smokers aged ≥80 years were 1.63 and 5.49, respectively, in comparison to nonsmokers aged < 80 years [58]. Cigarette smoke causes oxidative damage directly and indirectly. Toxins in smoke cause damage directly by generating a large number of free radicals [59] and indirectly by depleting endogenous circulating antioxidants [14].

This study has several limitations. First, the KNHANES is a cross-sectional study, so we cannot explain the causal relationship between dietary nutrient intake and AMD. Second, our dietary data was derived from a single 24-h dietary recall survey, which may provide an inaccurate estimate of normal diet. However, according to the KNHANES report, variations in data from a single day and 2–10 days of 24-h dietary recall were not much different (3.9% for energy, 14.2% for vitamin A, and 7.8% for fiber) [60]. Furthermore, the difference (30.3%) in vitamin A intake between nonsmokers and smokers is much greater than the within-person variation for vitamin A intake. Third, we examined only dietary intake of antioxidant nutrients, but not dietary supplement intake. We analyzed only the intakes of vitamin A and vitamin C from dietary supplements. There was no significant difference for vitamin A and C from dietary supplements according to smoking status (vitamin A: 292.8 ± 161.6 for nonsmokers, 153.2 ± 31.7 for former smokers, and 89.2 ± 41.6 for current smokers; vitamin C: 121.5 ± 32.8 for nonsmokers, 137.2 ± 20.1 for former smokers, and 93.5 ± 29.8 for current smokers). However, we have limited data on nutrient intakes from dietary supplements [515 subjects (36.4%)] and these data were available for 2010 and 2011 years, but not 2012. Therefore, we were unable to estimate nutrient intakes from foods and supplements.

Nevertheless, to the best of our knowledge, this is the first study to find that the AMD prevalence among cigarette smokers is inversely associated with consumption of F&V and antioxidant nutrients. This observation implies that future studies investigating the protective effect of fruit and vegetable consumption on AMD should consider smoking status. We estimated the association between β-carotene intake and AMD. Several studies have observed associations between carotenoids, particularly lutein/zeaxanthin, and AMD [26, 27, 56]. Thus, further studies are needed to elucidate this relationship between antioxidant nutrients and AMD.

Conclusions

In conclusion, we found that intake of fruits and vegetables, vitamin C, α-carotene, and β-carotene may protect against AMD in elderly male smokers. Future studies are warranted to explore the mechanisms related to the beneficial role of fruits and vegetables and antioxidant nutrients against AMD in smokers. The current results also suggest that public health interventions for elderly smokers should focus on improving dietary habits, including increasing fruit and vegetable consumption, as well as on smoking cessation.

Abbreviations

AMD: Age-related macular degeneration; CAREDS: Carotenoids in Age-Related Eye Disease Study; CSCS: China Seven Cities Study; F&V: Fruits and vegetables; HEI: Healthy Eating Index; KNHANES: Korea National Health and Nutrition Examination Survey; NHANES: National Health and Nutrition Examination Survey; OECD: Organization for economic cooperation and development; ROS: Reactive oxygen species; RPE: Retinal pigment epithelium

Acknowledgements

Not applicable

Funding

This research was supported by the Brain Korea 21 Plus.

Authors' contributions

EK analyzed the data and wrote the manuscript; HK interpreted data and revised the manuscript; AV revised the manuscript; OK constructed the carotenoid database; NC designed the research. All the authors read and approved the final manuscript.

Competing interests

The authors declare that they have no competing interests.

References

1. Foran S, Wang JJ, Mitchell P. Causes of visual impairment in two older population cross-sections: the Blue Mountains eye study. Ophthalmic Epidemiol. 2003;10:215–25.
2. Cho BJ, Heo JW, Kim TW, Ahn J, Chung H. Prevalence and risk factors of age-related macular degeneration in Korea: the Korea National Health and nutrition examination survey 2010-2011. Invest Ophthalmol Vis Sci. 2014;55:1101–8.
3. Shahid H, Khan JC, Cipriani V, Sepp T, Matharu BK, Bunce C, Harding SP, Clayton DG, Moore AT, Yates JR. Age-related macular degeneration: the importance of family history as a risk factor. Br J Ophthalmol. 2012;96:427–31.
4. Cho BJ, Heo JW, Shin JP, Ahn J, Kim TW, Chung H. Epidemiological association between systemic diseases and age-related macular degeneration: the Korea National Health and nutrition examination survey 2008-2011. Invest Ophthalmol Vis Sci. 2014;55:4430–7.

5. Piermarocchi S, Tognetto D, Piermarocchi R, Masetto M, Monterosso G, Segato T, Cavarzeran F, Turrini A, Peto T. Risk factors and age-related macular degeneration in a Mediterranean-Basin population: the PAMDI (prevalence of age-related macular degeneration in Italy) study - report 2. Ophthalmic Res. 2016;55:111–8.
6. Myers CE, Klein BE, Gangnon R, Sivakumaran TA, Iyengar SK, Klein R. Cigarette smoking and the natural history of age-related macular degeneration: the beaver dam eye study. Ophthalmology. 2014;121: 1949–55.
7. Woodell A, Rohrer B. A mechanistic review of cigarette smoke and age-related macular degeneration. In: Retinal degenerative diseases. Advances in experimental medicine and biology (Volume 801). New York: Springer; 2014. p. 301–7.
8. Gopinath B, Liew G, Russell J, Cosatto V, Burlutsky G, Mitchell P. Intake of key micronutrients and food groups in patients with late-stage age-related macular degeneration compared with age-sex-matched controls. Br J Ophthalmol. 2017;101(8):1027–31.
9. Amirul Islam FM, Chong EW, Hodge AM, Guymer RH, Aung KZ, Makeyeva GA, Baird PN, Hopper JL, English DR, Giles GG, Robman LD. Dietary patterns and their associations with age-related macular degeneration: the Melbourne collaborative cohort study. Ophthalmology. 2014;121:1428–34. e1422
10. Koushan K, Rusovici R, Li W, Ferguson LR, Chalam KV. The role of lutein in eye-related disease. Nutrients. 2013;5:1823–39.
11. Schleicher M, Weikel K, Garber C, Taylor A. Diminishing risk for age-related macular degeneration with nutrition: a current view. Nutrients. 2013;5:2405–56.
12. Smith W, Assink J, Klein R, Mitchell P, Klaver CC, Klein BE, Hofman A, Jensen S, Wang JJ, de Jong PT. Risk factors for age-related macular degeneration: pooled findings from three continents. Ophthalmology. 2001;108:697–704.
13. Jarrett SG, Boulton ME. Consequences of oxidative stress in age-related macular degeneration. Mol Asp Med. 2012;33:399–417.
14. Moriarty SE, Shah JH, Lynn M, Jiang S, Openo K, Jones DP, Sternberg P. Oxidation of glutathione and cysteine in human plasma associated with smoking. Free Radic Biol Med. 2003;35:1582–8.
15. Ozawa Y. Oxidative stress in the RPE and its contribution to AMD pathogenesis: implication of light exposure. In: Neuroprotection and Neuroregeneration for retinal diseases. Japan: Springer; 2014. p. 239–53.
16. Cho E, Seddon JM, Rosner B, Willett WC, Hankinson SE. Prospective study of intake of fruits, vegetables, vitamins, and carotenoids and risk of age-related maculopathy. Arch Ophthalmol. 2004;122:883–92.
17. Gopinath B, Flood VM, Louie JC, Wang JJ, Burlutsky G, Rochtchina E, Mitchell P. Consumption of dairy products and the 15-year incidence of age-related macular degeneration. Br J Nutr. 2014;111:1673–9.
18. Zhu W, Wu Y, Meng YF, Xing Q, Tao JJ, Lu J. Fish consumption and age-related macular degeneration incidence: a meta-analysis and systematic review of prospective cohort studies. Nutrients. 2016;8(11):e743.
19. Aoki A, Inoue M, Nguyen E, Obata R, Kadonosono K, Shinkai S, Hashimoto H, Sasaki S, Yanagi Y. Dietary n-3 fatty acid, alpha-tocopherol, zinc, vitamin D, vitamin C, and beta-carotene are associated with age-related macular degeneration in Japan. Sci Rep. 2016;6:20723.
20. Evans JR, Lawrenson JG. Antioxidant vitamin and mineral supplements for slowing the progression of age-related macular degeneration. Cochrane Database Syst Rev. 2012;11:Cd000254.
21. Ma L, Yan SF, Huang YM, XR L, Qian F, Pang HL, XR X, Zou ZY, Dong PC, Xiao X, et al. Effect of lutein and zeaxanthin on macular pigment and visual function in patients with early age-related macular degeneration. Ophthalmology. 2012;119:2290–7.
22. Krinsky NI, Landrum JT, Bone RA. Biologic mechanisms of the protective role of lutein and zeaxanthin in the eye. Annu Rev Nutr. 2003;23:171–201.
23. Eisenhauer B, Natoli S, Liew G, Flood VM. Lutein and Zeaxanthin-Food sources, bioavailability and dietary variety in age-related macular degeneration protection. Nutrients. 2017;9(2):e120.
24. Pisoschi AM, Pop A. The role of antioxidants in the chemistry of oxidative stress: a review. Eur J Med Chem. 2015;97:55–74.
25. Chichili GR, Nohr D, Frank J, Flaccus A, Fraser PD, Enfissi EM, Biesalski HK. Protective effects of tomato extract with elevated beta-carotene levels on oxidative stress in ARPE-19 cells. Br J Nutr. 2006;96:643–9.
26. Wu J, Cho E, Willett WC, Sastry SM, Schaumberg DA. Intakes of lutein, zeaxanthin, and other carotenoids and age-related macular degeneration during 2 decades of prospective follow-up. JAMA Ophthalmol. 2015;133:1415–24.
27. Chew EY, Clemons TE, Sangiovanni JP, Danis RP, Ferris FL 3rd, Elman MJ, Antoszyk AN, Ruby AJ, Orth D, Bressler SB, et al. Secondary analyses of the effects of lutein/zeaxanthin on age-related macular degeneration progression: AREDS2 report no. 3. JAMA Ophthalmol. 2014;132:142–9.
28. Kaarniranta K, Machalinska A, Vereb Z, Salminen A, Petrovski G, Kauppinen A. Estrogen signalling in the pathogenesis of age-related macular degeneration. Curr Eye Res. 2015;40:226–33.
29. Beatty S, Koh H, Phil M, Henson D, Boulton M. The role of oxidative stress in the pathogenesis of age-related macular degeneration. Surv Ophthalmol. 2000;45:115–34.
30. Michikawa T, Ishida S, Nishiwaki Y, Kikuchi Y, Tsuboi T, Hosoda K, Ishigami A, Iwasawa S, Nakano M, Takebayashi T. Serum antioxidants and age-related macular degeneration among older Japanese. Asia Pac J Clin Nutr. 2009;18:1–7.
31. Yao Y, Qiu QH, XW W, Cai ZY, Xu S, Liang XQ. Lutein supplementation improves visual performance in Chinese drivers: 1-year randomized, double-blind, placebo-controlled study. Nutrition. 2013;29:958–64.
32. Nidhi B, Mamatha BS, Padmaprabhu CA, Pallavi P, Vallikannan B. Dietary and lifestyle risk factors associated with age-related macular degeneration: a hospital based study. Indian J Ophthalmol. 2013;61:722–7.
33. Kellen E, Zeegers M, Paulussen A, Van Dongen M, Buntinx F. Fruit consumption reduces the effect of smoking on bladder cancer risk. The Belgian case control study on bladder cancer. Int J Cancer. 2006;118:2572–8.
34. Korea Centers for Disease Control and Prevention. In: Ministry oHaW, editor. Korea National Health and Nutrition Examination Survey 2015 (KNHANES VI-3). Seoul: Korea Centers for Disease Control and Prevention; 2016.
35. How's Life? 2015 Measuring Well-being [http://www.oecd-ilibrary.org/content/graph/how_life-2015-graph61-en].
36. Park SJ, Lee JH, Woo SJ, Ahn J, Shin JP, Song SJ, Kang SW, Park KH. Age-related macular degeneration: prevalence and risk factors from Korean National Health and nutrition examination survey, 2008 through 2011. Ophthalmology. 2014;121:1756–65.
37. Korea Centers for Disease Control and Prevention. In: Ministry oHaW, editor. The Fifth Korea National Health and Nutrition Examination Survey (KNHANES V). Seoul: Korea Centers for Disease Control and Prevention; 2013.
38. Yoon K-C, Mun G-H, Kim S-D, Kim S-H, Kim CY, Park KH, Park YJ, Baek S-H, Song SJ, Shin JP, et al. Prevalence of eye diseases in South Korea: data from the Korea national health and nutrition examination survey 2008-2009. Korean J Ophthalmol. 2011;25:421–33.
39. Cho BJ, Heo JW, Shin JP, Ahn J, Kim TW, Chung H. Association between reproductive factors and age-related macular degeneration in postmenopausal women: the Korea National Health and nutrition examination survey 2010-2012. PLoS One. 2014;9:e102816.
40. Bird AC, Bressler NM, Bressler SB, Chisholm IH, Coscas G, Davis MD, de Jong PT, Klaver CC, Klein BE, Klein R, et al. An international classification and grading system for age-related maculopathy and age-related macular degeneration. The international ARM epidemiological study group. Surv Ophthalmol. 1995;39:367–74.
41. Palaniappan U, Jacobs Starkey L, O'Loughlin J, Gray-Donald K. Fruit and vegetable consumption is lower and saturated fat intake is higher among Canadians reporting smoking. J Nutr. 2001;131:1952–8.
42. Haibach JP, Homish GG, Giovino GA. A longitudinal evaluation of fruit and vegetable consumption and cigarette smoking. Nicotine Tob Res. 2013;15:355–63.
43. Masood S, Cappelli C, Li Y, Tanenbaum H, Chou CP, Spruijt-Metz D, Palmer PH, Johnson CA, Xie B. Cigarette smoking is associated with unhealthy patterns of food consumption, physical activity, sleep impairment, and alcohol drinking in Chinese male adults. Int J Public Health. 2015;60:891–9.
44. Endoh K, Kuriki K, Kasezawa N, Tohyama K, Goda T. Association between smoking status and food and nutrient consumption in Japanese: a large-scale cross-sectional study. Asian Pac J Cancer Prev. 2015;16:6527–34.
45. Mares JA, Voland RP, Sondel SA, Millen AE, Larowe T, Moeller SM, Klein ML, Blodi BA, Chappell RJ, Tinker L, et al. Healthy lifestyles related to

subsequent prevalence of age-related macular degeneration. Arch Ophthalmol. 2011;129:470–80.
46. Merle BM, Silver RE, Rosner B, Seddon JM. Adherence to a Mediterranean diet, genetic susceptibility, and progression to advanced macular degeneration: a prospective cohort study. Am J Clin Nutr. 2015;102:1196–206.
47. Xie H-L, B-H W, Xue W-Q, He M-G, Fan F, Ouyang W-F, S-I T, Zhu H-L, Chen Y-M. Greater intake of fruit and vegetables is associated with a lower risk of osteoporotic hip fractures in elderly Chinese: a 1: 1 matched case-control study. Osteoporos Int. 2013;24:2827–36.
48. Cheong S, Jasvindar K, Lim K, Surthahar A, Ambigga D. Prevalence and factors influencing fruit and vegetable consumption among Malaysian elderly. Int J Public Health Clin Sci. 2017;4:28–39.
49. Benetou V, Orfanos P, Feskanich D, Michaëlsson K, Pettersson-Kymmer U, Eriksson S, Grodstein F, Wolk A, Bellavia A, Ahmed LA. Fruit and vegetable intake and hip fracture incidence in older men and women: the CHANCES project. J Bone Miner Res. 2016;31:1743–52.
50. Sharkey JR, Johnson CM, Dean WR. Food access and perceptions of the community and household food environment as correlates of fruit and vegetable intake among rural seniors. BMC Geriatr. 2010;10:32.
51. Hyman L, Schachat AP, He Q, Leske MC. Hypertension, cardiovascular disease, and age-related macular degeneration. Age-related macular degeneration risk factors study group. Arch Ophthalmol. 2000;118:351–8.
52. Barbosa-Filho JM, Alencar AA, Nunes XP, Tomaz AC, Sena-Filho JG, Athayde-Filho PF, Silva MS, Souza MF, Da-Cunha EVL. Sources of alpha-, beta-, gamma-, delta-and epsilon-carotenes: a twentieth century review. Rev Bras. 2008;18:135–54.
53. Diana JN. Tobacco smoking and nutrition. Ann N Y Acad Sci. 1993;686:1–11.
54. Frei B. Ascorbic acid protects lipids in human plasma and low-density lipoprotein against oxidative damage. Am J Clin Nutr. 1991;54:1113s–8s.
55. Hininger I, Chopra M, Thurnham DI, Laporte F, Richard MJ, Favier A, Roussel AM. Effect of increased fruit and vegetable intake on the susceptibility of lipoprotein to oxidation in smokers. Eur J Clin Nutr. 1997;51:601–6.
56. Mares-Perlman JA, Fisher AI, Klein R, Palta M, Block G, Millen AE, Wright JD. Lutein and zeaxanthin in the diet and serum and their relation to age-related maculopathy in the third national health and nutrition examination survey. Am J Epidemiol. 2001;153:424–32.
57. Thornton J, Edwards R, Mitchell P, Harrison RA, Buchan I, Kelly SP. Smoking and age-related macular degeneration: a review of association. Eye (Lond). 2005;19:935–44.
58. Coleman AL, Seitzman RL, Cummings SR, Yu F, Cauley JA, Ensrud KE, Stone KL, Hochberg MC, Pedula KL, Thomas EL, Mangione CM. The association of smoking and alcohol use with age-related macular degeneration in the oldest old: the study of osteoporotic fractures. Am J Ophthalmol. 2010;149:160–9.
59. Church DF, Pryor WA. Free-radical chemistry of cigarette smoke and its toxicological implications. Environ Health Perspect. 1985;64:111–26.
60. Korea MoHaWo. In: Prevention KCfDCa, editor. Report presentation of Korea National Health and Nutrition Examination Survey IV, 2009. Osong: Korea Centers for Disease Control and Prevention; 2010.

PERMISSIONS

All chapters in this book were first published in NUTRITION, by BioMed Central; hereby published with permission under the Creative Commons Attribution License or equivalent. Every chapter published in this book has been scrutinized by our experts. Their significance has been extensively debated. The topics covered herein carry significant findings which will fuel the growth of the discipline. They may even be implemented as practical applications or may be referred to as a beginning point for another development.

The contributors of this book come from diverse backgrounds, making this book a truly international effort. This book will bring forth new frontiers with its revolutionizing research information and detailed analysis of the nascent developments around the world.

We would like to thank all the contributing authors for lending their expertise to make the book truly unique. They have played a crucial role in the development of this book. Without their invaluable contributions this book wouldn't have been possible. They have made vital efforts to compile up to date information on the varied aspects of this subject to make this book a valuable addition to the collection of many professionals and students.

This book was conceptualized with the vision of imparting up-to-date information and advanced data in this field. To ensure the same, a matchless editorial board was set up. Every individual on the board went through rigorous rounds of assessment to prove their worth. After which they invested a large part of their time researching and compiling the most relevant data for our readers.

The editorial board has been involved in producing this book since its inception. They have spent rigorous hours researching and exploring the diverse topics which have resulted in the successful publishing of this book. They have passed on their knowledge of decades through this book. To expedite this challenging task, the publisher supported the team at every step. A small team of assistant editors was also appointed to further simplify the editing procedure and attain best results for the readers.

Apart from the editorial board, the designing team has also invested a significant amount of their time in understanding the subject and creating the most relevant covers. They scrutinized every image to scout for the most suitable representation of the subject and create an appropriate cover for the book.

The publishing team has been an ardent support to the editorial, designing and production team. Their endless efforts to recruit the best for this project, has resulted in the accomplishment of this book. They are a veteran in the field of academics and their pool of knowledge is as vast as their experience in printing. Their expertise and guidance has proved useful at every step. Their uncompromising quality standards have made this book an exceptional effort. Their encouragement from time to time has been an inspiration for everyone.

The publisher and the editorial board hope that this book will prove to be a valuable piece of knowledge for researchers, students, practitioners and scholars across the globe.

LIST OF CONTRIBUTORS

Ina Olmer Specht and Peder Frederiksen
Parker Institute, Research Unit for Dietary Studies, Frederiksberg and Bispebjerg Hospital, Frederiksberg, Denmark

Berit Lilienthal Heitmann
Parker Institute, Research Unit for Dietary Studies, Frederiksberg and Bispebjerg Hospital, Frederiksberg, Denmark
Department of Public Health, Section for general Medicine, University of Copenhagen, Copenhagen, Denmark
National Institute of Public health, University of Southern Denmark, Odense, Denmark

Inge Huybrechts and Veronique Chajes
International Agency for Research on Cancer (IARC), Nutrition and Metabolism Section, Lyon, France

Eva Steliarova-Foucher
International Agency for Research on Cancer (IARC), Cancer Surveillance Section (CSU), Lyon, France

Zach Conrad, LuAnn K. Johnson, James N. Roemmich and Lisa Jahns
Grand Forks Human Nutrition Research Center, US Department of Agriculture, Agricultural Research Service, 2420 2nd Ave. N, Grand Forks, ND 58203, USA

WenYen Juan
Center for Food Safety and Applied Nutrition, US Department of Health and Human Services, Food and Drug Administration, 5001 Campus Drive, College Park, MD 20740, USA

Marcus Maringer, Pieter van't Veer and Anouk Geelen
Division of Human Nutrition, Wageningen University & Research, Wageningen, The Netherlands

Naomi Klepacz, Lada Timotijevic and Monique M. Raats
Food, Consumer Behaviour and Health Research Centre, University of Surrey, Guildford, Surrey, United Kingdom

Muriel C. D. Verain
Wageningen Economic Research, Wageningen University & Research, Wageningen, The Netherlands

Anne Normann and Suzanne Ekman
Division of Bioscience and Materials, Agrifood and Bioscience, RISE Research Institutes of Sweden, Gothenburg, Sweden

Michel Coutinho dos Santos, Ana Paula Cicci de Castro Coutinho, Mônica de Souza Dantas and Letícia Ayran Medina Yabunaka
University Hospital of the Federal University of Grande Dourados, Dourados, MS, Brazil

Dartagnan Pinto Guedes
Northern University of Paraná, Londrina, PR, Brazil

Silvia Aparecida Oesterreich
Faculty of Health Sciences, Federal University of Grande Dourados, Dourados, MS, Brazil

Helen Eyles, Yannan Jiang, Jennifer Crowley and Cliona Ni Mhurchu
National Institute for Health Innovation, School of Population Health, The University of Auckland, Private Bag 92019, Auckland Mail Centre, Auckland 1142, New Zealand

Tony Blakely and Christine Cleghorn
Department of Public Health, University of Otago, Wellington, New Zealand

Bruce Neal
The George Institute for Global Health, The University of Sydney, Sydney, Australia

Lana Vanderlee
Department of Nutritional Sciences, University of Toronto, Toronto, Canada

Erin P. Hobin
Department of Nutritional Sciences, University of Toronto, Toronto, Canada
Public Health Ontario, Toronto, Canada
Dalla Lana School of Public Health, University of Toronto, Toronto, Canada

Jessica L. Reid, Christine M. White, Rachel B. Acton, Amanda C. Jones, Sharon I. Kirkpatrick and David Hammond
School of Public Health and Health Systems, University of Waterloo, 200 University Ave W, Waterloo, ON, Canada

Meghan O'Neill
School of Public Health and Health Systems, University of Waterloo, 200 University Ave W, Waterloo, ON, Canada
Dalla Lana School of Public Health, University of Toronto, Toronto, Canada

Emmanuel Grellety
Research Center Health Policy and Systems - International Health, School of Public Health, Université Libre de Bruxelles, Bruxelles, Belgium

Michael H. Golden
Department of Medicine and Therapeutics, University of Aberdeen, Aberdeen, Scotland

Armando García-Guerra
Instituto Nacional de Salud Publica (INSP), Cuernavaca, Morelos, Mexico

Gabriela Añorve-Valdez
Instituto Nacional de Salud Publica (INSP), Cuernavaca, Morelos, Mexico
Autonomous University of the State of Morelos, Cuernavaca, Morelos, Mexico

Fabiola Mejía-Rodríguez
Instituto Nacional de Salud Publica (INSP), Cuernavaca, Morelos, Mexico Center for Nutrition and Health Research, INSP, Avenida Universidad 655, Colonia
Santa María Ahuacatitlán, Cuernavaca, Morelos, Mexico

Lynnette Marie Neufeld
Global Alliance for Improved Nutrition, Geneva, Switzerland

Amado David Quezada-Sánchez
Center for Evaluation and Surveys Research, National Institute of Public Health, INSP, Cuernavaca, Morelos, Mexico

Usha Dhingra, Pratibha Dhingra, Arup Dutta, Saikat Deb, Jitendra Kumar and Prabhabati Devi
Center for Public Health Kinetics, 214A, Vinoba Puri, Lajpat Nagar-II, New Delhi 110024, India

Sunil Sazawal
Center for Public Health Kinetics, 214A, Vinoba Puri, Lajpat Nagar-II, New Delhi 110024, India
Department of International Health, Johns Hopkins Bloomberg School of Public Health, Baltimore, MD, USA
Department of Pediatrics, Subharti Medical College, Meerut, Uttar Pradesh, India

Ashish Prakash
Department of Pediatrics, Subharti Medical College, Meerut, Uttar Pradesh, India

Huiqing Shi, Xiaodong Yang, Dan Wu, Xiulian Wang, Tingting Li, Guangjun Yu and Jinjin Chen
Shanghai Children's Hospital, Shanghai Jiao Tong University, Luding Road 355, Putuo district, Shanghai 200062, China

Honghua Liu
Dongying People's Hospital, Dongcheng South First Road 317, Dongying 257091, China

Chong Guo
Maternal and Children Hospital, Daoshan Road 18, Gulou District, Fuzhou 350001, China

Jian Wang and Xiangying Hu
Jing'an District Maternal and Child Healthcare Center of Shanghai, 1297 Kangding Road, Shanghai 200072, China

Won Jang, Hyesook Kim and Namsoo Chang
Department of Nutritional Science and Food Management, Ewha Womans University, Seoul, South Korea

Bo-Eun Lee
Environmental Health Research Division, National Institute of Environmental Research, Incheon, South Korea

Julie L. Woods
Institute for Physical Activity and Nutrition (IPAN), School of Exercise and Nutrition Sciences, Deakin University, Geelong 3220, Australia

Beth Gilham
Institute for Physical Activity and Nutrition (IPAN), School of Exercise and Nutrition Sciences, Deakin University, Geelong 3220, Australia
Centre for Advanced Sensory Science, School of Exercise and Nutrition Sciences, Deakin University, 221 Burwood Highway, Burwood, VIC 3125, Australia

Ramon Hall
Centre for Advanced Sensory Science, School of Exercise and Nutrition Sciences, Deakin University, 221 Burwood Highway, Burwood, VIC 3125, Australia

Helene Bohnert, Max Maurer, Johann Pratschke, Paul Thul and Verena Müller
Charité-Universitätsmedizin Berlin, Department of Surgery, Campus Charité Mitte | Campus Virchow-Klinikum, Chariteplatz, 10117 Berlin, Germany

Philip C. Calder
Human Development and Health, Faculty of Medicine, University of Southampton, Southampton, UK
NIHR Southampton Biomedical Research Centre, University Hospital Southampton NHS Foundation Trust and University of Southampton, Southampton, UK

Wenli Ni, Tian Tian, Le Zhang, Zhiwen Li, Linlin Wang and Aiguo Ren
Peking University Institute of Reproductive and Child Health, National Health Commission Key Laboratory of Reproductive Health, Beijing 100191, China
Department of Epidemiology and Biostatistics, School of Public Health, Peking University Health Science Center, Beijing 100191, China

Jufen Liu, Rongwei Ye and Jianmeng Liu
Institute of Reproductive and Child Health / Key Laboratory of Reproductive
Health, National Health Commission of the People's Republic of China,
Peking University, Beijing 100191, People's Republic of China
Department of Epidemiology and Biostatistics, School of Public Health, Peking University, Beijing 100191, People's Republic of China

Edyta Adamska-Patruno and Joanna Goscik
Clinical Research Centre, Medical University of Bialystok, Sklodowskiej 24A, 15-276, Bialystok, MC, Poland

Adam Kretowski
Clinical Research Centre, Medical University of Bialystok, Sklodowskiej 24A, 15-276, Bialystok, MC, Poland
Department of Endocrinology, Diabetology and Internal Medicine, Medical University of Bialystok, Sklodowskiej 24A, 15-276, Bialystok, MC, Poland

Lucyna Ostrowska and Barbara Pietraszewska
Department of Dietetics and Clinical Nutrition, Medical University of Bialystok, Mieszka I-go 4B, 15-054, Bialystok, Poland

Maria Gorska
Department of Endocrinology, Diabetology and Internal Medicine, Medical University of Bialystok, Sklodowskiej 24A, 15-276, Bialystok, MC, Poland

Asli Akyol, Aylin Ayaz, Elif Inan-Eroglu, Cansu Cetin and Gulhan Samur
Department of Nutrition and Dietetics, Hacettepe University, Sihhiye, 06100 Ankara, Turkey

Marie Vermote, Vickà Versele, Eva D'Hondt, Peter Clarys and Tom Deliens
Department of Movement and Sport Sciences, Vrije Universiteit Brussel, Pleinlaan 2, 1050 Brussels, Belgium

Patrick Mullie
Department of Movement and Sport Sciences, Vrije Universiteit Brussel, Pleinlaan 2, 1050 Brussels, Belgium
International Prevention Research Institute (iPRI), 15 chemin du Saquin, 69130 Ecully (Lyon), France

Benedicte Deforche
Department of Movement and Sport Sciences, Vrije Universiteit Brussel, Pleinlaan 2, 1050 Brussels, Belgium
Department of Public Health, Ghent University, De Pintelaan 185, 9000 Ghent, Belgium

Marijn Stok
Department of Interdisciplinary Social Sciences, Utrecht University, Heidelberglaan 1, 3584 CS Utrecht, Netherlands
Department of Psychological Assessment and Health Psychology, University of Konstanz, Universitätsstraße 10, D-78464 Konstanz, Germany

Hyesook Kim, Hyejin Kim and Namsoo Chang
Department of Nutritional Science and Food Management, Ewha Womans University, Seoul, South Korea

Eunjung Lee
Department of Nutritional Science and Food Management, Ewha Womans University, Seoul, South Korea
Department of Nutrition Consultation, Seoul National University Hospital, Healthcare System Gangnam Center, Seoul, South Korea

Eun-Hee Ha
Department of Occupational and Environmental Medicine, Ewha Womans University, College of Medicine, Seoul, South Korea

Jie Xu
Department of Clinical and Experimental Medicine, Linköping University, Linköping, Sweden

Tommy Jönsson
Center for Primary Health Care Research, Lund University, Skåne University Hospital, Malmö, Sweden

Merichel Plaza
Department of Analytical Chemistry, Physical Chemistry and Chemical Engineering, Faculty of Biology, Environmental Sciences and Chemistry, Universidad de Alcalá, Ctra. Madrid-Barcelona Km. 33.600, Alcalá de Henares, Madrid, Spain
Department of Chemistry, Lund University, Lund, Sweden

Charlotta Turner and Peter Spégel
Department of Chemistry, Lund University, Lund, Sweden

Åsa Håkansson and Yvonne Granfeldt
Department of Food Technology, Engineering and Nutrition, Lund University, Lund, Sweden

Martin Antonsson
ProViva AB, Lunnarp, Sweden

Irini Lazou Ahrén
Probi AB, Lund, Sweden

Angélica Ochoa-Avilés, Susana Andrade, Silvana Donoso and Patricia Liliana Ramírez
Departmento de Biociencias, Grupo Nutrición Alimentación y Salud, Facultad de Ciencias Químicas, Universidad de Cuenca, Avenida 12 de Abril y Avenida Loja, 0101168 Cuenca, Ecuador

Lieven Huybregts
Poverty, Health and Nutrition Division, International Food Policy Research Institute, 2033 K St, NW, Washington, DC, USA

Eun-kyung Kim, Hyesook Kim, Aswathy Vijayakumar, Oran Kwon and Namsoo Chang
Department of Nutritional Science and Food Management, Ewha Womans University, Seoul 120-750, Republic of Korea

Emma L. Wilkins, Duncan Radley and Claire Griffiths
Carnegie, Leeds Beckett University, Headingley Campus, Headingley, Leeds LS6 3QS, UK

Michelle A. Morris
Leeds Institute for Data Analytics, School of Medicine, University of Leeds, Leeds LS2 9JT, UK

Claudia Flemming Colussi
Department of Public Health, Federal University of SC, Florianópolis, Santa Catarina, Brazil

Margaret D. Condrasky
Department of Food, Nutrition, and Packaging Sciences, Clemson University, Clemson, South Carolina, USA

Index